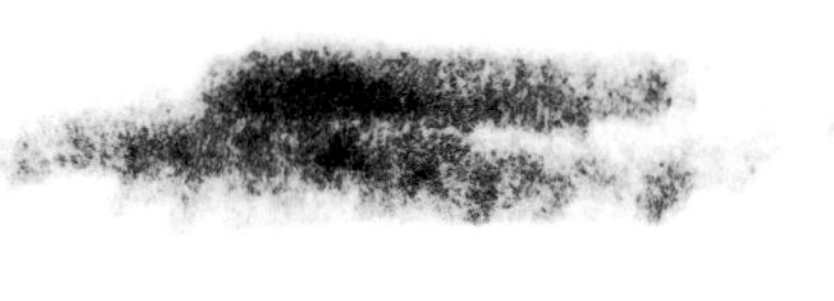

Essentials of the U.S. Health Care System

Second Edition

Leiyu Shi, DrPH, MBA, MPA
Professor
Department of Health Policy and Management
Bloomberg School of Public Health
Johns Hopkins University
Baltimore, Maryland

Douglas A. Singh, PhD, MBA
Associate Professor
School of Business and Economics
and the Department of Political Science
Indiana University–South Bend
South Bend, Indiana

JONES AND BARTLETT PUBLISHERS
Sudbury, Massachusetts
BOSTON TORONTO LONDON SINGAPORE

World Headquarters
Jones and Bartlett Publishers
40 Tall Pine Drive
Sudbury, MA 01776
978-443-5000
info@jbpub.com
www.jbpub.com

Jones and Bartlett Publishers
Canada
6339 Ormindale Way
Mississauga, Ontario L5V 1J2
Canada

Jones and Bartlett Publishers
International
Barb House, Barb Mews
London W6 7PA
United Kingdom

Jones and Bartlett's books and products are available through most bookstores and online booksellers. To contact Jones and Bartlett Publishers directly, call 800-832-0034, fax 978-443-8000, or visit our website www.jbpub.com.

Substantial discounts on bulk quantities of Jones and Bartlett's publications are available to corporations, professional associations, and other qualified organizations. For details and specific discount information, contact the special sales department at Jones and Bartlett via the above contact information or send an email to specialsales@jbpub.com.

Production Credits
Publisher: Michael Brown
Production Director: Amy Rose
Associate Editor: Katey Birtcher
Editorial Assistant: Catie Heverling
Senior Production Editor: Tracey Chapman
Marketing Manager: Sophie Fleck
Associate Marketing Manager: Jessica Cormier
Manufacturing and Inventory Control Supervisor: Amy Bacus
Composition: Cape Cod Compositors, Inc.
Illustrator: Accurate Artists, Inc.
Cover Design: Kate Ternullo
Cover Image: © Condor 36/ShutterStock, Inc.
Printing and Binding: Malloy, Inc.
Cover Printing: Malloy, Inc.

Library of Congress Cataloging-in-Publication Data
Shi, Leiyu.
Essentials of the U.S. health care system / Leiyu Shi, Douglas A. Singh.—2nd ed.
p. ; cm.
Includes bibliographical references and index.
ISBN-13: 978-0-7637-6380-0 (pbk.)
ISBN-10: 0-7637-6380-2 (pbk.)
1. Medical care—United States. 2. Medical policy—United States. I. Singh, Douglas A., 1946– II. Title. III. Title: Essentials of the United States health care system.
[DNLM: 1. Delivery of Health Care—United States. 2. Health Policy—United States.
W 84 AA1 S512e 2009]
RA395.A3S486 2005
362.10973—dc22

2008041625

6048

Printed in the United States of America
13 12 11 10 10 9 8 7 6 5 4

Contents

Preface

This book is a condensed and simplified version of our standard textbook on the U.S. health care system, *Delivering Health Care in America: A Systems Approach*, which has been widely used for teaching senior-level undergraduate and graduate courses. While retaining the main themes of the standard book, this version covers the essential elements of U.S. health care but leaves out much of the data and technical details provided in the standard book. This simplified format is produced for two main audiences: junior college students taking a basic course in U.S. health care and those who need a condensed text to supplement materials in another course, such as an advanced course in health policy or various courses taught in allied health settings in which a section of a course is devoted to the health care delivery system.

This book retains the systems model to organize the major themes of U.S. health care delivery into 14 chapters. The first three chapters lay the foundation that is necessary for understanding the U.S. health care delivery system, which is distinct from any other system in the world. Chapter 1 gives an overview of U.S. health care and contrasts the American system with the three most commonly used models of health care delivery in other advanced nations, such as Canada, Britain, and Germany. Chapter 2 explains the different models for understanding health and its determinants. In the context of American beliefs and values, this chapter also discusses the issue of equity using the concepts of market justice and social justice, and explains how health services are rationed in both market-justice– and social-justice–based systems. Chapter 3 traces the history of U.S. health care from colonial times to the present. The key to understanding the nature of the current health care system and its likely future direction is to understand its evolutionary past.

This chapter also includes current trends in corporatization, information revolution, and globalization as they pertain to health care delivery.

The next three chapters are about the resources—both human and nonhuman—employed in delivering health care. Chapter 4 addresses the roles played by some of the major personnel in health care delivery. The chapter also discusses some key issues pertaining to the number and distribution of physicians and the effect these factors have on the delivery of health care. Chapter 5 discusses medical technology and the various issues related to its development and dissemination. Chapter 6 explains the concept of health insurance, the major private and public health insurance programs in the United States, and methods of reimbursing providers.

Chapters 7 through 11 describe the system processes, beginning with outpatient and primary care services discussed in Chapter 7. Hospitals are the focus of Chapter 8. Chapter 9 is devoted to managed care, which has revolutionized health care delivery in recent years. This chapter also discusses different types of arrangements for organizational integration. Chapter 10 provides an overview of community-based and institution-based long-term care services. The direction of long-term care in the context of a rapidly growing elderly population is also explored. Chapter 11 highlights vulnerable populations and their special health care needs. This chapter also includes a section on mental health.

Chapters 12 and 13 deal with the main outcomes of the health care system and how those outcomes are addressed through health policy. The main outcomes associated with health care—costs, access to care, and quality of care—are presented in Chapter 12. Chapter 13 gives an overview of health policy in the United States. Chapter 14 extrapolates upon the past and present to explore the likely future directions. Expansion of health insurance to accommodate the uninsured is an ongoing concern. How this issue might be addressed during the Obama presidency is explored. An increased cost burden and a division among Americans on radical changes are major constraints that are likely to prevent systemwide reform. Apart from the challenges at home, the chapter also discusses emerging global challenges as they affect the health and well-being of Americans.

New in the Second Edition

This *Second Edition* has been updated with the latest health statistics and pertinent information available at the time the manuscript was prepared.

Some key additions to the text include the Veteran's Administration health care system, U.S. government-sponsored health insurance programs such as Medicare, Medicaid, and SCHIP, selected international health care systems (Chapter 1); public health system, interventions to improve performance (Chapter 2); discussion of corporatization of health care, the information revolution, and globalization (Chapter 3); role of hospitalists (Chapter 4); expanded coverage of information technology that includes electronic health records and e-health (Chapter 5); high-deductible health plans and health savings accounts, and an organized presentation of the four parts of Medicare (Chapter 6); an updated and revised discussion of long-term care and its services (Chapter 10); a comparison of health care spending among industrialized countries, electronic health records (Chapter 12); health policy issues such as 2008 presidential candidates' positions on health care reform, universal health coverage, smoking and tobacco use, fighting HIV/AIDS (Chapter 13); a discussion on conflicting realities of cost and coverage in the context of Massachusetts' health plan and universal health insurance; system reform in the context of 2008 presidential victory of Barack Obama; and a new section on evidence-based health care (Chapter 14).

Acknowledgment

We gratefully acknowledge Sylvia Shi for creating the cartoons for this book. We are also grateful for the valuable assistance of Angeli Bueno and Normalie Barton from Johns Hopkins University. Of course, all errors and omissions remain the responsibility of the authors.

Leiyu Shi
Douglas A. Singh

About the Authors

Dr. Leiyu Shi is Professor of health policy and health services research in the Department of Health Policy and Management at the Johns Hopkins University Bloomberg School of Public Health. He is Co-Director of Johns Hopkins Primary Care Policy Center. He received his doctoral education from the University of California Berkeley, majoring in health policy and services research. He also has a master's in business administration focusing on finance. Dr. Shi's research focuses on primary care, health disparities, and vulnerable populations. He has conducted extensive studies about the association between primary care and health outcomes, particularly on the role of primary care in mediating the adverse impact of income inequality on health outcomes. Dr. Shi is also well known for his extensive research on the nation's vulnerable populations, in particular community health centers that serve vulnerable populations, including their sustainability, provider recruitment and retention experiences, financial performance, experience under managed care, and quality of care. Dr. Shi is the author of seven textbooks and over 100 journal articles.

Dr. Douglas A. Singh teaches graduate and undergraduate courses in health care delivery, policy, finance, and management in the School of Business and Economics and in the Department of Political Science at Indiana University–South Bend. He has authored/coauthored four books and has published in peer-reviewed journals.

List of Exhibits

List of Tables

List of Figures

List of Abbreviations

CT	Computed Tomography
NIH	National Institutes of Health
R&D	Research and Development
DME	Durable Medical Equipment
SSI	Supplemental Security Income
CAM	Complementary and Alternative Medicine
ALOS	Average Length of Stay
JCAHO	Joint Commission on Accreditation of Healthcare Organizations
CEO	Chief Executive Officer
HMO	Health Maintenance Organization
MCO	Managed Care Organization
MD	Doctor of Medicine
COGME	Council on Graduate Medical Education
DO	Doctor of Osteopathic Medicine
PPO	Preferred Provider Organization
NOAA	National Oceanographic and Atmospheric Association
VA	Veterans Administration
BPHC	Bureau of Primary Health Care
DHHS	Department of Health and Human Services
SAEM	Society for Academic Emergency Medicine
WHO	World Health Organization
AMA	American Medical Association
AHA	American Hospital Association
AIDS	Acquired Immunodeficiency Syndrome

SARS	Severe Acute Respiratory Syndrome
DDS	Doctor of Dental Surgery
DMD	Doctor of Dental Medicine
PharmD	Doctor of Pharmacy
OD	Doctor of Optometry
PhD	Doctor of Philosophy
PsyD	Doctor of Psychology
DPM	Doctor of Podiatric Medicine
DC	Doctor of Chiropractic
RN	Registered Nurse
BSN	Bachelor of Science in Nursing
ADN	Associate's Degree in Nursing
LVN	Licensed Vocational Nurse
NCQA	National Committee for Quality Assurance
HEDIS	Healthcare Effectiveness Data and Information Set
LPN	Licensed Practical Nurse
APN	Advanced Practice Nurse
CNS	Clinical Nurse Specialist
CRNA	Certified Registered Nurse Anesthetist
NP	Nurse Practitioner
CNM	Certified Nurse-Midwife
PA	Physician Assistant
AAPA	American Academy of Physician Assistants
PT	Physical Therapist
MHA	Master of Health Administration
MHSA	Master of Health Services Administration
MBA	Master of Business Administration
MPH	Master of Public Health
MPA	Master of Public Administration
NAB	National Association of Boards of Examiners of Long-Term Care Administrators
MRI	Magnetic Resonance Imaging
HIPAA	Health Insurance Portability and Accountability Act
FDA	Food and Drug Administration
AHRQ	Agency for Healthcare Research and Quality
HIV	Human Immunodeficiency Virus
CMS	Centers for Medicare and Medicaid Services
SNF	Skilled Nursing Facility

SCHIP	State Children's Health Insurance Program
CPT	Current Procedural Terminology
DRG	Diagnosis Related Group
APC	Ambulatory Payment Classification
IPA	Independent Practice Association
POS	Point-of-Service
PHO	Physician-Hospital Organization
LTC	Long-Term Care
IADL	Instrumental Activities of Daily Living
PERS	Personal Emergency Response System
CCRC	Continuing Care Retirement Community
PRO	Peer Review Organization
CON	Certificate of Need
PORT	Patient Outcome Research Team
MSA	Medical Savings Account
EPA	Exclusive Provider Organization
RUG	Resource Utilization Group
HHRG	Home Health Resource Group
GDP	Gross Domestic Product
CPI	Consumer Price Index
ED	Emergency Department

Chapter 1

Major Characteristics of U.S. Health Care Delivery

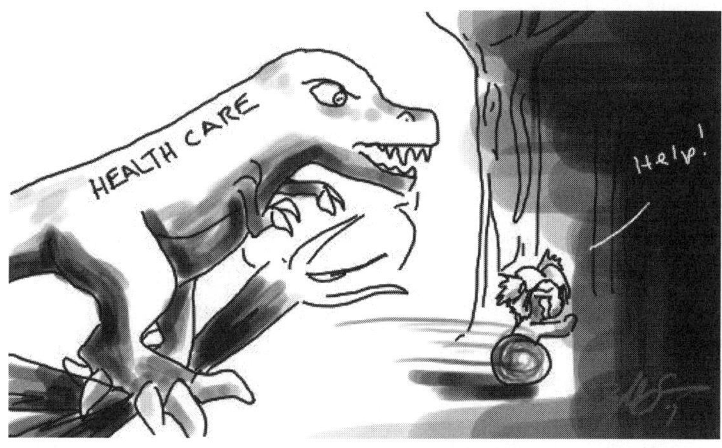

INTRODUCTION

The United States has a unique system of health care delivery. For the purposes of this discussion, "health care delivery" and "health services delivery" can have slightly different meanings, but in a broad sense, both terms refer to the major components of the system and the processes that enable people to receive health care. In a more restricted sense, the terms refer to the act of providing health care services to patients. The reader can identify which meaning is intended by paying attention to context.

In contrast to the United States, most developed countries have national health insurance programs that are run by the government and financed through general taxes. Almost all of the citizens in such countries are entitled to receive health care services that include routine and basic health care. These countries have what is commonly referred to as universal access. All American citizens, on the other hand, are not entitled to routine and basic health care services. Although the U.S. health care delivery system has evolved in response to concerns about cost, access, and quality, the system has been unable to provide universally a basic package of health care at an affordable cost. One barrier to universal coverage is the unnecessary fragmentation of the U.S. delivery system, which is perhaps its central feature (Shortell et al., 1996); however, the enormous challenge of expanding access to health care while containing overall costs and maintaining expected levels of quality continues to intrigue academics, policy makers, and politicians.

To make learning the structural and conceptual bases for the delivery of health services easier, this book is organized by the systems framework, which is presented at the end of this chapter. One of the main objectives of Chapter 1 is to provide a broad understanding of how health care is delivered in the United States.

The following overview introduces the reader to several concepts that are treated more extensively in later chapters. The U.S. health care delivery system is complex and massive. Interestingly, it is not actually a system in the true sense, although it is called a system when its various features, components, and services are referenced. Hence, it may be somewhat misleading to talk about the American health care delivery "system" (Wolinsky, 1988, p. 54), but the term will nevertheless be used throughout this book.

Organizations and individuals involved in health care range from educational and research institutions, medical suppliers, insurers, payers, and claims processors to health care providers. Total employment in various health delivery settings is almost 14.4 million, including professionally active doctors of medicine (MDs), doctors of osteopathy (DOs), active nurses, dentists, pharmacists, and administrators. Approximately 382,000 physical, occupational, and speech therapists provide rehabilitation services. The vast array of institutions includes 5,700 hospitals, 15,900 nursing homes, almost 2,900 inpatient mental health facilities, and 11,000 home health agencies and hospices. Close to 800 programs include basic health services for migrant workers and the homeless, community health centers, black lung clinics, human immunodeficiency virus (HIV) early intervention services, and integrated primary care and substance abuse treatment programs. Various types of health care professionals are trained in 144 medical and osteopathic schools, 56 dental schools, 109 schools of pharmacy, and more than 1,500 nursing programs located throughout the country.

There are 201.7 million Americans with private health insurance coverage, 40.3 million Medicare beneficiaries, and 38.3 million Medicaid recipients. Health insurance can be purchased from approximately 1,000 health insurance companies and 70 Blue Cross/Blue Shield plans. The managed care sector includes approximately 405 licensed health maintenance organizations (HMOs) and 925 preferred provider organizations (PPOs). A multitude of government agencies are involved with the financing of health care, medical and health services research, and regulatory oversight of the various aspects of the health care delivery system (Aventis Pharmaceuticals, 2002; Bureau of Primary Health Care, 1999; National Center for Health Statistics, 2007; U.S. Bureau of the Census, 1998; U.S. Census Bureau, 2007; Bureau of Labor Statistics, 2008).

SUBSYSTEMS OF U.S. HEALTH CARE DELIVERY

The United States does not have a universal health care delivery system enjoyed by everyone. Instead, multiple subsystems have developed, either through market forces or the need to take care of certain population segments. Discussion of the major subsystems follows.

Managed Care

Managed care is a system of health care delivery that (1) seeks to achieve efficiency by integrating the basic functions of health care delivery, (2) employs mechanisms to control (manage) utilization of medical services, and (3) determines the price at which the services are purchased and, consequently, how much the providers get paid. It is the most dominant health care delivery system in the United States today and is available to most Americans (for more details on managed care, please refer to Chapter 9).

The employer or government is the primary financier of the managed care system. Instead of purchasing coverage from a traditional insurance company, the financier contracts with a managed care organization (MCO), such as an HMO or a PPO, to offer a selected health plan to employees. In this case, the MCO functions like an insurance company and promises to provide health care services contracted under the health plan to the enrollees of the plan.

The term enrollee (member) refers to the individual covered under the plan. The contractual arrangement between the MCO and the enrollee—including the collective array of covered health services that the enrollee is entitled to—is referred to as the health plan (or "plan" for short). The health plan uses selected providers from whom the enrollees can choose to receive routine services. Primary care providers or general practitioners typically manage routine services and determine appropriate referrals for higher level or specialty services, often earning them the name of gate-keeper. The choice of major service providers, such as hospitals, is also limited. Some of the services may be delivered through the plans own hired physicians, but most are delivered through contracts with providers such as physicians, hospitals, and diagnostic clinics.

Although the employer finances the care by purchasing a plan from an MCO, the MCO is then responsible for negotiating with providers. Providers are typically paid either through a capitation (per head) arrangement, in which providers receive a fixed payment for each patient or employee under their care, or a discounted fee. Providers are willing to discount their services for MCO patients in exchange for being included in the MCO network and being guaranteed a patient population. Health plans rely on the expected cost of health care utilization, which always runs the risk of costing more than the premiums collected. By underwriting this risk, the plan assumes the role of insurer.

Figure 1.1 illustrates the basic functions and mechanisms that are necessary for the delivery of health services within managed care. The key functions of financing, insurance, delivery, and payment make up the quad-function model. Managed care arrangements integrate the four functions to varying degrees.

Military

The military medical care system is available free of charge to active-duty military personnel of the U.S. Army, Navy, Air Force, and Coast Guard and also to certain uniformed nonmilitary services such as the Public Health Service and the National Oceanographic and Atmospheric Association (NOAA). It is a well-organized, highly integrated system. It is comprehensive and covers preventive as well as treatment services that are provided by salaried health care personnel, many of whom are themselves in the military or uniformed services. This system combines public health

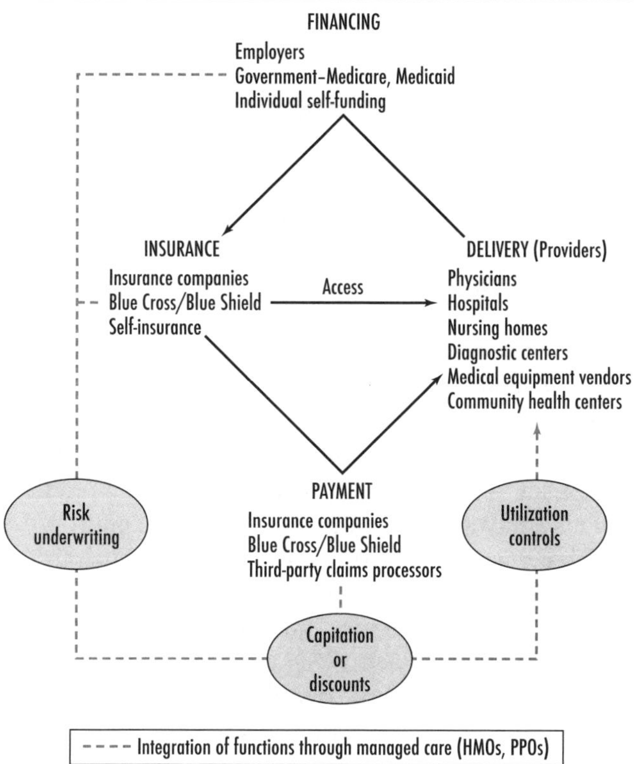

Figure 1.1 Managed Care: Integration of Functions

with medical services. Routine ambulatory care is provided close to the military personnel's place of work at the dispensary, sick bay, first-aid station, or medical station. Routine hospital services are provided at base dispensaries, in sick bays aboard ship, and at base hospitals. Complicated hospital services are provided in regional military hospitals. Long-term care is provided through Veterans Administration (VA) facilities to certain retired military personnel. Although patients have little choice regarding how services are provided, in general, the military medical care system provides high-quality health care.

Families and dependents of active-duty or retired career military personnel are either treated at the hospitals or dispensaries or are covered by

TRICARE, a program that is financed by the military. This insurance plan permits the beneficiaries to receive care from private medical care facilities as well as military ones.

The VA health care system is available to retired veterans of previous military service, with priority given to those who are disabled. The VA system focuses on hospital care, mental health services, and long-term care. It is one of the largest and oldest (1946) formally organized health care systems in the world. Its mission is to provide medical care, education and training, research, contingency support, and emergency management for the Department of Defense medical care system. It provides health care to more than 5.5 million persons at over 1,100 sites, including 153 hospitals, 732 ambulatory and community-based clinics, 135 nursing homes, 209 counseling centers, 47 domiciliaries (residential care facilities), 73 home health care programs, and various contract care programs. The VA budget is over $30 billion, and it employs a staff of 263,350 as of 2007 (National Center for Veterans Analysis and Statistics, 2007). The entire VA system is organized into 22 geographically distributed Veterans Integrated Service Networks (VISNs). Each VISN is responsible for coordinating the activities of the hospitals, outpatient clinics, nursing homes, and other facilities located within its jurisdiction. Each VISN receives an allocation of federal funds and is responsible for equitable distribution of those funds among its hospitals and other providers. VISNs are also responsible for improving efficiency by reducing unnecessarily duplicative services, by emphasizing preventive services, and by shifting services from costly inpatient care to less costly outpatient care.

Subsystem for Vulnerable Populations

Vulnerable populations, particularly those who are poor and uninsured or of minority and immigrant status, live in geographically or economically disadvantaged communities and receive care from "safety net" providers. These providers include health centers, physicians' offices, and hospital outpatient and emergency departments; of these, health centers are expressly designed to serve the underserved. Consistent with their unique role and mission, safety net providers offer comprehensive medical and enabling (e.g., language translation, transportation, outreach, nutrition and health education, social support services, case management, and child care) services targeted to the needs of vulnerable populations.

For example, for over 30 years, federally funded health centers have provided primary and preventive health services to rural and urban underserved populations. The Bureau of Primary Health Care (BPHC), located in the Health Resources and Services Administration in the Department of Health and Human Services (DHHS), provides federal support for community-based health centers that include programs for migrant and seasonal farm workers and their families, homeless persons, public housing residents, and school-aged children. These services facilitate regular access to care for patients who are predominantly minority, low-income, uninsured, or receiving Medicaid. By the end of calendar year 2002, the nationwide network of 843 reporting health centers delivered essential primary and preventive care at more than 3,500 sites, serving more than one fifth (more than 11 million) of the nation's 50 million underserved persons (Bureau of Primary Health Care, 2002). Health centers have contributed to significant improvements in health outcomes for the uninsured and Medicaid populations and have reduced disparities in health care and health status across socioeconomic and racial/ethnic groups (Politzer et al., 2003; Shi et al., 2001).

In addition to health centers, government health insurance programs, such as Medicare, Medicaid, and State Children's Health Insurance Program (SCHIP), provide vulnerable populations with access to health care services.

Medicare is one of the largest sources of health insurance in the country, serving nearly 39 million people, who are either 65 years old or older and who are suffering from certain disabilities or are diagnosed with end-stage renal disease. Managed by the Health Care Financing Administration (HCFA), another division within the DHHS, Medicare is composed of three parts, Part A, Part B, and most recently Part D. Part A and Part B were the original divisions of the Medicare program. Part A covers health care received in hospitals, nursing facilities, hospice care, and some home health care with no monthly premiums, while Part B covers doctors' services and other outpatient care not included in Part A with an additional monthly premium, which in 2008 cost about $96.40 per month. Part D, or the Medicare Prescription Drug Plan, provides coverage for brand-name and generic prescription drugs at pharmacies involved in the program. The program is designed to protect those in Medicare burdened with very high drug costs or unexpected prescription bills in the future.

In addition, Medicaid, the third largest source of health insurance in the country, provides coverage for low-income women, children, elderly people, and individuals with disabilities, covering 12% of the U.S. population. The program offers these vulnerable populations health insurance and long-term care for older Americans and individuals with disabilities and also provides additional coverage for low-income Medicare recipients for services not provided in the Medicare Part A Plan, such as outpatient care and prescription drugs.

Finally, with the growing uninsured population, the government has taken the initiative to provide insurance to children in uninsured families through SCHIP. Established in 1997, it expands coverage to children in families who do not qualify for Medicaid but who have a modest income, although each state has its own rules of eligibility. For little or no cost, the insurance pays for the child's physician visits, immunizations, hospitalizations, and emergency room visits.

America's safety net, however, is by no means secure, and the availability of safety net providers varies from community to community. Vulnerable populations residing in communities without safety net providers have to forego care or seek care from hospital emergency departments if one is nearby. Safety net providers face enormous pressure from the increasing number of uninsured and poor in their communities. The inability to shift costs for uncompensated care onto private insurance has become a significant problem as revenues from Medicaid, the primary source of third-party financing for core safety net providers, are restricted.

Integrated Delivery

Over the last decade, the hallmark of the U.S. health care industry has been organizational integration to form integrated delivery systems (IDSs) or networks. An IDS represents various forms of ownership and other strategic linkages among hospitals, physicians, and insurers. Its objective is to have one health care organization deliver a range of services. An IDS can be defined as a network of organizations that provides or arranges to provide a coordinated continuum of services to a defined population and that is willing to be held clinically and fiscally accountable for the outcomes and health status of the population. From the standpoint of integration, the major participants or players in the health care delivery system are physicians, hospitals, and insurers. The key strategic position that physicians, hospitals, and insurers hold gives rise to different forms of IDSs (see Chapter 9).

CHARACTERISTICS OF THE U.S. HEALTH CARE SYSTEM

The health care system of a nation is influenced by external factors, including the political climate, stage of economic development, technologic progress, social and cultural values, the physical environment, and population characteristics such as demographic and health trends. It follows, then, that the combined interaction of these environmental forces influences the course of health care delivery in the United States. This section summarizes the basic characteristics that differentiate the U.S. health care delivery system from that of other countries. There are eight main areas of distinction (see **Exhibit 1.1**).

No Central Governing Agency; Little Integration and Coordination

The U.S. health care system stands in conspicuous contrast to the health care systems of other developed countries. The centrally controlled universal health care system that most developed countries have authorizes the financing, payment, and delivery of health care to all residents. The U.S. system, however, is not centrally controlled and therefore has a variety of payment, insurance, and delivery mechanisms, and health care is financed both publicly and privately. Private financing, which is predominantly through employers, accounts for approximately 55% of total health care expenditures; the government finances the remaining 45% (National Center for Health Statistics, 2002).

Exhibit 1.1 Main Characteristics of the U.S. Health Care System

- No central governing agency and little integration and coordination
- Technology-driven delivery system focusing on acute care
- High on cost, unequal in access, average in outcome
- Delivery of health care under imperfect market condition
- Legal risks influence practice behaviors
- Government as subsidiary to the private sector
- Market justice vs. social justice: conflict throughout health care
- Multiple players and balance of power
- Quest for integration and accountability
- Access to health care services is selectively based on insurance coverage

Centrally controlled health care systems are less complex. They are also less costly because they can manage total expenditures through global budgets and can govern the availability and utilization of services. Because the United States has such a large private system of financing as well as delivery, the majority of hospitals and physician clinics are private businesses, independent of the government. Nevertheless, the federal and state governments in the United States play an important role in health care delivery. They determine public sector expenditures and reimbursement rates for services provided to Medicaid and Medicare patients. The government also formulates standards of participation through health policy and regulation, which means that providers must comply with the standards established by the government in order to deliver care to Medicaid and Medicare patients. Certification standards are also regarded as minimum standards of quality in most sectors of the health care industry.

Technology Driven and Focusing on Acute Care

The United States has been the hotbed of research and innovation in new medical technology. Growth in science and technology often creates a demand for new services despite shrinking resources to finance sophisticated care. Other factors contribute to increased demand for expensive technological care: Patients assume that current technologies offer the best care; physicians want to try the latest gadgets. Even hospitals compete on the basis of having the most modern equipment and are often under pressure to recoup capital investments made in technology by using it. Legal risks for providers and health plans alike may also play a role in the reluctance to deny new technology.

Although technology has ushered in a new generation of successful interventions, the negative outcomes resulting from its overuse are many. For example, the cost of highly technical interventions adds to the rising costs of health care, making it more difficult for employers to extend insurance to part-time workers or for insurance companies to lower their premiums. Because there are limited resources to invest in the American health care system, it is essential to think twice before assuming that the best solution always involves technology. Considering the broad benefits of primary care in preventing acute conditions that ultimately require technological intervention, it seems essential to strive for a balanced investment in both high- and low-technology medicine.

High on Cost, Unequal in Access, and Average in Outcome

The United States spends more than any other developed country on health care (primarily medical care), and costs continue to rise at an alarming rate. Despite spending such a high percentage (13%) of the nation's gross domestic product on health care, many U.S. residents have limited access to even the most basic care (Anderson et al., 2003).

Access means the ability of an individual to obtain health care services when needed. In the United States, access is restricted to those who (1) have health insurance through their employers, (2) are covered under a government health care program, (3) can afford to buy insurance out of their own private funds, and (4) are able to pay for services privately. Health insurance is the primary means for ensuring access. In 2000, the number of uninsured Americans—those without private or public health insurance coverage—was estimated to be 40.5 million or 16.8% of the U.S. population (National Center for Health Statistics, 2002). For consistent basic and routine care, commonly referred to as primary care, the uninsured are unable to see a physician unless they can pay the physician's fees. Those who cannot afford to pay generally wait until health problems develop, at which point they may be able to receive services free of charge in a hospital emergency department. Uninsured Americans therefore are able to obtain medical care for acute illness. Hence, one can say that the United States does have a form of universal catastrophic health insurance even for the uninsured (Altman & Reinhardt, 1996, p. xxvi).

It is well acknowledged that the absence of insurance inhibits the patient's ability to receive well-directed, coordinated, and continuous health care through access to primary care services and, when needed, referral to specialty services. Experts generally believe that the inadequate access to basic and routine primary care services is the main reason that the United States, in spite of being the most economically advanced country, lags behind other developed nations in measures of population health such as infant mortality and overall life expectancy.

Imperfect Market Conditions

Under national health care programs, patients have varying degrees of choice in selecting their providers; however, true economic market forces are virtually nonexistent. In the United States, even though the delivery of services is largely in private hands, health care is only partially governed by free market forces. The delivery and consumption of health care in the United States do not quite meet the basic tests of a free market. Hence, the system is best described as a quasi-market or an imperfect market. The following key characteristics of free markets help explain why U.S. health care is not a true free market.

In a free market, multiple patients (buyers) and providers (sellers) act independently. In a free market, patients should be able to choose their provider based on price and quality of services. If it were this simple, patient choice would determine prices by the unencumbered interaction of supply and demand. Theoretically, at least, prices are negotiated between payers and providers; however, in many cases, the payer is not the patient but an MCO, Medicare, or Medicaid. Because prices are set by agencies external to the market, they are not freely governed by the forces of supply and demand.

For the health care market to be free, unrestrained competition must occur among providers on the basis of price and quality. Generally speaking, free competition exists among health care providers in the United States. The consolidation of buying power into the hands of private health plans, however, is forcing providers to form alliances and IDSs on the supply side. As explained earlier, IDSs are networks that offer a range of health care services. In certain geographic sectors of the country, a single giant medical system has taken over as the sole provider of major health care services, restricting competition. As the health care system continues to move in this direction, it appears that only in large metropolitan areas will there be more than one large integrated system competing to get the business of the health plans.

A free market requires that patients have information about the availability of various services. Free markets operate best when consumers are educated about the products they are using, but patients are not always well informed about the decisions that need to be made regarding their care. Choices involving sophisticated technology, diagnostic methods, interventions, and pharmaceuticals can be difficult and often require physician input. Acting as an advocate, primary care providers can reduce this information gap for patients. Recently, health care consumers have taken the initiative to educate themselves with the use of Internet resources for gathering medical information. Pharmaceutical product advertising is also having an impact on consumer expectations and increasing awareness of available medications.

In a free market, patients have information on price and quality for each provider. Current pricing methods for health care services further confound free market mechanisms. Hidden costs make it difficult for patients to gauge the full expense of services ahead of time. *Item-based pricing*, for example, refers to the costs of ancillary services that often accompany major procedures such as surgery. Patients are usually informed of the surgery's cost ahead of time but cannot anticipate the cost of anesthesiologists and pathologists or hospital supplies and facilities, thus making it extremely difficult to ascertain the total price before services have actually been received. Package pricing and capitated fees can help overcome these drawbacks by providing a bundled fee for a package of related services. Package pricing covers services bundled together for one episode of care, which is less encompassing than capitation. Capitation covers all services an enrollee may need during an entire year.

In recent years, the quality of care has received much attention. Performance rating of health plans has met with some success; however, apart from sporadic news stories, the public generally has scant information on the quality of health care providers.

In a free market, patients must directly bear the cost of services received. The purpose of insurance is to protect against the risk of unforeseen major events. Because the fundamental purpose of insurance is to meet major expenses when unlikely events occur, having insurance for basic and routine health care undermines the principle of insurance. Health insurance coverage for minor services such as colds, coughs, and earaches amounts to prepayment for such services. There is a moral hazard that after enrollees have purchased health insurance they will use health care services to a greater extent than if they were without health insurance. Even certain referrals to higher level services may be foregone if the patient has to bear the full cost of these services.

In a free market for health care, patients as consumers make decisions about the purchase of health care services. The main factors that severely limit the patient's ability to make health care purchasing decisions have already been discussed. At least two additional factors limit the ability of patients to make decisions. First, decisions about the utilization of health care are often determined by need rather than price-based demand. Need has generally been defined as the amount of medical care that medical experts believe a person should have to remain or become healthy (Feldstein, 1993, p. 74–75). Second, the delivery of health care can result in creation of demand. This follows from self-assessed need that, coupled with moral hazard, leads to greater utilization. This creates an artificial demand because prices are not taken into consideration. Practitioners who have a financial interest in additional treatments also create artificial demand (Hemenway & Fallon, 1985), commonly referred to as provider-induced demand.

Government as Subsidiary to the Private Sector

In most other developed countries, the government plays a central role in the provision of health care. In the United States, however, the private sector plays the dominant role. This can be explained to some degree by the American tradition of reliance on individual responsibility and a commitment to limiting the power of the national government. As a result, government spending for health care has been largely confined to filling in the gaps left open by the private sector. These gaps include environmental protections, support for research and training, and care of vulnerable populations.

Market Justice versus Social Justice: Conflict Throughout Health Care

Market justice and social justice are two contrasting theories that govern the production and distribution of health care services in the United States. The principle of market justice places the responsibility for the fair distribution of health care on the market forces in a free economy. Medical care and its benefits are distributed on the basis of people's willingness and ability to pay (Santerre & Neun, 1996, p. 7). In contrast, social justice emphasizes the well-being of the community over that of the individual; thus, the inability to obtain medical services because of a lack of financial resources would be considered unjust. A just distribution of benefits must be based on need, not simply one's ability to purchase them in the marketplace. In a partial public and private health care system, the two theories often work well hand in hand, contributing ideals from both theories; however, market justice principles tend to prevail. As mentioned before, Americans generally prefer market solutions to government intervention in health care financing and delivery. Unfortunately, market justice results in the unequal allocation of health care services, neglecting critical human concerns that are not confined to the individual but have broader, negative impacts on society (see Chapter 2 for contrast between market and social justice).

Multiple Players and Balance of Power

The U.S. health services system involves multiple players. The key players in the system have been physicians, administrators of health service institutions, insurance companies, large employers, and the government. Big business, labor, insurance companies, physicians, and hospitals make up the powerful and politically active special interest groups represented before lawmakers by high-priced lobbyists. Each player has a different economic interest to protect. The problem is that the self-interests of each player are often at odds. For example, providers seek to maximize government reimbursement for services delivered to Medicare and Medicaid patients, but the government wants to contain cost increases. The fragmented self-interests of the various players produce counteracting forces within the system. One positive effect of these opposing forces is that they prevent any single entity from dominating the system. In an environment that is rife with motivations to protect conflicting self-interests, achieving comprehensive system-wide reforms is next to impossible, and cost containment remains a major challenge. Consequently, the approach to health care reform in the United States is characterized as incremental or piecemeal and is sometimes regressive when administrations change followed by its ripple effect on government health agencies.

Quest for Integration and Accountability

Currently in the United States, there is a drive to use primary care as the organizing hub for continuous and coordinated health services. Although this model gained popularity with the expansion of managed care, the model's development stalled before reaching its full potential. The envisioned role for primary care would include integrated health care by offering comprehensive, coordinated, and continuous services with a seamless delivery. Furthermore, the model emphasizes the importance of the patient–provider relationship and how it can best function to improve the health of each individual and thus strengthen the population. Integral to the relationship is the concept of accountability. Accountability on the provider's behalf means ethically providing quality health care in an efficient manner. On the patient's behalf, it means safeguarding one's own health and using available resources sensibly.

Access to Health Care Services Is Selectively Based on Insurance Coverage

Unlike countries with national health plans providing universal access, the United States' access to health care services is limited. Access is granted only to individuals who (1) have health insurance through their employers, (2) are covered under a government health care program, (3) can afford to buy insurance with their own private funds, and (4) can pay for services privately. Although the United States offers some of the best medical care in the world, this care is often available only to individuals with health insurance plans that provide adequate coverage or sufficient resources to pay for the procedures themselves.

In addition, there is a relatively large population of uninsured in the country. In 2006, 47 million people (15.8% of the population) were uninsured, meaning they were not covered by any type of insurance program, public nor private (DeNavas-Walt et al., 2006). This statistic does not include individuals in the population who are underinsured or only intermittently insured in a given year.

The uninsured have limited options when seeking medical care. They can either (1) pay physicians out of pocket that are typically at higher rates than those paid by insurance plans, (2) access federally funded health centers, or (3) obtain treatment for acute illnesses at a hospital emergency department for which hospitals do not receive direct payments unless patients have the ability to pay. The Emergency Medical Treatment and Labor Act of 1986 requires screening and evaluation of every patient, necessary stabilizing treatment, and admitting when necessary, regardless of ability to pay. Unfortunately, the inappropriate use of emergency departments results in cost-shifting, where patients able to pay for services, privately insured individuals, employers, and the government ultimately cover the costs provided to the uninsured in the emergency room. Also, the lack of insurance restricts the patients' capability to receive well-directed, coordinated, and continuous health care through access to primary care services, and when necessary, referral to specialty services.

Legal Risks Influence Practice Behaviors

Americans as a society are quick to engage in lawsuits. Motivated by prospects of enormous jury awards, people are easily prompted to drag alleged offenders into the courtroom because of the slightest perceptions of incurred harm. Because private health care providers are increasingly becoming more susceptible to litigations, risk of malpractice lawsuits is a serious consideration in the practice of medicine. As a form of protection, most providers engage in what is known as defensive medicine by prescribing additional diagnostic tests, scheduling checkup appointments, and maintaining abundant documentation on cases. Many of these efforts are unnecessary and only drive up costs and inefficiency.

HEALTH CARE SYSTEMS OF OTHER DEVELOPED COUNTRIES

Most Western European countries have national health care programs that provide universal access. There are three basic models for structuring national health care systems. In a system under National Health Insurance, such as Canada, the government finances health care through general taxes, but the actual care is delivered by private providers. In the context of the quad-function model (see Figure 1.1), National Health Insurance requires a tighter consolidation of the financing, insurance, and payment functions, which are coordinated by the government. Delivery is characterized by detached private arrangements.

In a national health system, such as the one in Great Britain, in addition to financing a tax-supported national health insurance program, the government also manages the infrastructure for the delivery of medical care. Under such a system, most of the medical institutions are operated by the government. Most health care providers, such as physicians, are either government employees or are tightly organized in a publicly managed infrastructure. In the context of the quad-function model, a National Health System requires a tighter consolidation of all four functions, typically by the government.

In a socialized health insurance system, such as in Germany, health care is financed through government-mandated contributions by employers and employees. Health care is delivered by private providers. Private not-for-profit insurance companies, called sickness funds, are responsible for collecting the contributions and paying physicians and hospitals (Santerre & Neun, 1996, p. 134). In a socialized health insurance system, insurance and payment functions are closely integrated, and the financing function is better coordinated with the insurance and payment functions than it is in the United States. Delivery is characterized by independent private arrangements. The government exercises overall control.

Canada

Canada's National Health Insurance system, referred to as Medicare, was initially established in the Medical Care Act of 1966, providing 50/50 cost sharing for provincial or territorial medical insurance plans. The system provides universal coverage with free care at the point of contact and is publicly funded through taxes, although it is privately run. Most doctors are private practitioners who are paid fee-for-service and submit service claims directly to the health insurance plan for payment. The federal government is responsible for establishing the constitution that determines how health care is run, whereas provincial and territorial governments administer and deliver heath care services and health insurance plans. In 1984, the addition of the Canadian Health Act solidified and defined five principles and criteria for territorial and provincial governments to meet in order to receive full funding for health insurance plans. Care must be (1) available to all eligible residents of Canada, (2) comprehensive in coverage, (3) accessible without financial and other barriers, (4) portable within the country and while traveling abroad, and (5) publicly administered. Canada's health care system relies heavily on primary care physicians, who account for 51% of active physicians in the country. These physicians serve two key functions. First, they provide first contact health care services, and second, they coordinate patient health care services across the system to ensure continuity. Primary physicians arrange patient access to specialists, hospital admissions, and diagnostic testing and prescription drug therapy.

Great Britain

In Great Britain, universal health coverage is provided by the National Health Service (NHS), which is publicly funded and run, relying on the belief that every citizen is entitled to health care. Through this system, all basic services, visits to primary care physicians and specialists, inpatient care, or x-ray and pathology services are free, whereas other costs are covered by the patient in full or subsidized by the government. Additionally, the purchase of private health insurance is also a choice for individuals with 7 million, or 12%, of the population covered by these plans. The system comes with serious problems that vary in severity across the region involving funding, service, and staff. One of the largest concerns plaguing the NHS is referred to as "health tourism," which is when individuals go into the country to get treated, escaping monetary fees and costing the agency almost £200 million each year. There are also long wait times for care, especially elective procedures, with 41.2% reporting a wait period of 12 or more weeks to see a specialist or receive surgical care, and much of the equipment used is outdated, as there is little funding directed towards technological innovations.

Germany

Germany follows the Socialized Health Insurance system with the statutory health insurance (GKV) providing organizational framework for the delivery of public health care. Employees and employers are required to provide 50/50 contributions toward the system if the employed earns below a specific level of income (40,500 Euros per year in 2004). The health plan also covers the spouse and children (until a certain age) of the employee. If income is above the limit, the individual is given a choice between private health insurance or the state insurance. Over 90% of the population is covered by the national health insurance—the remainder is insured privately. Although this system prevents the growth of an uninsured population, it is met with mixed opinions. In 2003, the German health ministry concluded that the system suffers from lack of competition, superfluous, insufficient, or inappropriate care, and shrinking revenue, and an aging population.

Table 1.1 presents selected features of the national health care programs in Canada, Germany, and Great Britain and compares them with those in the United States.

Table 1.1 Health Care Systems of Selected Industrialized Countries

	United States	Canada	Great Britain	Germany
Type	Pluralisitic	National health insurance	National health system	Socialized health insurance
Ownership	Private	Public/Private	Public	Private
Financing	Voluntary, multipayer system (premiums or general taxes)	Single-payer (general taxes)	Single-payer (general taxes)	Employer–employee (mandated payroll contributions, and general taxes)
Reimbursement (hospital)	Varies (DRGs, negotiated fee-for-service, per diem, capitation)	Global budgets	Global budgets	Per diem payments
Reimbursement (physicians)	RBRVS, fee-for-service	Negotiated fee-for-service	Salaries and capitation payments	Negotiated fee-for-service
Consumer Copayment	Small to significant	Negligible	Negligible	Negligible

Note: DRGs, diagnosis-related groups; RBRVS, resource-based relative value scale.

SYSTEMS FRAMEWORK

A system consists of a set of interrelated and interdependent components designed to achieve some common goals. The components are logically coordinated. Even though the various functional components of the health services delivery structure in the United States are at best only loosely coordinated, the main components can be identified with a systems model. The systems framework used here helps one understand that the structure of health care services in the United States is based on some foundations, provides a logical arrangement of the various components, and demonstrates a progression from inputs to outputs. The main elements of this arrangement are system inputs (resources), system structure, system processes, and system outputs (outcomes). In addition, system outlook (future directions) is a necessary element of a dynamic system. This systems framework has been used as the conceptual base for organizing later chapters in this book (see Figure 1.2).

System Foundations

The current health care system is not an accident. Historical, cultural, social, and economic factors explain its current structure. These factors also affect forces that shape new trends and developments and those that impede change. Chapters 2 and 3 provide a discussion of the system foundations.

System Resources

No mechanism for the delivery of health services can fulfill its primary objective without the necessary human and nonhuman resources. Human resources consist of the various types and categories of workers directly engaged in the delivery of health services to patients. Such personnel—including physicians, nurses, dentists, pharmacists, other professionals trained at the doctoral level, and numerous categories of allied health professionals—usually have direct contact with patients. Numerous ancillary workers, such as those involved in billing and collection, marketing and public relations, and building maintenance, often play an important but indirect supportive role in the delivery of health care. Health care managers are needed to manage and coordinate various types of health care services. This book discusses primarily the personnel engaged in the direct delivery

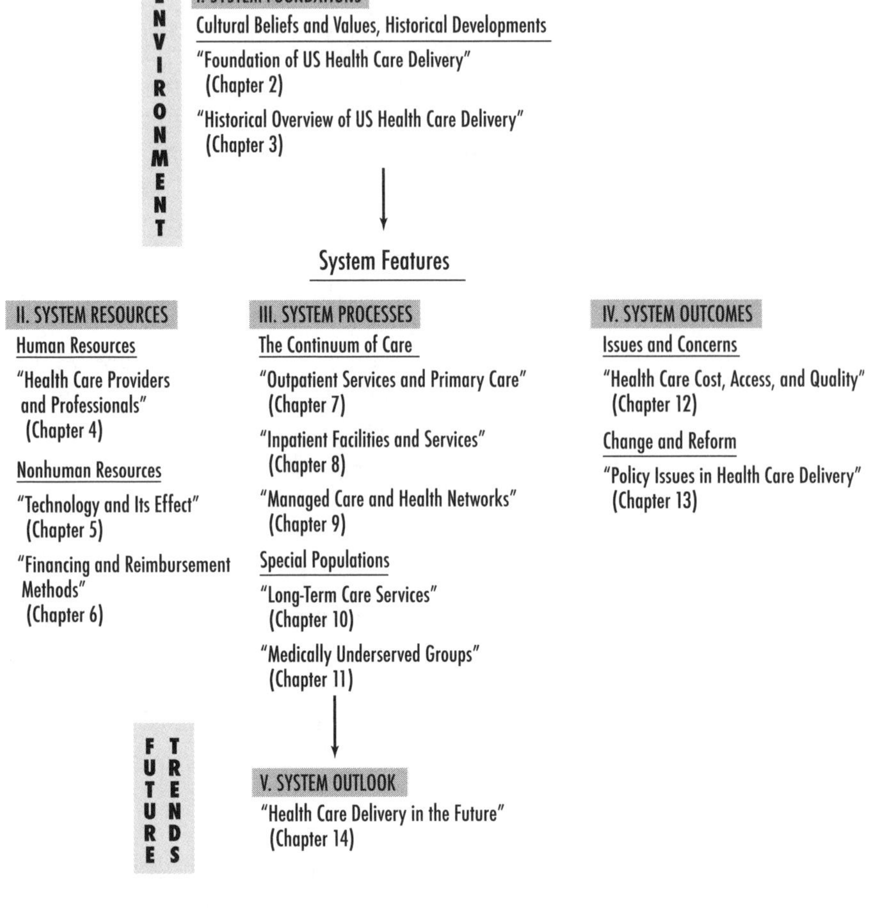

Figure 1.2 Systems Framework

of health care services (Chapter 4). The nonhuman resources include medical technology (Chapter 5) and health services financing (Chapter 6).

Resources are closely intertwined with access to health care. For instance, in certain rural areas of the United States, access is restricted because of a shortage of certain categories of health professionals. Development and diffusion of technology also determine the caliber of health care to which people may have access.

System Processes

The system resources influence the development and change in physical structures, such as hospitals, clinics, and nursing homes. These structures are associated with distinct processes of health services delivery, and the processes are associated with distinct health conditions. Most health care services are delivered in noninstitutional settings, which are mainly associated with processes referred to as outpatient care (Chapter 7). Institutional health services (inpatient care) are predominantly associated with acute care hospitals (Chapter 8). Managed care and integrated systems (Chapter 9) represent a fundamental change in the financing (including payment and insurance) and delivery of health care. Even though managed care represents an integration of the resource and process elements of the systems model, it is discussed as a process for the sake of clarity and continuity of the discussions. Special institutional and community-based settings have been developed for long-term care (Chapter 10) and mental health (Chapter 11).

System Outcomes

System outcomes refer to the critical issues and concerns surrounding what the health services system has been able to accomplish, or not accomplish, in relationship to its primary objective. The primary objective of any health care delivery system is to provide to an entire nation cost-effective health services that meet certain established standards of quality. The previous three elements of the systems model (foundations, resources, and processes) play a critical role in fulfilling this objective. Access, cost, and quality are the main outcome criteria for evaluating the success of a health care delivery system (Chapter 12). Issues and concerns regarding these criteria trigger broad initiatives for reforming the system through health policy (Chapter 13).

System Outlook

A dynamic health care system must look forward. In essence, it must project into the future the accomplishment of desired system outcomes in view of anticipated social, cultural, and economic changes. Chapter 14 discusses these future perspectives.

CONCLUSION

The United States has a unique system of health care delivery, but the system lacks universal access; therefore, continuous and comprehensive health care is not enjoyed by all Americans. Health care delivery in the United States is characterized by a patchwork of subsystems developed either through market forces or the need to take care of certain population segments. These include managed care, the military and VA systems, the system for vulnerable populations, and the emerging IDSs.

No country in the world has a perfect system. Most nations with a national health care program have a private sector that varies in size. The systems framework provides an organized approach to an understanding of the various components of the U.S. health care delivery system.

REFERENCES

Altman, S. H., and U. E. Reinhardt. 1996. Introduction: Where does health care reform go from here? An uncharted odyssey. In S. H. Altman and U. E. Reinhardt (eds.). *Strategic Choices for a Changing Health Care System* (pp. xxi–xxxii). Chicago: Health Administration Press.

Anderson, G. F., et al. 2003. It's the prices, stupid: Why the United States is so different from other countries. *Health Affairs* 22 (3):89–105.

Aventis Pharmaceuticals. 2002. *HMO-PPO Digest: Managed Care Digest Series.* Bridgewater, NJ: Aventis Pharmaceuticals.

Bureau of Labor Statistics. March 12, 2008. Health Care. U.S. Department of Labor. Retrieved July 11, 2008, from http://www.bls.gov/oco/cg/cgs035.htm.

Bureau of Primary Health Care. 1999. *Primary Care Programs Directory.* McLean, VA: National Clearinghouse for Primary Care Information.

Bureau of Primary Health Care. 2002. BPHC-UDS Annual Report. Rockville, MD: Bureau of Primary Health Care, Health Resources and Services Administration.

National Center for Health Statistics. 2002. *Health, United States, 2002.* Hyattsville, MD: Department of Health and Human Services.

National Center for Health Statistics. 2007. *Health, United States, 2007.* Hyattsville, MD: Department of Health and Human Services.

National Center for Veterans Analysis and Statistics. 2007. *FY07 VA Information Pamphlet.* Washington, DC: Department of Veterans Affairs.

Politzer, R. M., et al. 2003. The future role of health centers in improving national health. *Journal of Public Health Policy* 24 (3):296–306.

Santerre, R. E., and S. P. Neun. 1996. *Health Economics: Theories, Insights, and Industry Studies*. Chicago: Irwin.

Shi, L., et al. 2001. The impact of managed care on vulnerable populations served by community health centers. *Journal of Ambulatory Care Management* 24 (1):51–66.

Shortell, S. M., et al. 1996. Remaking health care in America: Building organized delivery systems. *Hospital Health Network* 70 (6):43–44, 46, 48.

U.S. Bureau of the Census. 1998. *Statistical Abstract of the United States: 1998*, 118th ed. Washington, DC: Bureau of the Census.

U.S. Census Bureau. 2007. Current Populations Report (pp. 60–233). *Income, Poverty, and Health Insurance Coverage in the United States: 2006*. Washington, DC: Government Printing Office.

Wolinsky, F. D. 1988. *The Sociology of Health: Principles, Practitioners, and Issues*, 2nd ed. Belmont, CA: Wadsworth Publishing Company.

Chapter 2

Foundation of U.S. Health Care Delivery

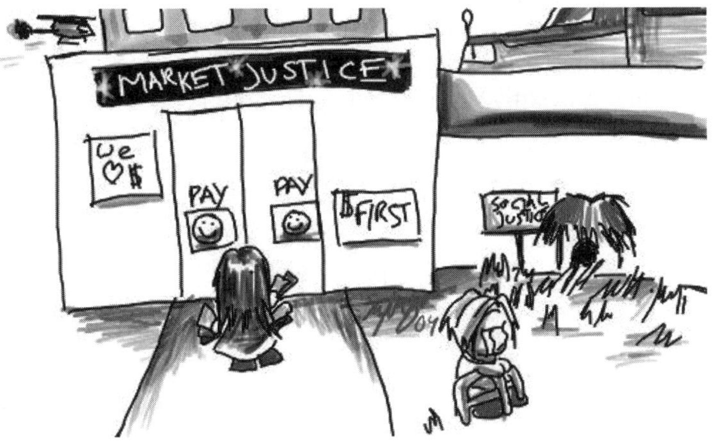

INTRODUCTION

From an economic perspective, curative medicine seems to produce decreasing returns in health improvement while health care expenditures increase (Saward & Sorensen, 1980). There is increased recognition of the benefits to society from the promotion of health and the prevention of disease, disability, and premature death. Although the financing of health care has focused primarily on curative medicine, some progress has been made toward an emphasis on health promotion and disease prevention; however, progress in this direction has been slow because of the social and institutional values and beliefs that emphasize disease rather than health. The common definitions of health, as well as measures for evaluating health status, reflect similar inclinations. This chapter proposes a holistic approach to health, although this may be an ideal that a health care delivery system may never fully achieve.

Beliefs and values ingrained in the American culture have also been influential in laying the foundations of a system that has remained predominantly private, as opposed to a tax-financed national health care program. This chapter further explores the issue of equity in the distribution of health services using the contrasting theories of market justice and social justice. The conflict between social and market justice is reflected throughout U.S. health care delivery. Justice and equity in making health care available to all Americans remains a lingering concern.

Planning of health services must be governed by demographic and health trends and initiatives toward reducing disease and disability. The concepts of health and its determinants should be used to design appropriate educational, preventive, and therapeutic initiatives.

WHAT IS HEALTH?

In the United States, the concepts of health and health care have largely been governed by the medical model or, more specifically, the biomedical model. The *medical model* presupposes the existence of illness or disease. It therefore emphasizes clinical diagnosis and medical intervention in the treatment of disease or its symptoms. Under the medical model, health is defined as the absence of illness or disease. The implication is that optimum health exists when a person is free of symptoms and does not require medical treatment; however, it is not a definition of health in the true sense but a definition of what is not ill health (Wolinsky, 1988, p. 76). Accordingly, prevention of disease and health promotion are relegated to a secondary status; therefore, when the term "health care delivery" is used, it actually refers to the delivery of medical care or illness care.

Medical sociologists have gone a step further in defining health as the state of optimum capacity of an individual to perform his or her expected social roles and tasks, such as work, school, and household chores (Parsons, 1972). A person who is unable (as opposed to unwilling) to perform his or her social roles in society is considered sick; however, this concept also tends to view health negatively because many people continue to engage in their social obligations despite suffering from pain, cough, colds, and other types of temporary disabilities, including mental distress. In other words, a person's engagement in social roles does not necessarily signify that the individual is in optimal health.

An emphasis on both the physical and mental dimensions of health is found in the definition of health proposed by the Society for Academic Emergency Medicine (SAEM), according to which health is "a state of physical and mental well-being that facilitates the achievement of individual and societal goals" (SAEM, 1992).

The World Health Organization's (WHO) definition of health has been most often cited as the ideal that health care delivery systems should try to achieve. The WHO defines health as "a complete state of physical, mental, and social well-being, and not merely the absence of disease or infirmity" (WHO, 1948). Because this definition includes physical, mental, and social dimensions, the WHO model can be referred to as the biopsychosocial model of health. The WHO has also recently defined a health care system as all of the activities whose primary purpose is to promote, restore, or maintain health (McKee, 2001). As this chapter points out, health care should include much more than medical care.

In recent years, there has been a growing interest in holistic health, which emphasizes the well-being of every aspect of what makes a person whole and complete. Thus, *holistic medicine* seeks to treat the individual as a whole person (Ward, 1995). Holistic health incorporates the spiritual dimension as a fourth element in addition to the physical, mental, and social aspects necessary for optimal health. Hence, the holistic model provides the most complete understanding of what health is (see **Exhibit 2.1** for some key examples of health indicators). A growing volume of medical literature now points to the healing effects of a person's religion and spirituality on morbidity and mortality (Levin, 1994). Numerous studies point to an inverse association between religious involvement and all-cause mortality (McCullough et al., 2000). Religious and spiritual beliefs and practices have been shown to have a positive impact on a person's physical, mental, and social well-being. They may affect the incidences,

Exhibit 2.1 Indicators of Health

- Self-reported health status
- Life expectancy
- Morbidity (disease)
- Mental well-being
- Social functioning
- Functional limitations
- Disability
- Spiritual well-being

experiences, and outcomes of several common medical problems (Maugans, 1996).

The spiritual dimension is often tied to one's religious beliefs, values, morals, and practices. More broadly, it is described as meaning, purpose, and fulfillment in life; hope and will to live; faith; and a person's relationship with God (Marwick, 1995; Ross, 1995; Swanson, 1995). The holistic approach to health also alludes to the need for incorporating alternative therapies (discussed in Chapter 7) into the predominant medical model.

Illness and Disease

The terms *illness* and *disease* are not synonymous, although they are often used interchangeably, as they are throughout this book. Illness is recognized by means of a person's own perceptions and evaluation of how he or she feels. For example, an individual may feel pain, discomfort, weakness, depression, or anxiety, but a disease may or may not be present; however, the determination that disease is present is based on a medical professional's evaluation rather than the patient's. It reflects the highest state of professional knowledge, particularly that of the physician, and it requires therapeutic intervention (May, 1993). Certain diseases, such as hypertension (high blood pressure), are asymptomatic and are not always manifested through illness. A hypertensive person has a disease but may not know it. Thus, it is possible to be diseased without feeling ill. Likewise, one may feel ill and not have a disease.

Disease can be classified as acute, subacute, or chronic. An *acute* condition is relatively severe, episodic (of short duration), and often treatable (Timmreck, 1994, p. 26). It is subject to recovery. Treatment is generally provided in a hospital. Examples of acute conditions are a sudden interruption of kidney function or a myocardial infarction (heart attack). A *subacute* condition is between acute and chronic but has some acute features. Subacute conditions can be postacute, requiring further treatment after a brief stay in the hospital. Examples include ventilator and head trauma care. A *chronic* condition is less severe but of long and continuous duration (Timmreck, 1994, p. 26). The patient may not fully recover. The disease may be kept under control through appropriate medical treatment, but if left untreated, the condition may lead to severe and life-threatening health problems. Examples are asthma, diabetes, and hypertension.

Quality of Life

The term *quality of life* is used in a denotative sense to capture the essence of overall satisfaction with life during and after a person's encounter with the health care delivery system. Thus, the term is used in two different ways. First, it is an indicator of how satisfied a person was with the experiences while receiving health care. Specific life domains such as comfort factors, dignity, privacy, security, degree of independence, decision-making autonomy, and attention to personal preferences are significant to most people. These factors are now regarded as rights that patients can demand during any type of health care encounter. Second, quality of life can refer to a person's overall satisfaction with life and with self-perceptions of health, particularly after some medical intervention. The implication is that desirable processes during medical treatment and successful outcomes would subsequently have a positive effect on an individual's ability to function and carry out social roles and obligations. It also can enhance a sense of fulfillment and self-worth.

DETERMINANTS OF HEALTH

The determinants of health have made a major contribution to the understanding that a singular focus on medical care delivery is unlikely to improve the health status of any given population. Instead, a more balanced approach must emphasize health determinants at an individual level, as well as broad policy interventions at the aggregate level (**Figure 2.1**).

The leading determinants of health (see examples in **Exhibit 2.2**) can be classified into four main categories:

- Environment
- Behavior and lifestyle
- Heredity
- Medical care

Environment

Environmental factors encompass the physical, socioeconomic, sociopolitical, and sociocultural dimensions. The physical environmental factors such as air pollution, food and water contaminants, radiation, and toxic chemicals

Exhibit 2.2 Examples of Health Determinants

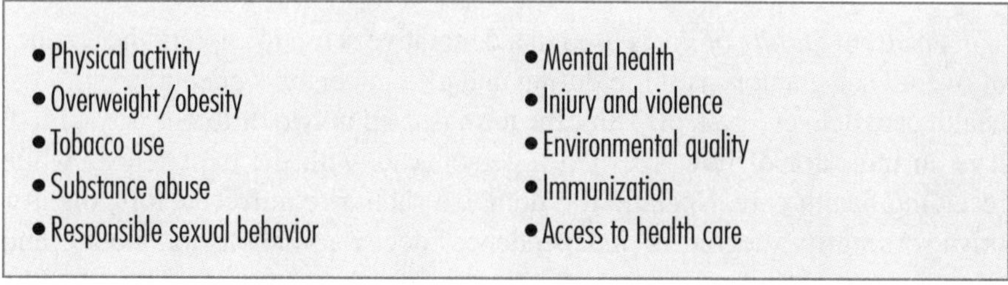

- Physical activity
- Overweight/obesity
- Tobacco use
- Substance abuse
- Responsible sexual behavior
- Mental health
- Injury and violence
- Environmental quality
- Immunization
- Access to health care

are easily identified as factors that can significantly influence health; however, the relationship of other environmental factors to health may not always be so obvious. For example, socioeconomic status is related to health and well-being. People who have higher incomes live in better homes and locations where they are less exposed to environmental risks and have better access to health care. The association of income inequality with a variety of health indicators such as life expectancy, age-adjusted mortality rates, and leading causes of death is well documented (Kaplan et al., 1996; Kawachi et al., 1997; Kennedy et al., 1996; Mackenbach et al., 1997). The greater the economic gap between the rich and the poor in a given geographic area, the worse the overall health status of the population of that area will be. It has been suggested that wide income gaps produce less social cohesion and greater psychosocial stress and, consequently, poorer health (Wilkinson, 1997).

The relationship between education and health status is also well established. Less educated Americans die younger than do their better educated counterparts. Better educated people are more likely to avoid risky behaviors such as smoking and drug abuse.

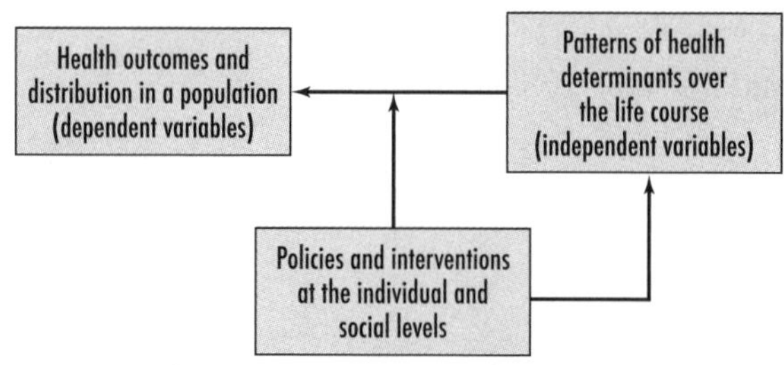

Figure 2.1 Schematic Definition of Population Health. Adapted from Kindig, D., and G. Stoddart. 2003. What is population health? *American Journal of Public Health* 93 (3):380–3.

The environment can also have a significant influence on developmental health. Neuroscientists have found that good nurturing and stimulation during the first three years of life—a prime time for brain development—activate the brain neural pathways that might otherwise atrophy and may even permanently increase the number of brain cells. Hence, the importance of the quality of child care provided in the first three years of life is monumental (Shellenbarger, 1997). Early childhood development influences a person's health in later years.

Behavior and Lifestyle

Individual lifestyles and behaviors are also a key determinant of health. For example, diet, exercise, stress-free lifestyle, promiscuous sex, and other individual choices such as smoking have been found to play a major role in most of the significant health problems of today. Heart disease, diabetes, stroke, sexually transmitted diseases, and cancer are just some of the ailments with direct links to individual choices and lifestyles.

Heredity

Heredity is a key determinant of health because genetic factors predispose individuals to certain diseases. There is little anyone can do about the genetic makeup he or she has already inherited, but a healthy lifestyle and health-promoting behaviors can have a significant influence on the development and severity of inherited disease in those predisposed to it, as well as on future generations.

Medical Care

Even though the other three factors are more important in the determination of health, well-being, and susceptibility to premature death, access to medical care is nevertheless a key determinant of health. Both individual health and population health are closely related to access to adequate preventive and curative health care services.

CULTURAL BELIEFS AND VALUES

A value system orients the members of a society toward defining what is desirable for that society. It has been observed that even a society as complex and highly differentiated as the United States can be said to have a relatively well-integrated system of institutionalized common values at the societal level (Parsons, 1972). Although such a view may still prevail, the current American society now has several different subcultures that have grown in size because of a steady influx of immigrants from different parts of the world. There are sociocultural variations in how people view their health and, more importantly, how such differences influence people's attitudes and behaviors concerning health, illness, and death (Wolinsky, 1988, p. 39). Cultural beliefs and values are strong forces against attempts to initiate fundamental changes in the financing and delivery of health care; therefore, enactment of major health system reforms would require consensus among Americans on basic values and ethics (Koop et al., 1993).

STRATEGIES TO IMPROVE HEALTH

Healthy People Initiatives

Since 1980, the United States has undertaken 10-year plans outlining certain key national health objectives to be accomplished during each of the 10-year time frames. These initiatives have been founded on the integration of medical care with preventive services, health promotion, and education; integration of personal and community health care; and increased access to integrated services. The current initiative, *Healthy People 2010: Healthy People in Healthy Communities*, was launched in January 2000. The context in which national objectives for *Healthy People 2010* have been framed take into account the realities of the 21st century: Advanced preventive therapies, vaccines and pharmaceuticals, and improved surveillance and data systems are now available. Demographic changes in the United States reflect an older and more racially diverse population. Global forces such as food supplies, emerging infectious diseases, and environmental interdependence present new public health challenges. The objectives also define new relationships between public health departments and health care delivery organizations (U.S. DHHS, 1998). *Healthy People 2010* specifically emphasizes the role of community partners such as businesses, local governments, and civic, professional, and religious organizations as effective agents for improving health in their local communities. Also, the objectives specifically focus on the determinants of health, as discussed earlier. The graphic framework for *Healthy People 2010* is presented in **Figure 2.2**.

Healthy People 2010 was designed to achieve two overarching goals (U.S. DHHS, 2000).

- *Increase quality and years of healthy life.* This first goal aims to help individuals of all ages increase life expectancy and improve their quality of life. Differences in life expectancy among populations especially suggest a substantial need and opportunity for improvement. At least 18 countries with populations of 1 million or more have life expectancies greater than those in the United States for both men and women. Similar to life expectancy, various population groups show dramatic differences in quality of life. A disproportionate number of women—those in low-income households and those living in rural areas—report their health status as fair or poor.

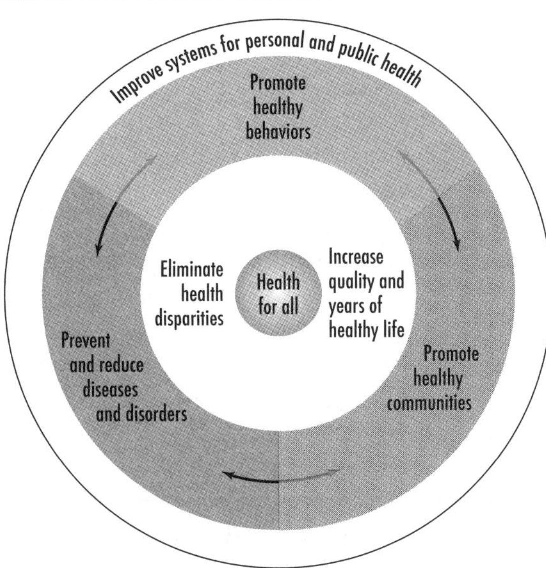

Figure 2.2 Healthy People 2010: Healthy People in Healthy Communities. From US DHHS. 2002. *Healthy People 2010.* Washington, DC: DHHS.

- *Eliminate health disparities.* The second goal of *Healthy People 2010* is to eliminate health disparities among different segments of the population. These include differences that occur because of gender, race or ethnicity, education or income, disability, living in rural localities, or sexual orientation. The greatest opportunities for reducing health disparities are in empowering individuals to make informed health care decisions and promoting community-wide safety, education, and access to health care.

To realize these two broad goals, measurable targets to be achieved by the year 2010 have been identified in 28 focus areas that span a variety of health status domains such as morbidity incidence and/or prevalence, injury, violence, and access to care.

Distribution of Health Care

The production, distribution, and subsequent consumption of health care must be perceived as equitable. No society has found a perfectly equitable method to distribute limited economic resources. In fact, any method of resource distribution leaves some inequalities. Societies, therefore, try to allocate resources according to some guiding principles acceptable to each society. Such principles are generally ingrained in a society's values and belief systems. It is generally recognized that not everyone can receive everything medical science has to offer. The fundamental question that deals with distributive justice or equity is who should receive the medical goods and services that society produces (Santerre & Neun, 1996, p. 7). By extension, this basic question about equity includes not only who should receive medical care but also what type of services and in what quantity.

A just and fair allocation of health care poses conceptual and practical difficulties; hence, a theory of justice is needed to resolve the problem of health care allocation (Jonsen, 1986). The principle of justice is derived from ethical theories, especially those advanced by John Rawls, who defined justice as fairness (Darr, 1991). Even though various ethical principles can be used to guide decisions pertaining to just and fair allocation of health care in individual circumstances, the broad concern about equitable access to health services is addressed by the theories referred to as *market justice* and *social justice*. These two contrasting theories govern the production and distribution of health care services.

Market Justice

The principle of market justice proposes that market forces in a free economy can best achieve a fair distribution of health care. Medical care and its benefits are distributed on the basis of people's willingness and ability to pay (Santerre & Neun, 1996, p. 7). In other words, people are entitled to purchase a share of the available goods and services that they value. They are to purchase these valued goods and services by means of wealth acquired through their own legitimate efforts. This is how most goods and services are distributed in a free market. The free market implies that giving people something they have not earned would be morally and economically wrong. The principle of market justice is based on the following key assumptions.

- Health care is like any other economic good or service, and therefore, it can be governed by free market forces of supply and demand.
- Individuals are responsible for their own achievements. When individuals pursue their own best interests, the interests of society as a whole are best served (Ferguson & Maurice, 1970).
- People make rational choices in their decisions to purchase health care products and services. People demand health care because it can rectify a health problem and restore health, can reduce pain and discomfort and make people feel better, and can reduce anxiety about health and well-being; therefore, people are willing to purchase health care services.
- People, in consultation with their physicians, know what is best for themselves. This assumption implies that people place a certain degree of trust in their physicians and that the physician–patient relationship is ongoing.
- The marketplace works best with minimum interference from the government. In other words, the market, rather than the government, can allocate health care resources in the most efficient and equitable manner.

Under market justice, the production of health care is determined by how much the consumers are willing and able to purchase at the prevailing market prices. It follows that in a pure market system individuals without sufficient income or who are uninsured face a financial barrier to obtaining health care (Santerre & Neun, 1996, p. 7). Thus, prices and ability to pay ration the quantity and type of health care services people consume. Such limitations to obtaining health care are referred to as *demand-side rationing* or price rationing.

The key characteristics of market justice and their implications are summarized in **Table 2.1**.

Table 2.1 Comparison of Market Justice and Social Justice

Market Justice	Social Justice
Characteristics	
• Views health care as an economic good	• Views health care as a social resource
• Assumes free market conditions for health services delivery	• Requires active government involvement in health services delivery
• Assumes that markets are more efficient in allocating health resources equitably	• Assumes that the government is more efficient in allocating health resources equitably
• Production and distribution of health care determined by market-based demand	• Medical resource allocation determined by central planning
• Medical care distribution based on people's ability to pay	• Ability to pay inconsequential for receiving medical care
• Access to medical care viewed as an economic reward of personal effort and achievement	• Equal access to medical services viewed as a basic right
Implications	
• Individual responsibility for health	• Collective responsibility for health
• Benefits based on individual purchasing power	• Everyone is entitled to a basic package of benefits
• Limited obligation to the collective good	• Strong obligation to the collective good
• Emphasis on individual well-being	• Community well-being supersedes that of the individual
• Private solutions to social problems	• Public solutions to social problems
• Rationing based on ability to pay	• Planned rationing of health care

Market justice emphasizes individual rather than collective responsibility for health. It proposes private rather than government solutions to the social problems of health.

The principles of market justice work well in the allocation of economic goods when their unequal distribution does not affect the larger society. For example, based on individual success, people live in different sizes and styles of homes, drive different types of automobiles, and spend their money on different things; however, market justice principles generally fail to rectify critical human concerns such as crime, illiteracy, and homelessness, which can significantly weaken the fabric of a society. Many Americans believe that health care is also a social concern.

Social Justice

The idea of social justice is at odds with the principles of capitalism and market justice. According to the principle of social justice, the equitable distribution of health care is a societal responsibility. This can best be achieved by letting a central agency, generally the government, take over the production and distribution functions. Social justice regards health care as a social good—as opposed to an economic good—that should be collectively financed and available to all citizens regardless of the individual recipient's ability to pay for that care. Canadians and Europeans, for example, long ago reached a broad social consensus that health care was a social good (Reinhardt, 1994). Public health also has a social justice orientation (Turnock, 1997). Under the social justice system, an inability to obtain medical services because of a lack of financial resources is considered unjust. A just distribution of benefits must be based on need, not simply on one's ability to purchase in the marketplace (demand). The need for health care is determined by either the patient or a health professional. The principle of social justice is also based on certain assumptions.

- Health care is different from most other goods and services. Health-seeking behavior is governed primarily by need rather than by how much it costs.
- Responsibility for health is shared. Individuals are not held totally responsible for their condition because factors outside of their control may have brought on the condition. Society feels responsible

for a lack of control over certain environmental factors such as economic inequalities, unemployment, unsanitary conditions, or air pollution.

- Society has an obligation to the collective good. The well-being of the community is superior to that of the individual. An unhealthy individual is a burden on society. A person carrying a deadly infection, for example, is a threat to society. Society, therefore, is obligated to cure the problem by providing health care to the individual because by doing so the whole society benefits.
- The government, rather than the market, can better decide through rational planning how much health care to produce and how to distribute it among all citizens.

Under social justice, how much health care to produce is determined by the government; however, no country can afford to provide unlimited amounts of health care to all of its citizens (Feldstein, 1994, p. 44). The government then also finds ways to limit the availability of certain health care services by deciding, for instance, how technology will be dispersed and who will be allowed access to certain types of high-tech services, even though basic services may be available to all. This concept is referred to as *planned rationing* or *supply-side rationing*. The government makes deliberate attempts, often referred to as "health planning," to limit the supply of health care services, particularly those beyond the basic level of care. The main characteristics and implications of social justice are summarized in Table 2.1.

Health Insurance

In the United States, the principles of market justice and social justice complement each other. Private, employer-based health insurance, mainly for middle-income Americans, falls under the heading of market justice. Publicly financed Medicaid and Medicare coverage for certain disadvantaged groups and the workers' compensation program for those injured at work fall under the heading of social justice. The two principles collide, however, regarding the large number of uninsured who cannot afford to purchase private health insurance and do not meet the eligibility criteria for Medicaid, Medicare, or other public programs. Americans have not been able to resolve the question of who should provide health insurance to the uninsured.

Organization of Health Care Delivery

In the United States, private and government health insurance programs enable the covered populations to have access to health care services delivered by private practitioners and private institutions (market justice). Tax-supported county and city hospitals, public health clinics, and community health centers can be accessed by the uninsured in areas where such services are available (social justice). Publicly run institutions generally operate in large inner cities and certain rural areas. Conflict between the two principles of justice arises in small cities and towns and in rural areas where such services are not available.

Public Health Systems

"Public health" is a reflection of society's desire and effort to improve the health and well-being of the total population, by relying on the role of government, the private sector, and the public in addition to focusing on the determinants of population health. The "public health system," then, reflects the organized effort to deliver public health services within a jurisdiction with the goal of improving health and well-being of the population.

Significant evidence indicates that public health contributes positively to population health. Indicators at the national, state, and local level should be developed to measure public health performance that improves population health and reduces health disparities along with a national surveillance system to track the indicators consistently in order to gain a better understanding of the system. In addition, the innovative effort of the states to improve their public health systems' infrastructure, practices, and performance should be encouraged and evaluated as most significant reforms take place at this level, more so than at the federal or municipal level.

Turning Point

Turning Point is an initiative of the Robert Wood Johnson Foundation to transform and strengthen the public health system with 21 states currently participating. Multisector partnerships to produce public health improvement plans employing strategies that include institutionalization within government, establishing "third-sector" institutions, cultivating relationships with significant allies, and enhancing communication and visibility among multiple communities (Shi, 2008).

Focusing on Determinants

To improve the nation's health and resolve disparities among its vulnerable populations, a framework embodying the social and medical determinants is warranted. This framework, presented in **Figure 2.3**, is built on the ballasts of both social and medical care determinants because it is the combination of these factors that ultimately shapes health and well-being. It synthesizes these multiple health influences and highlights points for intervention. Health, in this model, however, is not merely being free of disease and injury but includes the positive concept of well-being and encompasses the physical, mental, social, and spiritual aspects of health.

Social Determinants of Health

The framework acknowledges the confounding effects of demographics, socioeconomic status, personal behavior, and community-level inequalities and their defining influence on health. Personal demographics (e.g., race/ethnicity or age) directly contribute to vulnerability levels. Whether socioeconomic status is defined by education, employment, or income, both individual- and community-level socioeconomic status have independent effects on health. The health impact of personal behaviors (e.g., smoking or exercise) is well documented, but behavior is rarely isolated from the social and environmental contexts in which choices are made.

Social and income inequalities have also recently been shown to contribute to disparities in health. Underinvestment in human capital, erosion of social cohesion, and the consequences of relative deprivation are mechanisms by which income inequalities can lead to poorer health outcomes. Discrimination (the difference in one's actions toward an individual or group based on the innate personal characteristics of that group, such as race and/or ethnicity), for example, is an inequality prevalent in the United States that has direct consequences for individual health. Because many of the social factors of health care are the root causes of poor health, addressing them is vital to the improvement of population health and health disparities in the country.

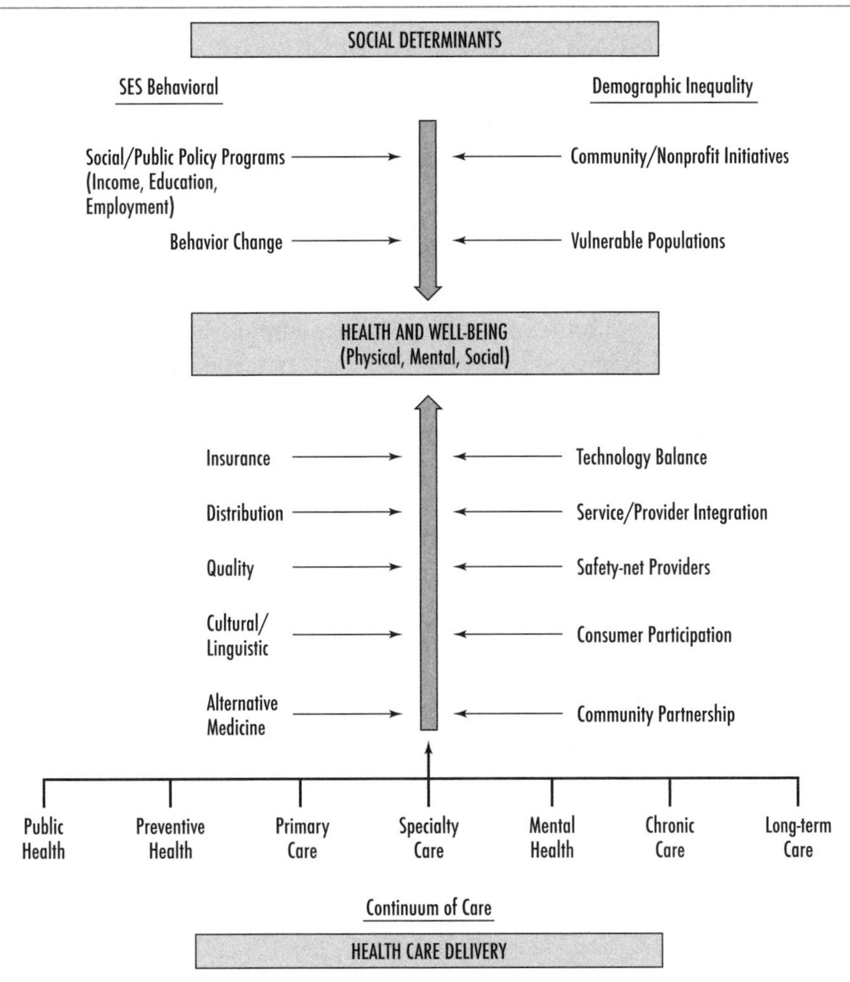

Figure 2.3 Health Determinants and Strategies to Improve Health

Medical Care Determinants of Health

Although social determinants influence the health status that patients bring to the health care system, the medical care system focuses primarily on treating illness or poor health. Preventive care is an exception to this rule, but understanding the influences of medical care on health should take into consideration disparities that exist in basic health care access and quality. The framework includes a broad spectrum of medical care services and interventions to improve health. Whereas some services (preventive and primary care) contribute to general health status, others are more influential in end-of-life situations (specialty and long-term care). Patients moving across the spectrum will contend with issues of fragmentation, poor continuity of care, and insufficient coordination of care for multiple health needs.

The relative value of each health service in the spectrum should be evaluated in determining health policy. For example, should equal investments be made in each service or are some investments better than others (e.g., primary versus specialty care)? How can we optimize the medical system's potential for eliminating disparities with limited resources (e.g., focusing on primary care for all or higher levels of technology care for certain populations)? Other health care factors such as the quality of care, access to alternative therapies, and technology will further affect the patient's health care experience and health outcomes.

Social and Medical Points of Intervention

Considering that social and medical determinants are responsive to numerous outside forces, the framework highlights important points for intervention. Dramatic reductions in health disparities are obtainable through interventions in both the social and medical domains and are grouped according to four main strategies: (1) social or medical care policy interventions, (2) community-based interventions, (3) health care interventions, and (4) individual interventions. The following sections elaborate on these strategies.

Policy Interventions Social or public policy affects the health of the population in many ways. Product safety regulations, screening food and water sources, and enforcing safe work environments are merely a few of the ways in which public policy directly guards the welfare of the nation. With fewer resources at their disposal, however, vulnerable populations are uniquely dependent on social and public policy to develop and implement programs that address basic nutritional, safety, social, and health care needs. Many of the mechanisms relating vulnerable status to poor health are amenable to policy intervention, and policy initiatives can be primary prevention strategies to alter the fundamental dynamics linking social factors to poor health.

Community-Based Interventions Disparities in health exist nationally, but they also vary substantially at the community level. This suggests that many of the sources of health disparities may be addressed at the community or local level. Neighborhood poverty, the presence of local health and social welfare resources, and societal cohesion and support are all likely to contribute to inequalities in a community. Armed with a greater understanding of these community-based challenges to health, those designing strategies to address disparities by race/ethnicity have adopted a renewed interest in tailoring interventions to address the multidimensional risks and needs in a particular community (see the examples in **Exhibit 2.3**). Because community partnerships reflect the priorities of a local population and are often managed by members of the community, they minimize cultural barriers and improve community buy-in to the program.

Community-based strategies have the particular benefit of mobilizing resources at the local level to address these problems. There are several other advantages to addressing disparities with community approaches. Community resources can be applied directly to community members, providing businesses and other local sources with greater incentive to contribute to local health causes. Communities should be seen as action centers for development, progress, and change, with local members and leaders playing a central role in planning and managing strategies for health improvement. Through community mobilization, skill-building, and resource sharing, communities can be empowered to identify and meet their own needs, making them stronger advocates in supporting the vulnerable populations within and across their community. Community solutions also benefit

Exhibit 2.3 Strategies to Improve Health and Reduce Disparities

- Nutrition programs
- Work/environment safety efforts
- Community-based partnerships
- Culturally appropriate care
- Patient safety/medical error reduction
- Prevention-oriented effort
- Coordinated care for chronically ill

from participatory decision making. Local researchers, health practitioners, social services, businesses, and community members are invited to contribute to the process of designing, implementing, evaluating, and sustaining the program. Moreover, many community programs are run by nonprofit organizations, and in exchange for providing services, these organizations are subsidized through federal, state, or local funds and receive tax exemptions. Thus, they are able to offer services at lower cost than private health organizations that are obligated to shareholders to price competitively.

Health Care Interventions Although social policy and community-level interventions are designed to address social disparities in health, billions of public and private dollars are spent annually to monitor and improve facets of the U.S. health care system. Interventions have been designed for health systems (e.g., integrated electronic medical records systems to better coordinate care for populations with multiple chronic and acute conditions), providers (e.g., continuing education for pediatricians to better target developmental services to children most in need), and patients (e.g., educating pregnant mothers to attend regular prenatal care visits).

Individual-Level Interventions Where policy and community-level interventions are unable to reduce either the occurrence of compromising social determinants or their consequences, individual-level initiatives can attempt to intervene and minimize the effects of negative social determinants on health status. Altering individual behaviors that influence health (e.g., reducing smoking and increasing exercise) is often the focus of these individual-targeted interventions, and numerous theories identify the complex pathways and barriers to eliciting changes or improvements in behavior. The integration of behavioral science into the public health field has been a valuable contribution, providing a toolbox of health-related behavior-changing strategies.

CONCLUSION

The system of health care delivery in the United States is predominantly private. Many of the peculiarities of this system can be traced back to the beliefs and values underlying the American culture. The delivery of health care is primarily driven by the medical model, which emphasizes illness rather than wellness. Even though major efforts and expenditures have been directed toward the delivery of medical care, they have failed to produce a proportionate impact on the improvement of health status. Holistic concepts of health care, along with integration of medical care with preventive and health promotional efforts, need to be adopted to significantly improve the health of Americans. Such an approach would require a fundamental change in how Americans view health. It would also require individual responsibility for one's own health-oriented behaviors, as well as community partnerships to improve both personal and community health. An understanding of the determinants of health, health education, community health assessment, and national initiatives such as *Healthy People 2010* are essential for accomplishing such goals. The emphasis on market justice in the U.S. health care delivery system, however, leaves the critical problem of access unaddressed. To improve the nation's health and resolve disparities among its vulnerable populations, it is critical to address both the social and medical determinants of health.

REFERENCES

Darr, K. 1991. *Ethics in Health Services Management*. Baltimore, MD: Health Professions Press.

Feldstein, P. J. 1994. *Health Policy Issues: An Economic Perspective on Health Reform*. Ann Arbor, MI: The Association of University Programs in Health Administration/Health Administration Press.

Ferguson, C. E., and S. C. Maurice. 1970. *Economic Analysis*. Homewood, IL: Richard D. Irwin.

Jonsen, A. R. 1986. Bentham in a box: Technology assessment and health care allocation. *Law, Medicine, and Health Care* 14 (3):172–174.

Kaplan, G. A., et al. 1996. Income inequality and mortality in the United States. *British Medical Journal* 312 (7037):999–1003.

Kawachi, I., et al. 1997. Social capital, income inequality, and mortality. *American Journal of Public Health* 87:1491–1498.

Kennedy, B. P., et al. 1996. Income distribution and mortality: Cross sectional ecological study of the Robin Hood Index in the United States. *British Medical Journal* 312 (7037):1004–1007.

Koop, C. E. Quoted in Kardos, B. C., and A. T. Allen. 1993. Healthy neighbors: Exploring the health care systems of the United States and Canada. *Journal of Post Anesthesia Nursing* 8 (1):48–51.

Levin, J. S. 1994. Religion and health: Is there an association, is it valid, and is it causal? *Social Science and Medicine* 38 (11):1475–1482.

Mackenbach, J. P., et al. 1997. Socioeconomic inequalities in morbidity and mortality in Western Europe. *Lancet* 349:1655–1660.

Marwick, C. 1995. Should physicians prescribe prayer for health? Spiritual aspects of well-being considered. *Journal of the American Medical Association* 273 (20):1561–1562.

Maugans, T. A. 1996. The SPIRITual history. *Archives of Family Medicine* 5 (1):11–16.

May, L. A. 1993. The physiologic and psychological bases of health, disease, and care seeking. In S. J. Williams and P. R. Torrens (eds.). *Introduction to Health Services*, 4th ed. (pp. 31–45). New York: Delmar Publishers.

McCullough, M. E., et al. 2000. Religious involvement and mortality: A meta-analytic review. *Health Psychology* 19 (3):211–222.

McKee, M. 2001. Measuring the efficiency of health systems. *British Medical Journal* 323 (7308):295–296.

Parsons, T. 1972. Definitions of health and illness in the light of American values and social structure. In E. G. Jaco (ed.). *Patients, Physicians and Illness: A Sourcebook in Behavioral Science and Health*, 2nd ed. New York: Free Press.

Reinhardt, U. E. 1994. Providing access to health care and controlling costs: The universal dilemma. In P. R. Lee and C. L. Estes (eds.). *The Nation's Health*, 4th ed. (pp. 263–278). Boston: Jones and Bartlett Publishers.

Ross, L. 1995. The spiritual dimension: Its importance to patients' health, well-being and quality of life and its implications for nursing practice. *International Journal of Nursing Studies* 32 (5):457–468.

Santerre, R. E., and S. P. Neun. 1996. *Health Economics: Theories, Insights, and Industry Studies*. Chicago: Irwin.

Saward, E., and A. Sorensen. 1980. The current emphasis on preventive medicine. In S. J. Williams (ed.). *Issues in Health Services* (pp. 17–29). New York: John Wiley & Sons.

Shellenbarger, S. 1997, April 9. Good, early care has a huge impact on kids, studies say. *Wall Street Journal*, B1.

Society for Academic Emergency Medicine. Ethics Committee. 1992. An ethical foundation for health care: An emergency medicine perspective. *Annals of Emergency Medicine* 21:1381–1387.

Swanson, C. S. 1995. A spirit-focused conceptual model of nursing for the advanced practice nurse. *Issues in Comprehensive Pediatric Nursing* 18 (4):267–275.

Timmreck, T. C. 1994. *An Introduction to Epidemiology*. Boston: Jones and Bartlett Publishers.

Turnock, B. J. 1997. *Public Health: What It Is and How It Works*. Gaithersburg, MD: Aspen Publishers.

U.S. Department of Health and Human Services. 1998. Objectives: Draft for public comment. In *Healthy People 2010: Healthy People in Healthy Communities*. Washington, DC: Department of Health and Human Services.

U.S. Department of Health and Human Services. 2000. *Healthy People 2010: Understanding and Improving Health*, 2nd ed. Washington, DC: U.S. Government Printing Office.

Ward, B. 1995. Holistic medicine. *Australian Family Physician* 24 (5):761–762, 765.

Wilkinson, R. G. 1997. Comment: Income, inequality, and social cohesion. *American Journal of Public Health* 87:1504–1506.

Wolinsky, F. 1988. *The Sociology of Health: Principles, Practitioners, and Issues*, 2nd ed. Belmont, CA: Wadsworth Publishing.

World Health Organization. 1948. *Preamble to the Constitution*. Geneva, Switzerland: World Health Organization.

Chapter 3

Historical Overview of U.S. Health Care Delivery

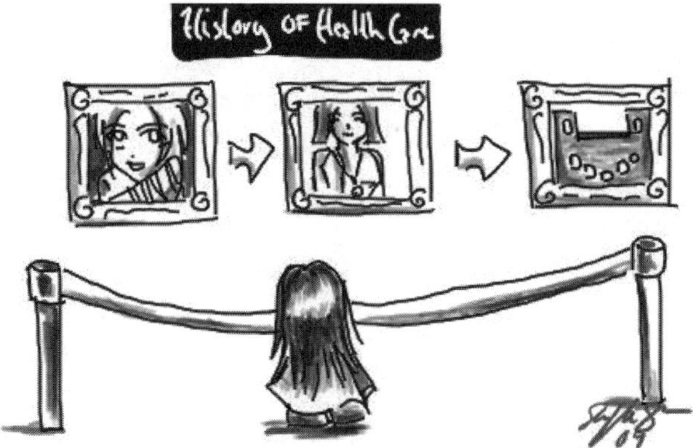

INTRODUCTION

This chapter discusses the main historical developments that have shaped the health care delivery system in the United States. Knowledge of the history of health care is essential for understanding the main characteristics of the system as it exists today. For example, the system's historical foundations explain why health care delivery in the United States has been resistant to national health insurance, which has been adopted by Canada and most European nations. Traditionally held American cultural beliefs and values, technological advances, social changes, economic constraints, and political opportunism are the main historical factors that have shaped health care delivery (see examples in **Exhibit 3.1**). Because of these factors, health care in the United States is mainly a private industry, but it also receives a fairly substantial amount of financing from the government. However, government financing is used mainly

Exhibit 3.1 Major Forces That Bring About Changes in Health Care Delivery

- Cultural beliefs and values
  - Self-reliance
  - Welfare assistance only for the most needy
- Social factors
  - Demographic shifts
  - Immigration
  - Health status
  - Urbanization
- Advances in science and technology
  - New treatments
  - Training of health professionals
  - Facilities and equipment
- Economic forces
  - Health care costs
  - Health insurance
  - Family incomes
- Political factors
  - President's agenda
  - Domestic and foreign priorities
  - Party politics
  - Power of interest groups
  - Laws and regulations

to help the very poor, the elderly, and the disabled receive health care services. Working middle-class Americans must depend on private health insurance, which for most people is obtained through their places of employment. Those who cannot afford the price of premiums and do not qualify for government insurance programs are left without any health insurance.

Major changes driven by social, cultural, technological, economic, and political forces will be instrumental in shaping the future of medical services in the United States. These forces interact in a complex manner. Therefore, it is not always easy to attribute a change in health policy or the creation of a new program to any single factor. The beliefs and values espoused by the majority of Americans, however, have been primarily responsible for shielding the health care system from a major overhaul. For example, most experts agree that at least one reason why past proposals to nationalize health care have failed is that Americans have a strong belief in capitalism, which promotes self-determination and discourages dependence on public welfare unless absolutely necessary. On the other hand, social, political, and economic forces have led to certain compromises, as seen in the creation of Medicare and Medicaid and other public programs to extend health insurance to certain defined groups of needy people.

American capitalism has also promoted entrepreneurship and innovation to champion advancements in science and technology. As a result, medical practice in the United States is highly specialized, whereas basic and routine care is given only secondary importance. Emphasis on the latest treatments and the frequency of their use has led to ever-increasing health care costs that experts do not think can be sustained in the longer term. These high costs are another reason why it has been impractical to expand health insurance to all residents of the United States.

Could a social or economic crisis eventually usher in a national health care program? It is anyone's guess. Although there is always a possibility that, given the right set of conditions, a national health care program could become a reality in the United States, no one seriously thinks that such a drastic change will take place anytime soon. Fundamental reforms in the financing and delivery of health care can occur only when the sizable American middle class develops a mindset based on social justice principles.

This chapter traces the evolution of health care delivery through three major historical periods, each demarcating a major change in the structure of the medical delivery system. The first phase is the *preindustrial* era, which lasted from the middle of the 18th century to the latter part of the 19th century. The second phase is the *postindustrial* era, which began in the late 19th century. The third, but by no means the final phase that we call the *corporate* era, covers developments that started around 1970 and continue into the 21st century.

MEDICAL SERVICES IN PREINDUSTRIAL AMERICA

From Colonial times to the middle to late 1800s, medical education and practice were far more advanced in Great Britain, France, and Germany than they were in the United States. The practice of medicine in the United States had a strong domestic rather than professional character because medical procedures were primitive. Medical education was not grounded in science. Consequently, medical practice was more a trade than a profession. The nation had only a handful of hospitals, and these existed in large cities such as New York, Boston, New Orleans, St. Louis, and Philadelphia. There was no health insurance, private or public. The main characteristics of health care delivery during this period are summarized in **Exhibit 3.2**.

Exhibit 3.2 Main Features of Health Care Delivery in Preindustrial America

- Primitive medical procedures were practiced.
- Medical training was lacking in science.
- Medical education was not standardized.
- Intense competition existed because any tradesman could practice medicine.
- People relied on family members, neighbors, and publications for domestic remedies.
- Hospitals were few and located only in big cities.
- Hospitals had poor sanitation and unskilled staff.
- Almshouses served the destitute and disruptive elements of society and provided some basic nursing care.
- Pesthouses quarantined people with contagious diseases.
- Dispensaries delivered outpatient charity care in urban areas.

Medical Training

Until around 1870, medical training was largely received through individual apprenticeship with a practicing physician rather than through university education. The irony is that many of the preceptors under whom medical students apprenticed were themselves poorly trained (Rothstein, 1972, p. 86). Only a small number of medical schools existed at this time. To train a larger number of students than what was possible through apprenticeship, American physicians began opening medical schools mainly because of economic necessity. By opening medical schools, physicians were also able to enhance their incomes because student fees were paid directly to the physicians. However, these physicians did not have classroom facilities at their disposal, nor did they have the authority to confer the Doctor of Medicine degree. Hence, they had to affiliate with local colleges. Four or more physicians would get together to form a faculty. Medical schools were inexpensive to operate and often quite profitable. It is estimated that there were 42 such schools in 1850 (Rothstein, 1972, p. 91).

Medical education at this point was still seriously lacking in science. The 2-year Doctor of Medicine degree required attending courses for 3 to 4 months during the first year and then essentially repeating the same coursework during the second year. Because fees were only paid as the student passed each course, low standards and a less-than-rigorous curriculum were necessary in order to attract and keep students. Even the best medical schools admitted students without a high school diploma. Training in the biological sciences was considered useful but not essential. Laboratories were nonexistent. Library facilities were inadequate, and clinical observation and practice were not part of the curriculum (Starr, 1982).

Medical Practice

The early practice of medicine was a trade without much significance or prestige. First, it did not require the rigorous course of study, clinical practice, residency training, board exams, and licensing without which it is impossible to practice today. Second, medical procedures were primitive because medical science was still in its infancy. Bleeding, use of emetics, and purging with enemas and purgatives were popular forms of clinical therapy in early medicine. Surgery was limited because anesthesia had not yet been developed, and antiseptic techniques were not known. The stethoscope and x-rays had not been discovered. The clinical thermometer was not in use, and the microscope was not available for medical diagnosis. Physicians mainly relied on their five senses and experience to diagnose and treat medical problems. Hence, in most cases, physicians did not possess technical expertise any more than family members at home and experienced neighbors in the local community.

One of the main consequences of nonprofessional medicine was that anyone, trained or untrained, could practice as a physician. The clergy, for example, often combined medical services and religious duties. The generally well-educated clergymen and government officials were actually more learned in medicine than many physicians (Shryock, 1966, p. 252). Tradesmen such as tailors, barbers, commodity merchants, and those engaged in numerous other trades also practiced the healing arts by selling herbal prescriptions, nostrums, elixirs, and cathartics. The red and white striped poles (symbolizing blood and bandages) outside barber shops today are reminders that barbers also functioned as surgeons at one time, using the same blade to cut hair, shave beards, and do blood letting.

Free entry into medical practice created intense competition. Physicians did not enjoy the status, influence, and income that they do today. Many physicians found it necessary to engage in a second occupation because income from medical practice alone was inadequate to support a family. It is estimated that most physicians' incomes in the mid 1800s put them at the lower end of the middle class (Starr, 1982, p. 84).

In the small communities of rural America, a spirit of strong self-reliance prevailed. Families and communities treated the sick using folk remedies that were passed on from one generation to the next. It was common for people to consult published books and pamphlets on home remedies (Rosen, 1983, p. 2). The market for physicians' services was also limited by economic conditions. Most families simply could not afford them because they had to purchase the services without the help of government or private insurance. Also, most Americans resided in small rural communities, and summoning a physician could require traveling for several hours and sometimes an entire day, which resulted in loss of work and income.

Medical Institutions

Before the 1880s, the United States had only a few isolated hospitals, and these were found only in big cities. Generally, American hospitals played only a small part in medical practice because most of them served a social welfare function by taking care of the poor, those without families, and those away from home on travel. In France and Britain, in contrast, general hospital expansion began much before the 1800s (Stevens, 1971, p. 9–10). In Europe, medical professionals were closely associated with hospitals and readily adopted new advances in medical science. Dispensaries were established as outpatient clinics to provide free care to those who could not afford to pay. The dispensaries provided basic medical care and dispensed drugs to ambulatory patients (Raffel, 1980, p. 239). Around 1900 in the United States, approximately 100 dispensaries were located in large cities (Madison, 1990). Generally, young physicians and medical students desiring clinical experience staffed the dispensaries (as well as hospital wards) on a part-time basis for little or no income (Martensen, 1996).

The forerunner of today's hospitals and nursing homes in the United States was the *almshouse* (also called a *poorhouse*). Almshouses existed in almost all cities of moderate size and were run by the local government. The almshouse was not a health care institution in the true sense. It was a place where the destitute and disruptive elements of society were confined. The inmates, as they were called, included many of the elderly, the homeless, orphans, the ill, and the disabled. They were given food, shelter, and some basic nursing care if needed. In many ways, the almshouse was an infirmary, old-age facility, mental asylum, homeless shelter, and orphanage all rolled into one institution. Living conditions in these institutions were squalid, and they were a far cry from today's health care facilities. Thus, the early health care institutions emerged mainly to take care of indigent people who could not be cared for by their own families.

Another type of institution, the *pesthouse*, was operated by local governments to isolate people who had contracted a contagious disease such as cholera, smallpox, typhoid, or yellow fever. Their main function was to contain the spread of communicable disease and protect the inhabitants of a city.

The few hospitals that did exist at this time had deplorable sanitation conditions and poor ventilation. Unhygienic practices prevailed because nurses were generally unskilled and untrained. It was far more dangerous to receive care in a hospital than at home. These hospitals had a popular image as houses of death and institutions of welfare. People went to hospitals only because of dire circumstances, not by personal choice.

MEDICAL SERVICES IN POSTINDUSTRIAL AMERICA

The postindustrial era was marked by the growth and development of a medical profession that benefited from urbanization, new scientific discoveries, and reforms in medical education. American physicians formed professional organizations, and to this day, they have been a powerful force in resisting proposals for a national health care program.

The system for delivering health care in America took its current shape during this period. The private practice of medicine became firmly entrenched as physicians became a cohesive profession, opted for specialization, and gained power and prestige. The hospital emerged as a repository for high-tech facilities and equipment. Private and public health insurance took roots. Notable developments of this era are summarized in Exhibit 3.3. Changes that revolutionalized health care delivery are discussed in subsequent sections.

Educational Reform

Advances in medical science necessitated the reform of medical education, which began around 1870 when medical schools began affiliating with universities. In 1871, Harvard Medical School completely revolutionized the system of medical education. The academic year was extended from 4 to 9 months, and the length of medical education was increased from 2 to 3

Exhibit 3.3 Notable Developments During the Postindustrial Era

- Urbanization
- Scientific discoveries and their applications in medicine
  - Advanced science-based treatments
  - Increased health care costs
  - Growing imbalance between specialists and generalists
- Medical education reform
- Power and prestige of physicians
- Organized medicine
  - Control over medical training
  - Powerful political interest group
  - Support of licensing laws
  - Opposition to national health insurance proposals
  - Support of private entrepreneurship in medical practice
- Hospitals became true medical care institutions
- Growth of private health insurance
- Creation of Medicare and Medicaid

years. Following the European model, laboratory instruction and clinical courses such as chemistry, physiology, anatomy, and pathology were added to the curriculum. Johns Hopkins University took the lead in further reforming medical education when it opened its medical school in Baltimore, Maryland in 1893. For the first time, medical education became a graduate training program requiring a college degree, not a high school diploma, as an entrance requirement. Johns Hopkins also pioneered the practice of complementing classroom education with residency training in its own teaching hospital. Standards at Johns Hopkins became the model of medical education in other leading institutions around the country. Still, in the early 1900s, less than half of the medical schools provided acceptable levels of training.

In 1910, a widely acclaimed report was published by Abraham Flexner under the auspices of the Carnegie Foundation for the Advancement of Teaching. The Flexner Report, as it came to be known, was based on an inspection of medical schools. It found widespread inconsistencies in medical education. By this time, the American Medical Association (AMA) had gained a firm foothold in medical training by creating the Council on Medical Education. It pushed for state laws that required graduation from a medical school accredited by the AMA as the basis for a license to practice medicine (Haglund & Dowling, 1993). Educational standards were formalized, and schools that did not meet the proposed standards were forced to close. As a note of interest, Howard

University School of Medicine (1869) and the Meharry Medical College (1876) were established at the end of the American Civil War specifically to prepare black physicians to practice medicine.

Medical Profession

Notably, much of the transformation in American medicine occurred in the aftermath of the American Civil War. During this period, America transitioned from a rural agricultural economy to a system of industrial capitalism. Urban development attracted more and more Americans to the growing towns and cities. In 1840, only 11% of the U.S. population lived in urban areas; by 1900, it was up to 40% (Stevens, 1971, p. 34).

Urbanization created increased reliance on the specialized skills of paid professionals as it distanced people from their families and neighborhood surroundings where family-based care had traditionally been given. At the same time, urbanization led to the concentration of medical practice in cities and towns where office-based practice began to replace house calls. Better geographic proximity of patients enabled physicians to see more patients in a given amount of time.

As medicine became increasingly driven by science and technology, lay people could no longer deliver legitimate medical care. Science-based medicine also created an increased demand for the advanced services that were no longer available through family and neighbors. Advances in bacteriology, antiseptic surgery, anesthesia, immunology, and diagnostic techniques, along with a growing array of new drugs, helped bring medical practice into the category of a legitimate profession. **Exhibit 3.4** summarizes some of the groundbreaking early scientific discoveries in medicine.

A preoccupation with science and technology in the American culture brought numerous benefits, but also produced some undesirable effects. For example, an overemphasis on the use of technology in medical care delivery created a bias toward specialization in medical training. It ended up creating far too many specialists in relation to generalists. Technology and specialization also increased the cost of medical care, but without significantly improving the health status of Americans. In contrast, other developed nations have emphasized primary care in which, apart from delivering routine and basic care, a primary care physician and trained nurses ensure the continuity, coordination, and appropriateness of medical services received by a patient.

Exhibit 3.4 Groundbreaking Medical Discoveries

- The discovery of anesthesia was instrumental in advancing the practice of surgery. Nitrous oxide (laughing gas) was first employed as an anesthetic around 1846 for tooth extraction by Horace Wells, a dentist. Later, ether and chloroform were used as anesthetics. Before the anesthetic properties of certain gases were discovered, strong doses of alcohol were used to dull the sensations. A surgeon who could do procedures, such as limb amputations, in the shortest length of time was held in high regard.
- Around 1847, Ignaz Semmelweis, a Hungarian physician practicing in a hospital in Vienna, implemented the policy of handwashing. Thus, an aseptic technique was born. Semmelweis was concerned about the high death rate from puerperal fever among women after childbirth. Even though the germ theory of disease was unknown at this time, Semmelweis surmised that there might be a connection between puerperal fever and the common practice by medical students of not washing their hands before delivering babies and right after doing dissections. Semmelweis' hunch was right.
- Louis Pasteur is generally credited with pioneering the germ theory of disease and microbiology around 1860. Pasteur demonstrated sterilization techniques, such as boiling to kill microorganisms and withholding exposure to air to prevent contamination.
- Joseph Lister is often referred to as the father of antiseptic surgery. Around 1865, Lister used carbolic acid to wash wounds and popularized the chemical inhibition of infection (antisepsis) during surgery.
- Advances in diagnostics and imaging can be traced to the discovery of x-rays in 1895 by Wilhelm Roentgen, a German professor of physics. Radiology became the first machine-based medical specialty. Some of the first training schools in x-ray therapy and radiography in the United States attracted photographers and electricians to become doctors in roentgenology (from the inventor's name).
- Alexander Fleming discovered the antibacterial properties of penicillin in 1929.

American Medical Association

Throughout the history of medicine, the AMA has played a critical role in galvanizing the profession and in protecting the interests of physicians. The concerted activities of physicians through the AMA are collectively referred to as *organized medicine* to distinguish them from the uncoordinated actions of individual physicians competing in the marketplace (Goodman & Musgrave, 1992, pp. 137, 139). Although it was founded in 1847, the AMA did not attain real strength until it delegated regional control by organizing its members into county and state medical societies. It first consolidated its power by controlling medical education, as stated earlier. The AMA also vigorously pursued its objectives by supporting states in the establishment of medical licensing laws.

Employment of physicians by hospitals and insurance companies was frowned upon. Physicians who attempted to seek salaried employment in a corporate setting were chastised by the medical profession and pressured into abandoning such practices. Independence from corporate control promoted private entrepreneurship and put American physicians in an envious strategic position in relation to organizations such as hospitals and insurance companies.

During and after World War I, physicians' incomes grew sharply, and their supremacy as a profession finally emerged. The sphere of their influence expanded into nearly all aspects of health care delivery. For example, laws were passed that prohibited individuals from obtaining certain classes of drugs without a physician's prescription. Health insurance paid for treatments only when they were rendered or prescribed by physicians.

Development of Hospitals

As had already occurred in Europe, the growth of hospitals in the United States came to symbolize the institutionalization of health care (Torrens, 1993). The hospital became the central core around which other medical services were organized.

Advancements in medical science created the need to centralize expensive facilities and equipment in a medical institution. The hospital became the center for advanced technology to be used in medical diagnosis and treatment and for the training of various types of health care personnel. Physicians could no longer afford to have the needed equipment and facilities in their own offices. Hospitals, on the other hand, depended on physicians to refer patients to keep the beds filled. These conditions created the need for informal alliances between hospitals and physicians. Alongside these developments came remarkable progress in sanitation practices. The professionalization of nursing promoted healing and improved patient recovery. Thus, the growing appeal of hospital services in communities, sick patients' increasing need for hospital care, and the increasing professionalization of medical practice became closely intertwined. Physicians began to play a dominant role in hospital affairs even though they were not employees of the hospitals. As hospitals grew in number, physicians' ability to decide where to hospitalize their patients gave them enormous influence over hospital policy. The expansion of surgery in particular had profound implications for hospitals, physicians, and the public.

HISTORY OF HEALTH INSURANCE

There are several reasons why private health insurance (also called voluntary health insurance) took root and expanded in the United States. Later, the medical needs of the elderly and the poor in an environment of rising health care costs prompted the U.S. Congress to create the publicly financed Medicare and Medicaid programs.

Workers' Compensation

The first broad-coverage health insurance in the United States emerged in the form of workers' compensation. It was originally designed to make cash payments to workers for wages lost because of job-related injuries and disease. Later, compensation for medical expenses and death benefits for survivors were added.

Between 1910 and 1915, workers' compensation laws made rapid progress in the United States (Stevens, 1971, p. 136). Looking at the trend, some reformers believed that because Americans had been persuaded to adopt compulsory insurance against industrial accidents they could also be persuaded to adopt compulsory insurance against sickness. Workers' compensation served as a trial balloon for the idea of government-sponsored health insurance. However, the growth of private health insurance, along with other key factors which will be discussed later, have prevented any proposals for a national health care program from taking hold in the United States.

Rise of Private Health Insurance

Private health insurance began in the form of disability coverage that provided income during temporary disability resulting from bodily injury or sickness. During the early 1900s, medical treatments and hospital care became more and more a part of American life. However, they also became increasingly more expensive, and people could not predict their future needs for medical care or its costs. These developments pointed to the need for some kind of insurance to spread an individual's financial risk over a large number of people. Between 1916 and 1918, 16 state legislatures, including New York and California, attempted to enact legislation compelling employers to provide health insurance, but the efforts were unsuccessful (Davis, 1996).

First Hospital Plan and the Birth of Blue Cross

It seems that the dire economic conditions of the Great Depression set the stage for innovation in health insurance. Hospitals faced economic instability by relying too much on philanthropic donations. On the other hand, individual patients faced not only loss of income from illness but also burdensome debt from medical care costs. In 1929, the blueprint for modern health insurance was conceived when Justin F. Kimball began a hospital insurance plan for teachers at the Baylor University Hospital in Dallas, Texas. Within a few years, it became the model for Blue Cross plans around the country (Raffel, 1980, p. 394). At first, other independent hospitals copied Baylor and started to offer single-hospital plans. Later, plans sponsored by groups of hospitals became more popular because they offered consumers a choice of hospitals. The American Hospital Association (AHA) supported these hospital plans and became the coordinating agency that united the plans into the Blue Cross network. The Blue Cross plans were nonprofit; that is, they had no shareholders to receive profit distributions. Later, control of the plans was transferred to a completely independent body, the Blue Cross Commission, which subsequently became the Blue Cross Association (Raffel, 1980, p. 395).

Private health insurance grew in popularity. In 1946, Blue Cross plans in 43 states served 20 million members. Between 1940 and 1950 alone, the proportion of the population covered by hospital insurance increased from 9% to 57% (Anderson, 1990, p. 128). Private health insurance had received the AMA's endorsement, but the AMA had also made it clear that private health insurance plans should include only hospital care. Within a few years, lured by the success of the Blue Cross plans, commercial insurance companies also started offering health insurance.

First Physician Plan and the Birth of Blue Shield

In 1939, the California Medical Association started the first Blue Shield plan, which was designed to pay physician fees. By endorsing hospital insurance and by actively developing the first plans that covered physicians' services, the medical profession protected its own financial interests. The AMA ensured that private health insurance would be preserved, and to this day, the AMA has remained opposed to a government-run national health insurance. Starting in 1974, Blue Cross and Blue Shield plans began to merge. Now, in nearly every state Blue Cross and Blue Shield plans are joint corporations or have close working relationships (Davis, 1996).

Employer-Based Health Insurance

Health insurance became a permanent feature of employment benefits during World War II. During this period, wages were frozen in an attempt to control wartime inflation, and employees accepted employer-paid health insurance to compensate for the loss of raises in their salaries. Congress amended the Internal Revenue Code to make employer-provided health coverage nontaxable. In economic value, employer-paid health insurance was equivalent to getting additional salary without having to pay taxes on it. Hence, U.S. tax policy provided an incentive to obtain health insurance as an employer-furnished benefit. Also, the U.S. Supreme Court ruled that employee benefits were a legitimate part of union–management negotiations. Health insurance thus became an important component of collective bargaining between unions and employers. Subsequently, employment-based health insurance expanded rapidly, and private health insurance became the primary vehicle for the delivery of health care services in the United States. It is estimated that private health insurance grew from a $1 billion industry in 1950 to an $8.7 billion industry by 1965.

Failure of National Health Care in the United States

In some of the Western European countries, national health care initiatives were closely associated with labor movements and worker sentiments. Notably in Germany and England, labor unrest threatened political stability. Universal health insurance for all citizens was seen as a means to obtain workers' loyalty and thwart any labor uprisings. By around 1912, national health insurance had spread throughout Europe, but political conditions in the United States were quite different. Unlike countries in Europe, the American government was highly decentralized and engaged in little direct regulation of social welfare. Despite this, Theodore Roosevelt ran for the United States presidency in 1912 on a platform of social reform. Not surprisingly, Roosevelt was defeated by Woodrow Wilson; however, the Progressive movement favoring national health insurance remained alive for several more years.

The entry of the United States into World War I in 1917 was a political blow to the national health care movement as anti-German feelings were aroused and the U.S. government denounced German social insurance. Opponents of national health care called it a "Prussian menace," inconsistent with American values (Starr, 1982, p. 240, 253).

The AMA has always been at the forefront of opposition to national health care because it is perceived as a potential threat to the private practice of medicine. Proposals for national health care have often been stigmatized as "government interference with the practice of medicine" or "socialized medicine." Such slogans are used to play on the psyche of middle-class Americans who have traditionally espoused beliefs and values that are consistent with capitalism, self-determination, distrust of big government, and reliance on the private sector to address social concerns. The AMA was instrumental in the demise of several bills on national health insurance that were introduced in Congress in the early 1940s during Franklin Roosevelt's presidency. In 1946, Harry Truman became the first president to make a direct appeal for a national health care program (Anderson, 1990, p. 119). The initial public reaction to Truman's plan was positive. However, when a government-controlled medical plan was compared with privately obtained insurance, polls showed a drastic decline in public support. The AMA was once again vehement in denouncing the plan. Other powerful health care interest groups such as the American Hospital Association also opposed the proposal. In 1948, Truman was reelected while promising national health insurance, which actually came as a surprise to many political observers. This time the AMA launched what was to become one of the most expensive lobbying efforts in American history. The campaign directly linked national health insurance with communism until the idea of socialized medicine was firmly implanted in the public's minds. By 1950, national health insurance was a dead issue, and it remained so for decades.

The most recent unsuccessful attempt to bring about a national health care program was initiated by the Clinton administration. While seeking the presidency in 1992, then-governor Bill Clinton made health system reform a major campaign issue. Public opinion polls at that time seemed to confirm that health care was a pressing concern on the minds of the American people. In one well-regarded national survey, a substantial number of insured and relatively affluent Americans said that they had not received the services they needed. The poll also suggested that the public was looking to the federal government, not the states or private sector, to contain rising health care costs (Smith et al., 1992).

Shortly after taking office in 1993, President Clinton made health system reform one of his top priorities, but his proposal was largely rejected by the American people. Defeat of the Clinton plan furnishes another lesson on the power of beliefs and values prevalent in the United States. On the one hand, as a matter of principle, Americans endorse tax-supported health insurance to help needy citizens, but they are unwilling to pay in higher taxes what a national health care program could realistically cost. Americans are also uneasy about more government regulation and interference with what many believe they have legitimately earned. In a 1999 national poll, half of the respondents—regardless of gender, race, age, or working status—indicated that employers would be their preferred source of health insurance. Only 18% said they would prefer to rely on the government (Commonwealth Fund, 2000). In 2006, almost 90% of those who had health insurance rated their coverage as excellent or good, and were satisfied with the quality of care they received. Only about a third of Americans favored a universal care system. On the other hand, health care costs have remained a major concern (Henry J. Kaiser Family Foundation, 2007). Grassroots sentiments evaluated by polls fluctuate according to the state of the economy and how secure Americans feel about their overall well-being. So far traditional American beliefs and values have succeeded in keeping at bay any large-scale proposals to tinker with the private health insurance system. The main reasons for the failure of national health care are summarized in **Exhibit 3.5**.

Creation of Medicaid and Medicare

Before 1965, private health insurance was the only widely available source of payment for health care, and it was available primarily to middle-class working people and their families. The elderly, the unemployed, and

Exhibit 3.5 Reasons Why National Health Care Has Failed in America

- Unlike Europe, it failed to get an early footing because of labor and political stability in the United States.
- A decentralized American system gives the federal government little direct control over social policy.
- The German social insurance system was denounced during World War I. Since then, the term "socialized medicine" has been used as a synonym for national health insurance.
- The AMA has historically opposed national health care initiatives.
- Middle-class Americans have traditionally espoused beliefs and values that are consistent with capitalism, self-determination, and distrust of big government.
- Middle-class Americans are averse to higher taxes that a national health care program would result in.

the poor had to rely on their own resources, on limited public programs, or on charity from hospitals and individual physicians.

The earlier debates over national health insurance had made one thing clear: Most Americans did not desire government intervention in how they received health care, with one exception. They would be less opposed to reform initiatives for the underprivileged classes. In principle, the poor were considered a special class who could be served through a government-sponsored program. The elderly—those 65 years of age and over—were another group that started to receive increased attention in the 1950s. On their own, most of the poor and the elderly could not afford the increasing cost of health care. Also, because the health status of these population groups was significantly worse than that of the general population, their medical needs were more critical. The elderly particularly had a higher incidence and prevalence of disease than did younger age groups. It was also estimated that less than half of the elderly were covered by private health insurance. By this time, the growing elderly middle class was also becoming a politically active force.

A bill introduced in Congress by Aime Forand in 1957 started the momentum for including necessary hospital and nursing home care as an extension of Social Security benefits (Stevens, 1971, p. 434). The AMA, however, undertook a massive campaign to portray a government insurance plan as a threat to the physician–patient relationship. The bill was stalled, but public hearings around the country, which were packed by the elderly, produced an intense grassroots support to push the issue onto the national agenda (Starr, 1982, p. 368). A compromise reform, the Medical Assistance Act, also known as the Kerr–Mills Act, went into effect in 1960. Under the Act, federal grants were given to the states so they could extend health services under their welfare programs to low-income elderly. However, putting the elderly under a welfare program became controversial. Liberal congressional representatives regarded it as a source of humiliation to the elderly (Starr, 1982, p. 369). Within 3 years, the program was declared ineffective because many states did not even implement it (Stevens, 1971, p. 438). In 1964, health insurance for the aged and the poor became a top priority of President Lyndon Johnson's Great Society programs.

After considering several different proposals, a three-part program was adopted. Part A and Part B of Medicare (also known as *Title 18* of the Social Security amendment of 1965) became the first two layers. Medicare provided publicly financed health insurance to all elderly regardless of their income. *Part A* of Medicare was designed to use Social Security funds to finance hospital insurance and short-term nursing home coverage after discharge from a hospital. *Part B* of Medicare was designed to cover physicians' bills through government-subsidized insurance in which the elderly would pay part of the premiums. The *Medicaid* program (*Title 19* of the Social Security amendment of 1965) was the third layer. It covered the eligible poor and was based on the earlier Kerr–Mills program. It would be financed through federal matching funds to the states based on financial needs determined by each state's per capita income.

Although adopted together, Medicare and Medicaid reflected sharply different traditions. Medicare was upheld by broad grassroots support and, being attached to Social Security, had no class distinction. Medicaid, on the other hand, carried the stigma of public welfare. Medicare had uniform national standards for eligibility and benefits; Medicaid varied from state to state in terms of eligibility and benefits. Medicare covered anyone at or over the age of 65 years. Medicaid became a *means-tested* program, which confined eligibility to people below a predetermined income level. Consequently, many of the poor did not qualify because their incomes exceeded the means-test limits. The main characteristics of Medicare and Medicaid are summarized in **Table 3.1**.

Table 3.1 Comparisons Between Medicare and Medicaid

Medicare	Medicaid
• Covers all elderly (as originally designed)	• Covers only the very poor
• No income/means test	• Income criteria established by states (means test)
• No class distinction	• Public welfare
• Part A for hospitalization and short-term nursing home stay	• All services are covered under one program
• Part B for physician and other outpatient services	• Program varies from state to state
• Nationally uniform program	• Title 19 of the SSA
• Title 18 of the SSA	• Financed by the states, with matching funds from the federal government according to each state's per capita income
• Part A financed through SS taxes	
• Part B subsidized through general taxes, but the participants pay part of the premium cost	

Note: SSA, Social Security Act; SS, Social Security.

The Medicare and Medicaid programs are financed by the government, but in most instances, the enrollees receive health care services from private hospitals, physicians, and other providers. As a major payer of health care services, the government uses numerous regulations to govern the delivery of services and determines how much the providers should be paid. As a result, the regulatory powers of government have increasingly encroached on the private sector. In 1997, the Health Care Financing Administration (now called the Centers for Medicare and Medicaid Services) was created to manage Medicare and Medicaid separately from the Social Security Administration.

Initially created to cover only the elderly, the Medicare program was expanded in 1973 after Congress extended coverage to nonelderly disabled people receiving social security and to people with end-stage renal disease (ESRD) who needed dialysis or a kidney transplant. In 1997, Medicare added coverage options under Part C, and in 2003 a new prescription drug benefit (Part D) was added—see Chapter 6. The creation of Medicare and Medicaid had a drastic impact on both federal and state budgets, but the federal government bore the brunt. As pointed out in Table 3.2, the gross domestic product—representing total economic consumption—grew at an average annual rate of 7.6% between 1965 and 1970. In contrast, total state and local government expenditures grew at an average annual rate of 13.6%, but health care expenditures grew at a somewhat slower rate of 12.5%. In the case of the federal government, however, health care expenditures increased at an average annual rate of 30%, whereas total federal expenditures increased at a rate of only 11.3%. Figure 3.1 shows the portion of federal government expenditures used for health care, which increased from 3% to 11% between 1965 and 1970.

MEDICAL SERVICES IN THE CORPORATE ERA

The latter part of the 20th century and the start of the 21st have been marked by the growth and consolidation of large business corporations and tremendous advances in global communications, transportation, and trade. These developments are starting to change the way health care is delivered in the United States and, indeed, around the world. The rise of multina-

Table 3.2 Average Annual Percent Increase in Gross Domestic Product and Federal and State Expenditures Between 1965 and 1970

	Total (%)	Health Care (%)
Gross domestic product	7.6	–
Federal government expenditures	11.3	30.0
State and local government expenditures	13.6	12.5

National Center for Health Statistics. Data from *Health, United States, 1995*, p. 239.

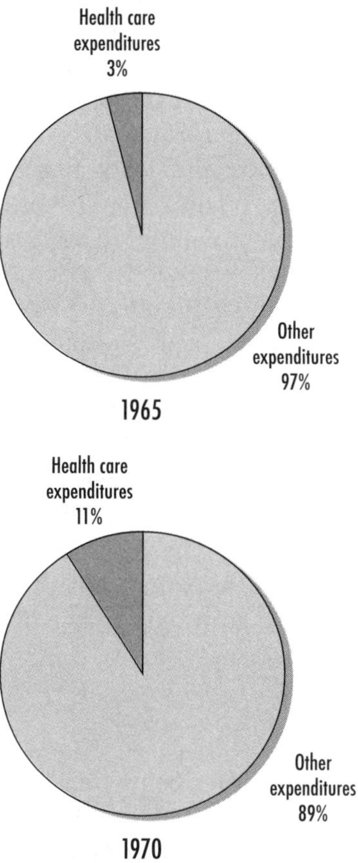

Figure 3.1 Portion of Total Federal Expenditures for Health Care: 1965 and 1970. Data from Statistical Abstract of the United States, 1976, p. 229, U.S. Census Bureau; *Health, United States, 1995*, p. 245, National Center for Health Statistics.

tional corporations, the information revolution, and globalization have been interdependent phenomena.

Corporatization of Health Care Delivery

Corporatization here refers to the ways in which health care delivery in the United States has become the domain of large organizations. Since the

1990s, managed care has emerged as a dominant force by becoming the primary vehicle for insuring and delivering health care to the majority of Americans. The rise of managed care organizations consolidated immense purchasing power to obtain health care services at discounted prices and to implement various types of controls to reduce the rising cost of health care. To counteract this imbalance, providers also began to consolidate, and larger, integrated health care organizations began forming. Large integrated delivery systems (IDSs) can provide a full array of health care services that include hospital inpatient care, surgical services in both inpatient and outpatient settings, primary care and multispecialty outpatient services, home health care, long-term care, and specialized rehabilitation services. Together, managed care organizations and IDSs have in reality corporatized the delivery of health care in the United States. They have also made the health care system extremely complex.

In a health care landscape that has been increasingly dominated by corporations, individual physicians have struggled to preserve their autonomy. As a matter of survival, many physicians had to consolidate into larger group practices, form strategic partnerships with hospitals, or start their own specialty hospitals. A growing number of physicians have become employees of large medical corporations.

Information Revolution

The delivery of health care is being transformed in unprecedented and irreversible ways by telecommunication. For example, telemedicine and E-health have been on the rise. *Telemedicine* came to the forefront in the 1990s with the technological advances in the distant transmission of image data. This technology has made it possible to provide health care at a distance, such as real-time transmission of video examinations as well as telesurgery. *E-health* has become an unstoppable force that is driven by consumer demand for health care information and services offered over the Internet by professionals and nonprofessionals alike (Maheu et al., 2001). The Internet has created a new revolution that is increasingly characterized by patient empowerment. Access to expert information is no longer strictly confined to the physician's domain, which in some ways has led to a dilution of the dependent role of the patient.

Globalization

Globalization refers to various forms of cross-border economic activities. It is driven by global exchange of information, production of goods and services more economically in developing countries, and increased interdependence of mature and emerging world economies. It confers many advantages, but also has some downsides.

From the standpoint of cross-border trade in health services, Mutchnick and colleagues (2005) identified four different modes of economic interrelationships: (1) Cross-country telemedicine and outsourcing of certain medical services has been made possible by advanced telecommunications technology. For example, teleradiology (the electronic transmission of radiological images over a distance) now enables physicians in the United States to transmit radiology images to Australia where they are interpreted and reported back the next day (McDonnell, 2006). (2) Consumers travel abroad to receive medical care (sometimes referred to as medical travel). For example, countries such as India and Thailand offer state-of-the-art medical facilities to foreigners at a fraction of what it would cost to have the same procedures done in the United States or Europe. (3) Foreign direct investment in health services enterprises. For example, Chindex International, a U.S. corporation, provides medical equipment, supplies, and clinical care in China. (4) Health professionals move to other countries that present high demand for their services and better economic opportunities than their native countries. Migration of physicians from developing countries helps alleviate at least some of the shortage in underserved locations in the developed world. On the downside, the developing world pays a price when emigration leaves these countries with shortages of trained professionals.

Globalization has also posed some new threats, for instance, the threat of diseases that were previously unknown in the United States, and the threat of bioterrorism that diverts resources from other needed health care services. Infectious diseases appearing in one country can spread rapidly to other countries. HIV/AIDS, hepatitis B, and hepatitis C infections have spread worldwide. New viral infections such as avian flu and SARS (severe acute respiratory syndrome) have at times threatened to create worldwide pandemics.

CONCLUSION

In a little over 100 years, health care delivery has come a long way from being a primitive and family-oriented craft to becoming a technology-driven service and the largest industry in the United States. In the process, many medical procedures and services have become increasingly unaffordable. Both private and public health insurance have become firmly entrenched mechanisms to pay for costly health care. However, public insurance programs cover only those individuals who meet established criteria for eligibility. Past efforts to create a national health insurance program have failed for various reasons. Perhaps the most important one is the beliefs and values that make Americans distrustful of government interference and a general mindset against paying higher taxes to expand social programs.

The 21st century has been marked by the corporate era in the delivery of medical care. Corporatization has put the delivery of health care into the hands of large managed care and integrated health care organizations. It has turned the delivery of health care into a complex enterprise. The information revolution has created advanced telecommunication technologies. The application of these technologies in health care has made the distant delivery of certain health care services possible. E-health has given consumers access to health care information over the Internet. Globalization has added a worldwide dimension to the delivery of medical care through telemedicine and outsourcing, availability of advanced services in foreign countries at reduced costs, foreign direct investment in health care enterprises, and migration of health care professionals from underdeveloped to developed countries. Globalization has conferred many advantages, but it has not been without its downsides. Spread of infectious diseases from one country to another and threat of bioterrorism are some of the main issues related to globalization.

REFERENCES

Anderson, O. W. 1990. *Health Services as a Growth Enterprise in the United States Since 1875*. Ann Arbor, MI: Health Administration Press.

Commonwealth Fund. 2000. *1999 National Survey of Workers' Health Insurance*. New York: Commonwealth Fund.

Davis, P. 1996. The fate of Blue Shield and the new Blues. *South Dakota Journal of Medicine* 49 (9):323–330.

Goodman, J. C., and G. L. Musgrave. 1992. *Patient Power: Solving America's Health Care Crisis*. Washington, DC: CATO Institute.

Haglund, C. L., and W. L. Dowling. 1993. The hospital. In S. J. Williams and P. R. Torrens (eds.). *Introduction to Health Services*, 4th ed. (pp. 135–176). New York: Delmar Publishers.

Henry J. Kaiser Family Foundation. 2007. *Health Care in America 2006 Survey*. Menlo Park, CA: The Henry J. Kaiser Family Foundation.

Madison, D. L. 1990. Notes on the history of group practice: The tradition of the dispensary. *Medical Group Management Journal* 37 (5):52–54, 56–60, 86–93.

Maheu, M. M., et al. 2001. *E-Health, Telehealth, and Telemedicine: A Guide to Start-Up and Success*. San Francisco: Jossey-Bass.

Martensen, R. L. 1996. Hospital hotels and the care of the "worthy rich." *Journal of the American Medical Association* 275 (4):325.

McDonnell, J. 2006. Is the medical world flattening? *Ophthalmology Times* 31 (19):4.

Mutchnick, I. S., et al. 2005. Trading health services across borders: GATS, markets, and caveats. *Health Affairs—Web Exclusive* 24 (Suppl 1):W5-42 to W5-51.

Raffel, M. W. 1980. *The U.S. Health System: Origins and Functions*. New York: John Wiley & Sons.

Rosen, G. 1983. *The Structure of American Medical Practice 1875–1941*. Philadelphia: University of Pennsylvania Press.

Rothstein, W. G. 1972. *American Physicians in the Nineteenth Century: From Sect to Science*. Baltimore, MD: Johns Hopkins University Press.

Shryock, R. H. 1966. *Medicine in America: Historical Essays*. Baltimore, MD: Johns Hopkins University Press.

Smith, M. D., et al. 1992. Taking the public's pulse on health system reform. *Health Affairs* 11 (2):125–133.

Starr, P. 1982. *The Social Transformation of American Medicine*. Cambridge, MA: Basic Books.

Stevens, R. 1971. *American Medicine and the Public Interest*. New Haven, CT: Yale University Press.

Torrens, P. R. 1993. Historical evolution and overview of health services in the United States. In S. J. Williams and P. R. Torrens (eds.). *Introduction to Health Services*, 4th ed. New York: Delmar Publishers.

Chapter 4

Health Care Providers and Professionals

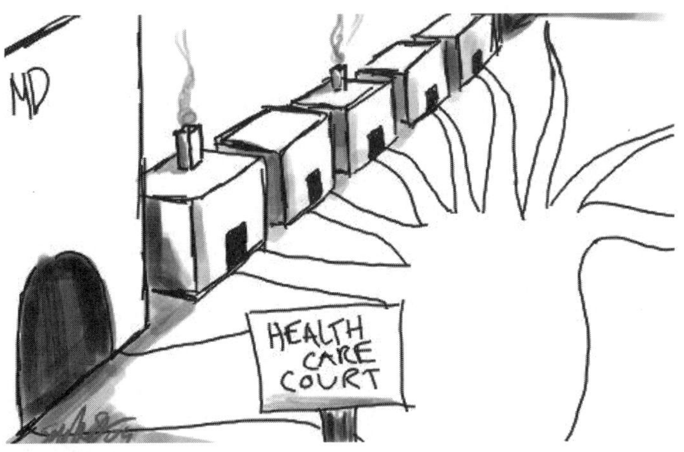

INTRODUCTION

The U.S. health care industry is the largest and most powerful employer in the nation. It employs more than 3% of the total labor force in the United States. In terms of total economic output, in the year 2000, the health care sector contributed 13.2% to the gross domestic product. The health care sector of the U.S. economy will continue to grow for two main reasons: (1) growth in population, mainly due to immigration, and (2) aging of the population, especially as the baby boom generation starts to hit retirement age in the year 2011 and beyond.

Health services professionals include physicians, nurses, dentists, pharmacists, optometrists, psychologists, podiatrists, chiropractors, non-physician practitioners (NPPs), health services administrators, and allied health professionals. Therapists, laboratory and radiology technicians, social workers, and health educators are referred to as allied health professionals. Health professionals are among the most well-educated and diverse of all labor groups. Almost all of these practitioner groups are now represented by professional associations.

Health services professionals work in a variety of health care settings that include hospitals, managed care organizations (MCOs), nursing care facilities, mental health centers, insurance firms, pharmaceutical companies, outpatient facilities, community health centers, migrant health centers, school clinics, physicians' offices, laboratories, voluntary health agencies, professional health associations, colleges of medicine and allied health professions, and research institutions. According to 2005 data (Table 4.1), the majority of health professionals are employed by hospitals (40.7%), followed by nursing care facilities (13.2%), and physicians' offices and clinics (12.8%).

The growth of health care services is closely linked to the demand for health services professionals. The expansion of the number and types of health services professionals closely follows population trends, advances in research and technology, disease and illness trends, and changes in health care financing and the delivery of services. Population growth and the aging of the population enhance the demand for health services. Advances in scientific research contribute to new methods of preventing, diagnosing, and treating illness. New and complex medical techniques and machines are constantly introduced. Health services professionals must then learn how to use them. Scientific research and technologic development have contributed to specialization in medicine and the proliferation of different types of medical technicians. The changing pattern of disease from acute to chronic has led to an increasing emphasis on behavioral risk factors and the need for health services professionals who are formally prepared to address these health risks, their consequences, and their prevention. The widespread availability of insurance from both the public and private sectors has contributed to the increase in medical care utilization, which has created a greater demand for health services providers. Changes in reimbursement from retrospective to prospective payment methods and increased enrollment in managed care have contributed to cost reductions, a shift from inpatient to outpatient care, and an emphasis on the role of primary care providers.

This chapter provides an overview of the large array of health services professionals employed in the vast assortment of health delivery settings. It briefly discusses the training and practice requirements for the various

Table 4.1 Persons Employed at Health Services Sites

Site	1994		2001		2005	
	Number of Persons (in thousands)	Percentage Distribution	Number of Persons (in thousands)	Percentage Distribution	Number of Persons (in thousands)	Percentage Distribution
All health services sites	10,587	100.0	12,211	100.0	14,052	100.0
Offices and clinics of physicians	1,404	13.3	1,387	11.4	1,801	12.8
Offices and clinics of dentists	596	5.6	672	5.5	792	5.6
Offices and clinics of chiropractors	105	1.0	120	1.0	163	1.2
Hospitals	5,009	47.3	5,202	42.6	5,716	40.7
Nursing care facilities	1,692	16.0	1,593	13.0	1,848	13.2
Other health services sites	1,781	16.8	3,273	26.5	3,729	26.5

Data are from the National Center for Health Statistics. 1999. *Health, United States* (p. 265); 2006. *Health, United States* (p. 353). Hyattsville, MD: U.S. Department of Health and Human Services.

health professionals, their major roles, the practice settings in which they are generally employed, and some critical issues concerning their professions. Emphasis is placed on physicians because they play a leading role in the delivery of health care. There has been increased recognition of the role NPPs (nurse practitioners [NPs], physician assistants, and certified nurse-midwives [CNMs]) play in the delivery of primary care services. As a group they have taken over some basic medical functions that have been traditionally performed by physicians only.

The U.S. health care delivery system is characterized by an imbalance between primary and specialty care services, which has contributed to an imbalance in the ratio of generalists to specialists. There is also a maldistribution of practitioners and an aggregate oversupply of physicians. This chapter describes these imbalances and explores their main causes. Although a detailed discussion of primary care is provided in Chapter 7, this chapter highlights some of the main differences between primary and specialty care.

PHYSICIANS

In the delivery of health services, physicians play a central role by evaluating a patient's health condition, diagnosing abnormalities, and prescribing treatment. Some physicians are engaged in medical education and research to find new and better ways to control and cure health problems. A growing number are involved in the prevention of illness.

All states require physicians to be licensed in order to practice. The licensure requirements include graduation from an accredited medical school that awards a Doctor of Medicine (MD) or Doctor of Osteopathic Medicine (DO) degree, successful completion of a licensing examination governed by either the National Board of Medical Examiners or the National Board of Osteopathic Medical Examiners, and completion of a supervised internship/residency program (Stanfield, 1995, p. 102–104). *Residency* is graduate medical education in a specialty that takes the form of paid on-the-job training, usually in a hospital. Most physicians serve a 1-year rotating internship after graduation before entering a residency, which may last 2 to 6 years.

The number of active physicians, both MDs and DOs, has steadily increased from 14.1 physicians per 10,000 population in 1950 to 27.4 physicians per 10,000 population in 2001 (**Table 4.2**). Of the 157 medical

Table 4.2 Active Physicians: Type and Number per 10,000 Population

Year	All Active Physicians	Doctors of Medicine	Doctors of Osteopathy	Active Physicians per 10,000 Population
1950	219,900	209,000	10,900	14.1
1960	259,500	247,300	12,200	14.0
1970	326,500	314,200	12,300	15.6
1980	457,500	440,400	17,100	19.7
1990	589,500	561,400	28,100	23.4
1995	672,859	637,192	35,667	25.6
2000	772,296	727,573	44,723	27,8
2001	793,263	751,689	41,574	27.4

Data are from the National Center for Health Statistics. 1995. *Health, United States* (p. 220); 2002. *Health, United States* (p. 274); 2006. *Health, United States* (p. 358). Hyattsville, MD: U.S. Department of Health and Human Services.

schools in the United States, 129 teach allopathic medicine (see next section for definition) and award the MD degree, and 28 teach osteopathic medicine and award the DO degree.

Similarities and Differences Between MDs and DOs

Both MDs and DOs use traditionally accepted methods of treatment, including drugs and surgery. The two differ mainly in their philosophies and approaches to medical treatment. Osteopathic medicine, practiced by DOs, emphasizes the musculoskeletal system of the body, such as correction of joints or tissues. In their treatment plans, DOs stress preventive medicine such as diet and the environment as factors that might influence natural resistance. They take a holistic approach to patient care. MDs are trained in allopathic medicine, which views medical treatment as active intervention to produce a counteracting reaction in an attempt to neutralize the effects of disease. MDs, particularly generalists, may also use preventive medicine along with allopathic treatments. About one third of MDs and more than half of DOs are generalists (U.S. Bureau of Labor Statistics, 2002a).

Generalists and Specialists

Whereas most DOs are generalists, most MDs are specialists. In the United States, physicians trained in family medicine/general practice, general internal medicine, and general pediatrics are considered primary care physicians or generalists (Rich et al., 1994). For the most part, primary care physicians provide preventive services (e.g., health examinations, immunizations, mammograms, Pap smears) and treat frequently occurring and less severe problems. Problems that occur less frequently or that require complex diagnostic or therapeutic approaches may be referred to specialists.

Physicians in nonprimary care specialties are referred to as specialists. Specialists must seek certification in an area of medical specialization, which commonly requires additional years of advanced residency training followed by several years of practice in the specialty. A specialty board examination is often required as the final step for becoming a board-certified specialist. The common medical specialties include anesthesiology, cardiology, dermatology, specialized internal medicine, neurology, obstetrics and gynecology, ophthalmology, pathology, pediatrics, psychiatry, radiology, and surgery. These specialties can be divided into six major functional groups: (1) the subspecialties of internal medicine; (2) a broad group of medical specialties; (3) obstetrics and gynecology; (4) surgery of all types; (5) hospital-based radiology, anesthesiology, and pathology; and (6) psychiatry (Cooper, 1994).

Hospitalist

One type of specialty not categorized by a specific organ, disease, or age is a hospitalist, a specialty organized around the site of care (the hospital) instead. Hospitalists are involved in inpatient medicine and parallel the roles of primary physicians in an outpatient setting in that they manage the care of hospitalized patients. Although this specialty has long served a significant role in urban hospitals in Canada and Great Britain, it has only surfaced in the U.S. health care system as a significant role player in the last decade when managed care began to predominate the health care system. Built around the idea of cost-efficiency, hospitalists may decrease overall cost and length of stay for patients, yet still maintain referring-physician satisfaction and the readmission rates of subspecialist colleagues. Currently, this specialty is not yet a formal one, lacking its own residency programs and board certification. Most practicing hospitalists train under various primary care concentrations such as general internal medicine, family practice, or general pediatrics.

Differences Between Primary and Specialty Care

Primary care can be distinguished from specialty care by the time, focus, and scope of the services provided to patients. The five main areas of distinction are as follows.

1. In linear time sequence, primary care is first-contact care and is regarded as the portal to the health care system (Kahn et al., 1994). Specialty care, when needed, generally follows primary care.
2. In a managed care environment where health services functions are integrated, primary care physicians serve as gatekeepers, an important role in controlling cost, utilization, and the rational allocation of resources. In the gatekeeping model, specialty care requires referral from a primary care physician.
3. Primary care is longitudinal (Starfield & Simpson, 1993). In other words, primary care providers follow through the course of treatment and coordinate various activities, including initial diagnosis, treatment, referral, consultation, monitoring, and follow-up. Specialty care is episodic and thus more focused and intense.
4. Primary care focuses on the person as a whole, whereas specialty care centers on particular diseases or organ systems of the body. Primary care is holistic in nature and provides an integrating function. Patients often have multiple problems, a condition referred to as comorbidity. Primary care, in essence, seeks to balance the multiple requirements a patient's condition may call for and refers patients to appropriate specialty care when needed. Specialty care, in contrast, tends to be limited to episodes of illness, specific organ systems, or the disease process involved. Specialty care is also associated with secondary and tertiary levels of services.
5. The difference in scope is reflected in how primary and specialty care providers are trained. Primary care medical students spend a significant amount of time in ambulatory care settings, familiarizing themselves with a variety of patient conditions and problems. Students in

medical subspecialties spend significant time in inpatient hospitals, where they are exposed to state-of-the-art medical technology.

Work Settings and Practice Patterns

Physicians practice in a variety of settings and arrangements. Some work in hospitals as medical residents or staff physicians. Others work in the public sector, such as federal government agencies, public health clinics, community and migrant health centers, schools, and prisons. Most physicians, however, are office-based practitioners, and most physician contacts occur in offices. An increasing number of physicians are partners or salaried employees under contractual arrangements, working in various outpatient settings such as group practices, freestanding ambulatory care clinics, diagnostic imaging centers, and MCOs.

Figure 4.1 shows that physicians in general/family practice accounted for the greatest proportion of ambulatory care visits (22.5%), followed by those in internal medicine and pediatrics (16.1%).

Imbalance and Maldistribution of Physicians

Aggregate Physician Oversupply

Aided by tax-financed subsidies, the United States has experienced a sharp increase in its physician labor force. Current numbers far surpass the estimated 145 to 185 physicians per 100,000 population that the United States

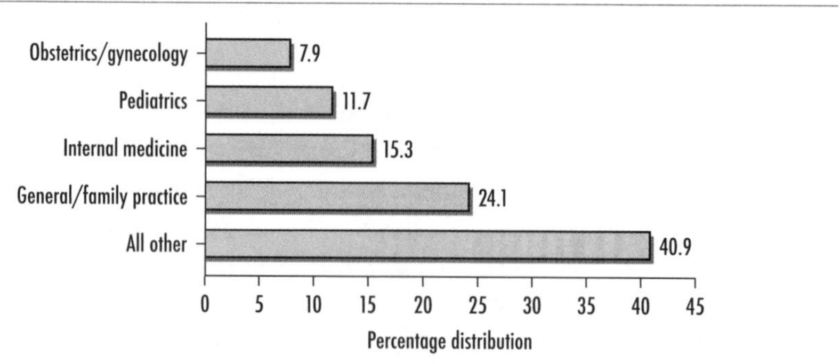

Figure 4.1 Ambulatory Visits to Physicians According to Specialty: 2000. Data from National Center for Health Statistics. *Health, United States, 2002,* p. 244–245. Hyattsville, MD: US DHHS.

actually needs, according to the Council on Graduate Medical Education (COGME). Current physician supply also exceeds previous projections and future growth projections, at least through the first decade of the 21st century.

A surplus of physicians leads to unnecessary increases in health care expenditures. A shortage, on the other hand, adversely affects the delivery of health services. The irony is that despite sharp increases in the aggregate surplus of physicians, physician shortages still exist in certain parts of the country. The shortages are caused by a maldistribution of physicians in terms of both geography and specialty. *Maldistribution* refers to either a surplus or a shortage of the type of physicians needed to maintain the health status of a given population at an optimum level.

Geographic Maldistribution

Physicians are more likely to concentrate in metropolitan and suburban areas rather than in rural and inner-city areas because the former generally offer greater prospects for high living standards, professional interaction, access to modern facilities and technology, continuing education, and professional growth. The basic source of the physician distribution problem in the United States, however, is a system that does not extend health care coverage to all Americans. The need for additional physicians is determined primarily on the basis of the population's health care needs. Medical services, on the other hand, are delivered in a market that links delivery of services to people's ability to pay for them, mainly through health insurance. The need-based model assumes an even distribution of physicians in the projection of labor force requirements, but the market-oriented model is based on consumer demand factors. The inconsistency between the two models largely contributes to provider surpluses in metropolitan and suburban areas and shortages in rural areas and inner cities. The problem of obtaining medical care in the underserved areas is further exacerbated by low rates of health insurance coverage; because of this, many such areas do not have the economic capacity to support additional physicians.

Specialty Maldistribution

Besides geographic maldistribution of physicians, a considerable imbalance exists between primary and specialty care in the United States. From 1965 to 1992, the number of primary care physicians increased by only 13%, whereas the number of specialists increased by 121% (Rivo & Kindig, 1996). The supply of primary care physicians dropped sharply between 1949 and 1970 and has been on a slow decline path since then. The number of positions filled in family practice residency programs showed an increase during the first few years of the 1990s, but there has been a slow decline since 1998 (Pugno et al., 2001). Other areas in primary care training show similar trends. The trends portray a declining interest in primary care among medical graduates.

In the United States, approximately 34.5% of physicians are generalists, and the remaining 65.5% are specialists, according to 1999 data from the American Medical Association (U.S. Bureau of Labor Statistics, 2002a). In other industrialized countries, only 25% to 50% of physicians are specialists (Schroeder, 1992).

The delivery of health care in the United States has been moving toward the managed care model, which reduces the demand for physician services, particularly those of specialists. Specialty maldistribution has become ingrained in the U.S. health care delivery system for three main reasons: medical technology, reimbursement methods and remuneration, and specialty-oriented medical education. On the other hand, the need for primary care physicians is determined mainly by the demographics of the general population.

The major driving force behind the increasing number of specialists is the development of medical technology. The rapid advances in medical technology have continuously expanded the diagnostic and therapeutic options at the disposal of physician specialists. Because the population increases at a significantly slower rate than technological advancements, the gap between primary and specialty care physician workforces continues to expand.

The higher incomes earned by specialists relative to primary care physicians have also contributed to an oversupply of specialists. Traditionally, physician payments by Medicare have been based on historically determined practice costs (Hsiao et al., 1993; Physician Payment Review Commission, 1993), which have been higher in specialty practice. It is only recently that reimbursement systems designed to increase payments to primary care physicians have been implemented.

Specialists not only earn higher incomes, but they also have more predictable work hours and enjoy higher prestige, both among their colleagues and from the public at large (Rosenblatt & Lishner, 1991; Samuels & Shi, 1993). High status and prestige are accorded to tertiary care and specialties employing high technology. Such considerations have influenced career decisions of medical students. Other factors affecting medical students' career choices are society's perception of value, intellectual challenge, and future financial rewards.

The imbalance between generalists and specialists has several undesirable consequences. Having too many specialists has contributed to the high volume of intensive, expensive, and invasive medical services and to the rise in health care costs (Greenfield & Nelson, 1992; Rosenblatt, 1992; Schroeder & Sandy, 1993; Wennberg et al., 1993). A greater supply of surgeons increases the demand for initial contacts with surgeons. In fact, the rate of surgery in the United States grew at twice the rate of the population from 1979 to 1986 (Kramon, 1991). Seeking care directly from specialists is often less effective than using primary care because the latter attempts to provide early intervention before complications develop (Starfield, 1992; Starfield & Simpson, 1993). Having higher numbers of primary care professionals is associated with lower overall mortality and lower death rates resulting from diseases of the heart and cancer (Shi, 1992, 1994). Primary care physicians have been the major providers of care to minorities, the poor, and people living in underserved areas (Ginzberg, 1994; Starr, 1982). Hence, the underserved populations suffer the most from shortages of primary care physicians.

DENTISTS

Dentists are the major providers of dental care. The major role of dentists is to diagnose and treat problems related to the teeth, gums, and tissues of the mouth. All dentists must be licensed to practice. The licensure requirements include graduation from an accredited dental school that awards a Doctor of Dental Surgery (DDS) or Doctor of Dental Medicine (DMD) degree and successful completion of both written and practical examinations. The median annual income of these salaried dentists was $129,030 in 2000 (U.S. Bureau of Labor Statistics, 2002b).

Some states require dentists to obtain a specialty license before practicing as a specialist in that state (Stanfield, 1995, p. 110–113). Eight specialty areas are recognized by the American Dental Association: orthodontics (straightening teeth), oral and maxillofacial surgery (operating on the mouth and jaws), pediatric dentistry (dental care for children), periodontics (treating gums), prosthodontics (making artificial teeth or dentures), endodontics (root canal therapy), public health dentistry (community dental health), and oral pathology (diseases of the mouth). The growth of dental specialties is influenced by technologic advances, including implant dentistry, laser-guided surgery, orthognathic surgery for the restoration of facial form and function, new metal combinations for use in prosthetic devices, new bone graft materials in "tissue-guided regeneration" techniques, and new materials and instruments.

Many dentists are involved in the prevention of dental decay and gum disease. Dental prevention includes regular cleaning of teeth and educating patients on proper dental hygiene. Water fluoridation programs have significantly reduced the rate of dental caries in children. Dentists also spot symptoms that require treatment by a physician. Dentists employ dental hygienists and assistants to perform many of the preventive and routine care services.

Most dentists practice in private offices, alone or in groups. As such, dental offices are operated as private businesses, and dentists often perform business tasks such as staffing, financing, purchasing, leasing, and work scheduling. Some dentists work in dental clinics in private companies, retail stores, franchised dental outlets, or MCOs. Group dental practices, offering lower overhead and increased productivity, have slowly grown. The federal government also employs dentists, mainly in the hospitals and clinics of the Department of Veterans Affairs and the U.S. Public Health Service.

The emergence of employer-sponsored dental insurance caused an increased demand for dental care because it enabled a greater segment of the population to afford it. The demand for dentists will continue to increase with the increase in populations having high dental needs, such as the elderly, the handicapped, the homebound, and patients with HIV. Other factors contributing to the increased demand for dentists include greater public awareness of the importance of dental care to general health status, the fairly widespread appeal of cosmetic and aesthetic dentistry, and the inclusion of dental care as part of many public-funded programs (Head Start, Medicaid, community and migrant health centers, maternal and infant care).

PHARMACISTS

The traditional role of pharmacists has been to dispense medicines prescribed by physicians, dentists, and podiatrists and to provide consultation on the proper selection and use of medicines. All states require a license to practice pharmacy. The licensure requirements include graduation from an accredited pharmacy program that awards a Bachelor of Pharmacy or Doctor of Pharmacy (PharmD) degree, successful completion of a state board examination, and practical experience or completion of a supervised internship (Stanfield, 1995, p. 142–147). After 2005, the bachelor's degree will be phased out, and a PharmD requiring six years of postsecondary education will become the standard. The median annual income of pharmacists in 2000 was $70,950.

Although most pharmacists are generalists, dispensing drugs and advising providers and patients, some become specialists. Pharmacotherapists specialize in drug therapy and work closely with physicians. Nutrition-support pharmacists determine and prepare drugs needed for nutritional therapy. Radiopharmacists or nuclear pharmacists produce radioactive drugs used for patient diagnosis and therapy.

Most pharmacists hold salaried positions and work in community pharmacies that are independently owned or are part of a national drugstore, supermarket, or department store chain. Pharmacists are also employed by hospitals, MCOs, home health agencies, clinics, government health services organizations, and pharmaceutical manufacturers.

The role of pharmacists has expanded over the last 2 decades from the preparation and dispensing of prescriptions to include drug product education and serving as experts on specific drugs, drug interactions, and generic drug substitution. Pharmacists play a critical role in promoting rational drug use and effective drug management (Passmore & Kailis, 1994). Under the Omnibus Budget Reconciliation Act of 1990, pharmacists are required to give consumers information about drugs and their potential misuse. This educating and counseling role of pharmacists is broadly referred to as *pharmaceutical care*. Pharmacists inform physicians of patient compliance, achievement of therapeutic outcome, and potential drug interactions (Marcrom et al., 1992, p. 50) and identify, prevent, and resolve drug-related problems (Morley & Strand, 1989, p. 328).

Another area in which pharmacists are receiving broadened clinical involvement is referred to as "disease management." In about half the 50 states, pharmacists now have the authority to initiate or modify drug treatment, as long as they have collaborative agreements with physicians.

OTHER DOCTORAL-LEVEL HEALTH PROFESSIONALS

In addition to physicians, dentists, and some pharmacists, other health professionals have doctoral educations, including optometrists, psychologists, podiatrists, and chiropractors. Optometrists provide vision care such as examination, diagnosis, and correction of vision problems. They must be licensed to practice. The licensure requirements include the possession of a Doctor of Optometry (OD) degree and the ability to pass a written and clinical state board examination. Most optometrists work in solo or group practices. Others work for the government, MCOs, optical stores, or vision care centers as salaried employees.

Psychologists provide patients with mental health care. They must be licensed or certified to practice. The ultimate recognition is the diplomate in psychology, which requires a Doctor of Philosophy (PhD) or Doctor of Psychology (PsyD) degree, a minimum of 5 years of postdoctoral experience and the successful completion of an examination by the American Board of Examiners in professional psychology. Psychologists may specialize in several areas, such as clinical, counseling, developmental, educational, engineering, personnel, experimental, industrial, psychometric, rehabilitation, school, and social domains (Stanfield, 1995, p. 280–282).

Podiatrists treat patients with diseases or deformities of the feet, including performing surgical operations, prescribing medications and corrective devices, and administering physiotherapy. They must be licensed. Requirements for licensure include completion of an accredited program that awards a Doctor of Podiatric Medicine (DPM) degree and a national examination by the National Board of Podiatry. Most podiatrists work in private practice. Some are salaried employees of health services organizations.

Chiropractors provide treatment to patients through chiropractic (Greek for "done by hand") manipulation, physiotherapy, and dietary counseling. They typically help patients with neurologic, muscular, and vascular disturbances. Chiropractic care is based on the belief that the body is a self-healing organism. Chiropractors do not prescribe drugs or perform surgery. Chiropractors must be licensed to practice. Requirements for licensure include completion of an accredited program that awards a 4-year Doctor of Chiropractic (DC) degree and an examination by the state chiropractic board. Most chiropractors work in a private solo or group practice.

NURSES

Nurses constitute the largest group of health care professionals. The nursing profession developed around hospitals after World War I, and it primarily attracted women. Before World War I, more than 70% of nurses worked in private duty, either in patients' homes or for private-pay patients in hospitals. Hospital-based nursing flourished after the war as the effectiveness of nursing care became apparent. Federal support of nursing education increased after World War II, represented by the Nursing Training Act of 1964, the Health Manpower Act of 1968, and the Nursing Training Act of 1971, but state funding remains the primary source of financial support for nursing schools.

Nurses are the major caregivers of sick and injured patients, addressing their physical, mental, and emotional needs. All states require that nurses be licensed in order to practice. The licensure requirements include graduation from an approved nursing program and successful completion of a national examination. Educational preparation distinguishes between two levels of nurses. Registered nurses (RNs) must complete an associate's degree (ADN), a diploma program, or a bachelor of science in nursing (BSN) degree. ADN programs take about two to three years and are offered by community and junior colleges. Diploma programs take two to three years and are offered by hospitals. Bachelor of science in nursing programs take four to five years and are offered by colleges and universities (Stanfield, 1995, p. 126–199). Licensed practical nurses (LPNs)—called licensed vocational nurses (LVNs) in some states—must complete a state-approved program in practical nursing and take a national written examination. Most practical nursing programs last about one year and include classroom study as well as supervised clinical practice.

Nurses work in a variety of settings, including hospitals, nursing homes, private practice, ambulatory care centers, community and migrant health centers, emergency medical centers, MCOs, work sites, government and private agencies, clinics, schools, retirement communities, rehabilitation centers, and as private-duty nurses in patients' homes. Nurses are often classified according to the settings in which they work: hospital nurses, long-term care nurses, public health nurses, private duty nurses, office nurses, and occupational health or industrial nurses. Head nurses act as supervisors of other nurses. RNs supervise LPNs.

Because hospitals now treat much sicker patients than before, more nurses are needed per unit, and their work has become more intensive. In addition, the remarkable growth in alternative settings has created new opportunities for nursing employment. The growing opportunities for RNs in supportive roles such as case management, utilization review, quality assurance, and prevention counseling have also expanded the demand for their services. Estimates show a current national shortfall of nurses, which is projected to increase (Sochalski, 2002). Sluggish wages, low levels of job satisfaction, and inadequate career mobility pose some major impediments to attracting and retaining nurses (Sochalski, 2002).

Advanced-Practice Nurses

The term *advanced-practice nurse* (APN) is a general name for nurses who have education and clinical experience beyond that required of an RN. There are four areas of specialization for APNs (Cooper et al., 1998): clinical nurse specialists (CNSs), certified registered nurse anesthetists (CRNAs), nurse practitioners (NPs), and certified nurse-midwives (CNMs). NPs and CNMs are also categorized as NPPs and are discussed in the next section. Besides being direct caregivers, APNs perform other professional activities such as collaborating and consulting with other health care professionals, educating patients and other nurses, collecting data for clinical research projects, and participating in the development and implementation of total quality management programs, critical pathways, case management, and standards of care (Grossman, 1995).

The main difference between CNSs and NPs is that CNSs work in hospitals, whereas NPs work mainly in primary care settings. CNSs can specialize in specific fields such as oncology, neonatal health, cardiac care, or psychiatric care.

NONPHYSICIAN PRACTITIONERS

The terms "nonphysician practitioner" (NPP), "nonphysician clinician," and "midlevel provider" refer to clinical professionals who practice in many of the areas in which physicians practice but who do not have an MD or a DO degree. NPPs receive less advanced training than physicians but more training than RNs. They are also referred to as physician extenders because in the delivery of primary care they can, in many instances, substitute for physicians. They do not, however, engage in the entire range of primary care or deal with complex cases requiring the expertise of a physician (Cooper et al., 1998). Hence, NPPs often work in close consultation with physicians. NPPs typically include physician assistants (PAs), NPs, and CNMs. NPs work predominantly in primary care, whereas PAs are evenly divided between primary care and specialty care. In 2001, there were an estimated 103,600 NPs and PAs in clinical employment (Hooker & Berlin, 2002). In addition, there are roughly 8,000 CNMs in the United States.

The American Academy of Physician Assistants (1986, p. 3) (AAPA) defines PAs as "part of the healthcare team . . . [who] work in a dependent relationship with a supervising physician to provide comprehensive care." PAs are licensed to perform medical procedures only under the supervision of a physician. PAs assist physicians in the provision of care to patients. The supervising physician may be either onsite or offsite. The major services provided by PAs include evaluation, monitoring, diagnostics, therapeutics, counseling, and referral (Fizgerald et al., 1995). They practice in offices, hospitals, MCOs, clinics, nursing homes, mental health facilities, rehabilitation centers, community and migrant health centers, and government institutions. As of 2001, there were 132 accredited PA training programs in the United States, with a steady growth in enrollment (Hooker & Berlin, 2002). PA programs award bachelor's degrees, certificates, associate degrees, or master's degrees. In most states, PAs have the authority to prescribe medications.

NPs constitute the largest group of NPPs and the group that has undergone the most growth (Cooper et al., 1998); however, since 1997, enrollments have gradually dropped. The American Nurses Association defines NPs as individuals who have completed a program of study leading to competence as RNs in an expanded role. The training of NPs may be a certificate program (at least 9 months in duration) or a master's degree program

(2 years of full-time study). States vary with regard to licensure and accreditation requirements. Most NPs are now trained in master's- or post–master's-level nursing programs. In addition, NPs must complete clinical training in direct patient care. The primary function of NPs is to promote wellness and good health through patient education. NPs spend extra time with patients to help them understand the need to take responsibility for their own health. NPs are particularly valuable in outpatient settings where, for many patients, they are the first point of contact with the health care system. Another area where they provide service is nursing homes (Brody et al., 1976). NPs have statutory prescribing authority in almost all states.

CNMs are RNs with additional training from a nurse-midwifery program in areas such as maternal and fetal procedures, maternal and child nursing, and patient assessment (Endicott, 1976). CNMs deliver babies, provide family planning education, and manage gynecologic and obstetric care. They are often used as substitutes for obstetricians/gynecologists in prenatal and postnatal care. They refer abnormal or high-risk patients to obstetricians or jointly manage the care of such patients. Patients of CNMs are less likely to have continuous electronic monitoring, induced labor, or anesthesia. These differences are associated with lower Caesarean section rates and less resource use in areas such as hospital stay, operating room costs, and use of anesthesia staff (Rosenblatt et al., 1997).

Value of NPP Services

Efforts to formally establish the roles of NPs, PAs, and CNMs as nonphysician health care providers began in the late 1960s in recognition of the fact that they could improve access to primary care, especially in rural areas. Studies have confirmed the efficacy of NPPs as health care providers. Many studies have demonstrated that NPPs can provide both high-quality and cost-effective medical care because they show greater personal interest in patients and cost significantly less. Moreover, NPs have been noted to have better communication and interviewing skills than physicians. These skills are considered particularly important in community and migrant health centers in assessing patients who are predominantly of minority origin and often have little education (Brody et al., 1976). Clients are more satisfied with NPs than with physicians because NPs are more likely to do comprehensive examinations. NPPs are also more likely to be employed in rural and medically underserved areas than in urban areas (Moscovice & Rosenblatt, 1979), which alleviates some of the problems created by the geographic maldistribution of physicians. CNMs are considered effective in providing access to obstetrical and prenatal services in rural and poor communities.

Among the issues that need to be resolved before NPPs can be used to their full potential are legal restrictions on practice, reimbursement policies, and relationships with physicians (Samuels & Shi, 1993). The lack of autonomy to practice is a great legislative barrier facing midlevel providers. Most states require physician supervision as a condition for practice. In some states, midlevel providers lack prescriptive authority. NPPs also face reimbursement barriers. Reimbursement for their services is generally indirect; that is, payments are made to the physicians with whom they practice. Also, the opinions of NPPs are not actively sought in making medical policies and decisions. More evidence of the effect of their services, when compared with physicians, is also needed.

ALLIED HEALTH PROFESSIONALS

In the early part of the 20th century, the health care provider workforce consisted of physicians, nurses, pharmacists, and optometrists. The growth in technology and specialized interventions subsequently placed greater demands on the time physicians and nurses spent with their patients. Such time constraints as well as the limitations in learning new skills created a need to train other professionals who could serve as adjuncts to or as substitutes for physicians and nurses. These professionals received specialized training, and their clinical interventions were meant to complement the work of physicians and nurses. Thus, physicians and nurses were relieved of time pressures so that they could attend to functions that only they had the expertise to perform. The extra time also allowed them to keep abreast of the latest advances in their disciplines.

As noted in Section 701 of the Public Health Service Act, an allied health professional is someone who has received a certificate; associate's, bachelor's, or master's degree; doctoral level preparation; or postbaccalaureate training in a science related to health care and has responsibility for the delivery of health or related services. These services may include those associated with the identification, evaluation, and prevention of diseases and disorders, dietary and nutritional services, rehabilitation, or health system management. Furthermore, these professionals are different from those who have received a degree in medicine (MD or DO), dentistry, optometry, podiatry, chiropractic, or pharmacy; a graduate degree in health administration; a degree in clinical psychology; or a degree equivalent to one of these. In broad terms, allied health includes many health-related areas. Allied health professionals constitute approximately 60% of the U.S. health care work force. Formal requirements for allied health professionals range from certificates gained in postsecondary educational programs to postgraduate degrees for some professions. Allied health professionals can be divided into two broad categories: technicians and/or assistants and therapists and/or technologists.

Technicians and Assistants

Typically, technicians and assistants receive less than 2 years of post-secondary education and are trained to perform procedures. Assistants and technicians require supervision from therapists or technologists to ensure that care plan evaluation occurs as part of the treatment process. This group includes physical therapy assistants, certified occupational therapy assistants, medical laboratory technicians, radiological technicians, and respiratory therapy technicians.

Technologists and Therapists

Technologists and therapists receive more advanced training. They learn how to evaluate patients, diagnose problems, and develop treatment plans. They must also have the training to evaluate the appropriateness and the potential side effects of therapy treatments. Education at the technologist or therapist level includes skill development in teaching procedural skills to technicians.

Some key allied health professionals are graduates of programs accredited by their respective professional bodies. These programs train physical therapists (PTs), whose role is to provide care for patients with movement dysfunction. A bachelor's or a master's degree in physical therapy is required, as is passing a licensure examination administered by the American Physical Therapy Association. Certification, registration, or licensure is based on state requirements. Occupational therapists help people of all ages improve their ability to perform tasks in their daily living and working environments. They work with individuals who have conditions that are mentally, physically, developmentally, or emotionally disabling. Patients requiring occupational therapy services need specialized assistance to lead independent, productive, and satisfying lives. The basic education required is either a bachelor's or a master's degree in occupational therapy and a certification examination, which is administered by the National Board for Certification in Occupational Therapy.

Dietitians or nutritionists and dietetic technicians ensure that institutional foods and diets are prepared in accordance with acceptable nutritional standards. Dietitians are registered by the Commission on Dietetic Registration of the American Dietetic Association. Dispensing opticians fit eyeglasses and contact lenses. They are certified by the American Board of Opticianry and the National Contact Lens Examiners. Speech-language pathologists treat patients with speech and language problems. Audiologists treat patients with hearing problems. The American Speech-Language-Hearing Association is the credentialing association for audiologists and speech–language pathologists. Social workers help patients and families cope with the problems resulting from long-term illness, injury, and rehabilitation, among other things. The Council on Social Work Education accredits baccalaureate and master's degree programs in social work in the United States.

HEALTH SERVICES ADMINISTRATORS

Health services administrators are employed at the top, middle, and entry levels of various types of organizations that deliver health services. Top-level administrators provide leadership and strategic direction, work closely with the governing board, and are responsible for an organization's long-term success. They are responsible for the operational, clinical, and financial outcomes of the entire organization. Middle-level administrators may have leadership roles in major service centers such as outpatient, surgical services, or nursing services, or they may be departmental managers in charge of single departments such as diagnostics, dietary, rehabilitation, social services, environmental services, or medical records. Their jobs involve major planning and coordinating functions, organizing human and physical resources, directing and supervising, operational and financial controls, and decision making. They often have direct responsibility for implementing changes, creating efficiencies, and developing new procedures with respect to changes in the health care delivery system. Entry-level administrators may function as assistants to midlevel managers. They may supervise a small number of operatives. Their main function may be to oversee and assist with operations critical to the efficient operation of a departmental unit.

Health services administration is taught at the bachelor's and master's levels in a variety of settings, and the programs lead to several different degrees. The settings for such academic programs include schools of medicine, public health, public administration, business administration, and allied health sciences. Bachelor's degrees prepare students for entry-level positions. Mid- and senior-level positions require a graduate degree. The most common degrees are the Master of Health Administration (MHA) or Master of Health Services Administration (MHSA), Master of Business Administration (MBA, with a health care management emphasis), Master of Public Health (MPH), or Master of Public Administration (or Affairs; MPA) (Pew Health Professions Commission, 1998). The 32 or so graduate schools of public health in the United States, which are accredited by the Council on Education for Public Health, play a key role in training health services administrators in their MHA/MHSA and MPH programs.

Growth of the elderly population, along with a current shortage of qualified administrators, is creating attractive opportunities in long-term care management. The training of nursing home administrators has been influenced to a great extent by government licensing regulations. Passing a national examination administered by the National Association of Boards of Examiners of Long-Term Care Administrators (NAB) is a standard requirement; however, educational qualifications needed to obtain a license vary significantly from one state to another. Although the basic academic qualification required by most states is a bachelor's degree, acquiring adequate skills in nursing home administration requires a degree that specializes in long-term care administration or health care management (Singh, 2005).

CONCLUSION

Health services professionals in the United States constitute the largest portion of the labor force. The growth and development of these professions are influenced by demographic trends, advances in research and technology, disease and illness trends, and the changing environment of health care financing and delivery. Physicians play a leading role in the delivery of health services. In the United States, there is an overall surplus of physicians and a maldistribution of physicians by both specialty and geography. The basic physician labor force problem emanates from the fact that the supply of physicians is largely determined by population need, but medical services are actually delivered according to ability to pay. The inconsistency between supply and demand largely contributes to a provider surplus in certain metropolitan and suburban areas and to shortages in rural and inner-city areas. In addition to physicians, many other health services professionals also contribute significantly to the delivery of health care, including nurses, dentists, pharmacists, optometrists, psychologists, podiatrists, chiropractors, nonphysician providers, and other allied health professionals. These professionals require different levels of training and work in a variety of health care settings in roles complementary to or substituting for those of physicians.

REFERENCES

American Academy of Physician Assistants. 1986. *PA Fact Sheet*. Arlington, VA: Author.

Brody, S. J., et al. 1976. The geriatric nurse practitioner: A new medical resource in the skilled nursing home. *Journal of Chronic Diseases* 29 (8):537–543.

Cooper, R. A. 1994. Seeking a balanced physician workforce for the 21st century. *Journal of the American Medical Association* 272 (9):680–687.

Cooper, R. A., et al. 1998. Current and projected workforce of nonphysician clinicians. *Journal of the American Medical Association* 280 (9):788–794.

Endicott, K. M. 1976. Health and health manpower. In *Health in America: 1776–1976* (pp. 138–165). Health Resources Administration, U.S. Public Health Service. DHEW Pub. No. 76616. Washington, DC: U.S. Department of Health, Education, and Welfare.

Fizgerald, M. A., et al. 1995. The midlevel provider: Colleague or competitor? *Patient Care* 29 (1):20.

Ginzberg, E. 1994. Improving health care for the poor. *Journal of the American Medical Association* 271 (6):464–467.

Greenfield, S., and E. C. Nelson. 1992. Recent developments and future issues in the use of health status assessment measures in clinical settings. *Medical Care* 30 (5 Suppl):MS23–MS41.

Grossman, D. 1995. APNs: Pioneers in patient care. *American Journal of Nursing* 95 (8):54–56.

Hooker, R. S., and L. E. Berlin. 2002. Trends in the supply of physician assistants and nurse practitioners in the United States. *Health Affairs* 21 (5):174–181.

Hsiao, W., et al. 1993. Assessing the implementation of physician-payment reform. *New England Journal of Medicine* 328 (13):928–933.

Kahn, N. B., et al. 1994. AAFP constructs definitions related to primary care. *American Family Physician* 50 (6):1211–1215.

Kramon, G. 1991, February 24. Medical second-guessing: In advance. *New York Times*, 12.

Marcrom, R., et al. 1992. Create value-added services to meet patient needs. *American Pharmacy* S32 (7):48–57.

Morley, P., and L. Strand. 1989. Critical reflections of therapeutic drug monitoring. *Journal of Clinical Pharmacy* 2 (3):327–334.

Moscovice, I., and R. Rosenblatt. 1979. The viability of midlevel practitioners in isolated rural areas. *American Journal of Public Health* 69 (5):503–505.

Passmore, P., and S. Kailis. 1994. In pursuit of rational drug use and effective drug management: Clinic and public health viewpoint. *Asia-Pacific Journal of Public Health* 7 (4):236–241.

Pew Health Professions Commission. Pew Commission urges increased action to cut U.S. physician supply. 1998, November 10. *PT Bulletin*, 10.

Physician Payment Review Commission. 1993. *Annual Report to Congress*. Washington, DC: Author.

Pugno, P. A., et al. 2001. Results of the 2001 national resident matching program: Family practice. *Family Medicine* 33:594–601.

Rich, E. C., et al. 1994. Preparing generalist physicians: The organizational and policy context. *Journal of General Internal Medicine* 9 (1 Suppl):S115–S122.

Rivo, M. L., and D. Kindig. 1996. A report on the physician work force in the United States. *New England Journal of Medicine* 334 (13):892–896.

Rosenblatt, R. A. 1992. Specialists or generalists: On whom should we base the American health care system? *Journal of the American Medical Association* 267 (12):1665–1666.

Rosenblatt, R.A., and D. M. Lishner. 1991. Surplus or shortage? Unraveling the physician supply conundrum. *Western Journal of Medicine* 154 (1):43–50.

Rosenblatt, R. A., et al. 1997. Interspecialty differences in the obstetric care of low-risk women. *American Journal of Public Health* 87 (3):344–351.

Samuels, M. E., and L. Shi. 1993. *Physician Recruitment and Retention: A Guide for Rural Medical Group Practice*. Englewood, CO: Medical Group Management Press.

Schroeder, S. A. 1992. Physician supply and the U.S. medical marketplace. *Health Affairs* (Spring):235–243.

Schroeder, S., and L. G. Sandy. 1993. Specialty distribution of U.S. physicians: The invisible driver of health care costs. *New England Journal of Medicine* 328 (13):961–963.

Shi, L. 1992. The relation between primary care and life chances. *Journal of Health Care for the Poor and Underserved* 3 (2):321–335.

Shi, L. 1994. Primary care, specialty care, and life chances. *International Journal of Health Services* 24 (3):431–458.

Singh, D. A. 2005. *Effective Management of Long-Term Care Facilities*. Boston: Jones and Bartlett Publishers.

Sochalski, J. 2002. Nursing shortage redux: Turning the corner on an enduring problem. *Health Affairs* 21 (5):157–164.

Stanfield, P. S. 1995. *Introduction to the Health Professions*. Boston: Jones and Bartlett Publishers.

Starfield, B. 1992. *Primary Care: Concepts, Evaluation, and Policy*. New York: Oxford University Press.

Starfield, B., and L. Simpson. 1993. Primary care as part of US health services reform. *Journal of the American Medical Association* 269:3136–3139.

Starr, P. 1982. *The Social Transformation of American Medicine: The Rise of a Sovereign Profession and the Making of a Vast Industry*. New York: Basic Books.

U.S. Bureau of Labor Statistics. 2002a. Accessed January 18, 2002, from http://www.bls.gov/oco/text/ocos074.txt/.

U.S. Bureau of Labor Statistics. 2002b. Accessed September 23, 2002, from http://www.bls.gov/oco/content/ ocos072.stm/.

Wennberg, J. E., et al. 1993. Finding equilibrium in U.S. physician supply. *Health Affairs* (Summer):89–103.

Chapter 5

Technology and Its Effects

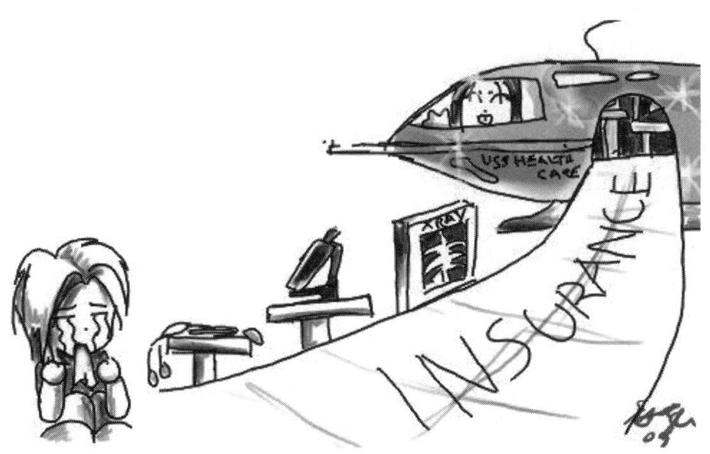

INTRODUCTION

Medical technology has brought numerous benefits to modern civilization. These benefits, however, come at a price that society has to pay. Research and development (R & D) and the production of new technology are costly. Sophisticated advanced diagnostic procedures have reduced health complications and disability. New medical cures have increased longevity, and new drugs have helped stabilize chronic conditions and have given an improved quality of life to many. Technology, however, has also enabled critically ill patients to be put on life support with little hope of full recovery and has raised complex moral and ethical dilemmas in medical research and decision making. The fact that life expectancy almost doubled from 1900 to 1965 was as a result of advances in social conditions—improved sanitation, nutrition, and living conditions—rather than advances in medical treatment. The continuing rise in longevity since then, however, has been largely attributed to advances in medical technology as well as continued improvement in living conditions.

With the rising cost of medical care, at some point, society will have to face the conflict between a commitment to medical innovation and the growth of new technology on the one hand and cost containment on the other. One reason why the United States has not been able to afford universal health care for all Americans is the tremendous cost of health care and the demands placed by Americans on the use of all available technology.

Canadians and residents of other advanced nations in Europe, who have enjoyed universal health care for several decades, have been able to place limits on the availability and use of costly technology through supply-side rationing, as discussed in Chapter 2. But, the notion of medical rationing is not palatable to Americans. Hence, the idea of extending basic health care to all Americans presents a major predicament. Access to only basic health care for some and availability of technologically advanced services for others are impractical in the United States.

In Chapter 3, it was pointed out that developments in science and technology were instrumental in drastically changing the nature of health care delivery during the postindustrial era. Since then, the ever-increasing proliferation of new technology has continued to profoundly alter many facets of health care delivery. Following are some of the major changes triggered by technology.

- It has raised consumer expectations about what may be possible. Patients' expectations have considerable influence on their health care–seeking behavior, leading to greater demand for and utilization of the latest and best that technology can offer.
- Technology influences the organization and financing of medical services.
- It has driven the scope and content of medical training and the practice of medicine. It has also influenced the way status is ascribed to various medical workers.
- Although some medical technology may reduce costs, as a whole, technology has contributed to health care cost inflation. For both the consumer and provider, the cost of excessive treatment has generally been of no concern as long as a third party—either an insurance plan or the government—pays for it.

Economic globalization has also enveloped biomedical knowledge and technology. This is particularly true of the developed and developing nations where leading physicians have access to the same scientific knowledge through medical journals and the Internet. Most drugs and medical devices available in the United States are also available in many other parts of the world.

WHAT IS MEDICAL TECHNOLOGY?

In a confined sense, medical technology refers to the practical application of the scientific body of knowledge produced by biomedical research. Medical science, in turn, has benefited from developments in other applied sciences, such as chemistry, physics, engineering, and pharmacology. For example, advances in organic chemistry made it possible to identify and extract the active ingredients found in natural plants to produce drugs and anesthetics. Developments in electrical and mechanical engineering led to such medical advances as radiology, cardiology, and encephalography (Bronzino et al., 1990, p. 11). Magnetic resonance imaging (MRI), a technology that had its origins in basic research on the structure of the atom, later was transformed into a major diagnostic tool (Gelijns & Rosenberg, 1994). The disciplines of computer science and communication systems find their application in information technology and telemedicine (Tan, 1995, p. 4).

In its narrow sense, medical technology includes sophisticated machines, pharmaceuticals, and biologicals. In a broader sense, however, it also covers medical and surgical procedures used in rendering medical care, ultramodern facilities and settings of care delivery, computer-supported information systems, and management and operational systems that make health care delivery more efficient (**Exhibit 5.1**).

INFORMATION TECHNOLOGY

Information technology (IT) has become an integral part of health care delivery. It is indispensable for managing information used in patient care delivery, quality improvement, cost containment, billing and collections,

Exhibit 5.1 Examples of Medical Technology

- Diagnostic equipment
  - CT (computed tomography) scanner
  - MRI (magnetic resonance imaging)
- Equipment and devices to render treatment
  - Lithotripter
  - Heart and lung machine
  - Kidney dialysis machine
  - Pacemaker
- Pharmaceuticals
- Medical procedures
  - Open-heart surgery
  - Tissue transplants
  - Hip and knee replacements
- Facilities and organizational systems
  - Medical centers and systems
  - Laboratories
  - Managed care networks
  - Information systems
  - Patient care management
  - Internet
  - E-health
  - Telemedicine
  - Distance education
  - Electronic Medical records

and other aspects of operating health care organizations. Many large health care organizations have information systems departments and managers to maintain and improve the flow of information.

Major Categories

Specific IT system applications in health services delivery fall into four main areas:

1. *Clinical information systems* involve the organized processing, storage, and retrieval of information to support patient care delivery. Electronic medical records, for example, can provide quick and reliable information necessary to guide clinical decision making and to produce timely reports on the quality of care delivered. Computerized physician-order entry (CPOE) enables physicians to transmit orders electronically right from the bedside. Telemedicine is based on integrated applications of telecommunications and information technologies. *Medical informatics* (or health informatics) is the term now used for IT applications that are designed to improve clinical efficiency, accuracy, and reliability.

2. *Administrative information systems* are designed to assist in carrying out financial and administrative support activities such as payroll, patient accounting, staff scheduling, materials management, budgeting and cost control, and office automation.
3. *Decision support systems* provide information and analytical tools to support managerial decision making. Such tools are used to forecast patient volume, project staffing requirements, evaluate financial performance, analyze utilization, conduct clinical research, and improve quality and productivity.
4. Internet and E-health enable patients and practitioners to access information, facilitate interaction between consumers or between patients and providers, add certain conveniences for both physicians and patients, and enable the possibility of virtual visits.

Information technology is more than having a computer and a programmer. Information systems are integrative in nature because they interface with many components of the organization. Increasingly, they are also being linked to agencies outside an organization. The process of determining data needs and gathering, storing, analyzing, and reporting data affects almost all major departments of a health care delivery organization.

Electronic Health Records

Electronic health records (EHRs) replace the traditional paper medical records. EHR systems make it possible to access individual records online from many separate, interoperable automated systems within an electronic network. According to the Institute of Medicine (2003), a fully developed EHR system includes four key components: (1) collection and storage of health information on individual patients over time, where health information is defined as information pertaining to the health of an individual or health care provided to an individual; (2) immediate electronic access to person and population level information by authorized users; (3) provision of knowledge and decision support that enhance the quality, safety, and efficiency of patient care (medical informatics); and (4) support of efficient processes for health care delivery. In the United States, hospitals and physicians' clinics have been converting their medical records to EHRs, but little progress has been made in the development of information sharing networks.

In the minds of many providers and patients alike, confidentiality of patient information has been a major concern. The Health Insurance Portability and Accountability Act (HIPAA) of 1996 made it illegal to gain access to personal medical information for reasons other than health care delivery, operations, and reimbursement. HIPAA legislation mandated strict controls on the transfer of personally identifiable health data between two entities, provisions for disclosure of protected information, and criminal penalties for violation (Clayton, 2001). HIPAA also conferred certain patient rights such as the right of patients to inspect and have copies of their protected health information, to request corrections to the records, and to restrict the use of the information.

The Internet and E-Health

The Internet has continued to revolutionize certain aspects of health care delivery, and its use will continue to grow. "*E-health* refers to all forms of electronic health care delivered over the Internet, ranging from informational, educational, and commercial 'products' to direct services offered by professionals, nonprofessionals, businesses, or consumers themselves" (Maheu et al., 2001). An increasing number of Americans reported going on-line to look for health care information, and about half indicated that the information affected their decisions about treatment and care (Blumenthal, 2002). Among physicians, at least 80% are using the Internet, which is quite a leap from just 3% in 1995 (Mullan & Lundberg, 2000). Of these physicians, 90% indicated that they were using the Internet to find clinical information (Blumenthal, 2002).

By accessing information from the Internet, patients have become more active participants in their own health care. Information empowers patients, but it also has the potential to create conflict between patients and their physicians. Using the right source can provide valid and up-to-date information to both consumers and practitioners. For instance, departments of the U.S. government offer a wealth of current information based on their own publications.

The Internet is not merely a source of information; it offers new ways to create efficiency. In practice settings, the Internet is being used to register patients, direct them to alternative care sites, transmit diagnostic results, and order pharmaceuticals and other products. By accessing patient information through the Internet from their homes or hospital lounges, physicians can get a head start on their hospital rounds (Morrissey, 2002). Internet-facilitated virtual visits may be on the verge of entering mainstream medicine (Robeznieks, 2007). Although not appropriate in all instances, virtual visits can assist patients with the monitoring of certain health conditions and treatment follow-up when a face-to-face visit may not be necessary. Some positive aspects of virtual visits are their cost-saving potential, convenience, and patient satisfaction. Consequently, some health plans have started to reimburse for virtual visits.

Telemedicine

Telemedicine, or distance medicine, employs the use of telecommunications technology for medical diagnosis and patient care when the provider and client are separated by distance. It also enables a generalist to consult a specialist when a patient's illness and diagnosis are complex. General adoption of telemedicine has been slow. Some of the main barriers have been licensure of physicians and other providers across state lines, concerns about legal liability, and lack of reimbursement for services provided via telemedicine. Also, the cost-effectiveness of most telemedicine applications remains unsubstantiated. Diagnostic and consultative teleradiology, on the other hand, is almost universally reimbursed and has been proven to be cost-effective (Field & Grigsby, 2002). Despite the obstacles, several new applications are being studied. Remote in-home patient monitoring programs that monitor vital signs, blood pressure, and blood glucose levels are proving to be cost-effective.

USE OF MEDICAL TECHNOLOGY

High-tech procedures are more readily available in the United States than they are in most other countries, and little is done to limit the expansion of new medical technology. For example, compared with most European hospitals, American hospitals perform a far greater number of catheterizations, angioplasties, and heart bypass surgeries. The United States also has more high-tech equipment such as MRI and CT scanners available for its population than most countries do (Kim et al., 2001). To control medical costs, almost all other nations have tried to limit, mainly through central planning (supply-side rationing), the distribution and utilization of high-tech procedures. For instance, compared with the United States, Canada had 76% fewer MRI machines and performed 72% fewer coronary bypass procedures per 100,000 population; Great Britain had 55% fewer MRI machines and performed 82% fewer coronary bypass surgeries (Anderson & Hussey, 2001). Only Japan and Switzerland were estimated to have more MRI machines per 100,000 population than the United States. The rationing of medical technology through central planning curtails costs, but it also restricts access to care. For example, waiting times to receive cancer therapy are three times longer in Canada than in the United States. Similar waiting times often apply when seeking specialty services or scheduling surgery (Walker, 1999).

Because of the lack of controls on the development and use of technology, spending on biomedical research in the United States increased from $37 billion in 1994 to $94.3 billion in 2003. The 5.6% of the total health care expenditures spent on biomedical research was more than any other country's spending (Hamilton et al., 2005). In 2002, per capital expenditures in the United States on pharmaceutical R & D were 35% higher than in Europe and 232% higher than in Japan (Hay, 2006). Much of the R & D in the United States is funded by private corporations, such as pharmaceutical and medical equipment manufacturers.

The major reasons why the United States leads all other nations in the development and use of technology are (1) cultural beliefs and values, (2) medical training and practice, (3) payment methods, and (4) competition among providers. These factors are discussed in subsequent sections. **Exhibit 5.2** lists some interventions that the United States can undertake to curtail the growth of technology. Implementing these measures, however,

Exhibit 5.2 Mechanisms to Control the Growth of Technology

- Central planning to determine how much technology will be made available and where
- Withdraw federal funding for R & D
- Change the patterns of medical training, with a greater emphasis on primary care practice
- Reduce the number of specialty residency slots for medical graduates
- Curtail insurance payments for expensive medical treatments
- Impose controls on pharmaceutical prices, which in turn will make less money available for R & D and development of new drugs

would go against the fundamental beliefs and values of Americans and would generate much controversy.

Cultural Beliefs and Values

American beliefs and values have been instrumental in determining the nature of health care delivery in the United States. Capitalism and a lack of government intervention promote innovation. An environment in which innovation thrives creates opportunities for the scientists and manufacturers who develop technology. Americans have high expectations of finding cures through science and technology. Compared to Europeans, Americans generally think that it is absolutely essential for them to be able to get the most advanced tests, drugs, medical procedures, and equipment (Kim et al., 2001). The desire to have state-of-the-art technology available along with the desire to use it despite its cost is called the *technological imperative*.

Medical Training and Practice

The emphasis on specialty care over primary care and preventive services predominates in the medical culture of the United States. This emphasis is reflected in the training of physicians. American medical graduates persistently choose to specialize rather than go into primary care practice. For example, between 1995 and 2006, the number of U.S. medical graduates entering primary care residencies dropped by 7% compared with a 5% increase in those who opted to train as specialists (Evans, 2008). An oversupply of specialists has had important consequences for the development and use of new technology because primary care physicians use less technology than specialists, even for similar medical conditions.

Payment for Services

Evidence from several countries suggests that fixed provider payments (such as paying physicians a salary) and strong limits on payments to hospitals curtail the incentive to use high-tech procedures. Such payment arrangements, in turn, place limitations on how quickly new technology will be developed and how widely it will become available (McClellan & Kessler, 1999). Countries such as Canada have also implemented direct price controls over pharmaceuticals to keep their costs down.

In the United States, financing of health care through private insurance has insulated both patients and providers from any personal accountability for the utilization of high-cost services. As long as out-of-pocket costs are of little concern, patients expect their physicians to provide all that medical science has to offer. Knowing that the services demanded by their patients are covered by insurance, providers have shown little hesitation in providing the services. Traditionally, the U.S. health care delivery system has lacked internal checks and balances to determine when high-cost services are really appropriate.

Competition Among Providers

Specialization has been used by the medical establishment as an enticement to attract insured patients. State-of-the-art technology also plays a role in the ability of a hospital or clinic to recruit specialists. When hospitals develop new services and invest heavily in modernization programs, other hospitals in the area are generally forced to do the same. Such practices have resulted in a tremendous amount of duplication of services and equipment and have further contributed to medical specialization.

ROLE OF THE GOVERNMENT IN TECHNOLOGY DIFFUSION

The development and dissemination of technology is called *technology diffusion*. It determines which new technology will be developed, when it will be made available for use, and where it can be accessed. Once technology becomes available, its use is almost ensured. Hence, the diffusion and utilization of technology are closely intertwined.

Technology diffusion has been accompanied by issues of cost, safety, benefit, and risk. Federal legislation has been aimed at addressing these concerns. The government also plays a major role in carrying out research and providing funding for research to private organizations.

Regulation of Drugs and Devices

The Food and Drug Administration (FDA) is an agency of the U.S. Department of Health and Human Services (DHHS) and is responsible for ensuring that drugs and medical devices are safe and effective for their intended use. It also controls access to drugs by deciding whether a certain drug will be available by prescription only or as an over-the-counter purchase. In recent years, the FDA has approved the over-the-counter sale of several popular drugs previously obtained only with a prescription.

Legislation to Regulate Drugs

Exhibit 5.3 summarizes the main pieces of legislation that regulate drugs and medical devices. The regulatory functions of the FDA have evolved over time. According to the Food and Drugs Act of 1906, the FDA was authorized to take action only after drugs had been marketed to consumers. It was

Exhibit 5.3 Summary of FDA Legislation

Year	Legislation
1906	**Food and Drugs Act** FDA authorized to take action only after drugs sold to consumers cause harm
1938	**Federal Food, Drug, and Cosmetic Act** Evidence of safety required before new drugs or devices can be marketed
1962	**Drug Amendments** FDA takes charge of reviewing efficacy and safety of new drugs, which can be marketed only once approval is granted
1976	**Medical Devices Amendments** Premarket review of medical devices authorized; devices grouped into three classes
1983	**Orphan Drug Act** Drug manufacturers given incentives to produce new drugs for rare diseases
1990	**Safe Medical Devices Act** Health care facilities must report device-related injuries or illness of patients or employees to the manufacturer of the device and, if death is involved, the incident must also be reported to the FDA
1992	**Prescription Drug User Fee Act** FDA receives authority to collect application fees from drug companies to provide additional resources to shorten the drug approval process
1997	**Food and Drug Administration Modernization Act** Allows fast-track approvals for life-saving drugs when expected benefits exceed those of therapies that already exist

assumed that the manufacturer would conduct safety tests before marketing the product. If innocent consumers were harmed, only then could the FDA take action (Bronzino et al., 1990, p. 198). The drug law was strengthened by the passage of the Federal Food, Drug, and Cosmetic Act of 1938 in response to the infamous Elixir Sulfanilamide disaster, which caused almost 100 deaths in Tennessee because of poisoning from a toxic solvent used in the liquid preparation (Flannery, 1986). According to the revised law, drug manufacturers were required to provide scientific evidence about the safety of new products before putting them on the market.

The drug approval system was further transformed by the 1962 Drug Amendments to the Federal Food, Drug, and Cosmetic Act. The approval system authorized by these amendments is in place today for most new drugs. The law was tightened after the thalidomide tragedy. In the United States, thalidomide was a sleeping pill distributed as an experimental drug, but in Europe, it had been widely marketed. Thousands of deformed infants were born to mothers who had used this new drug. The 1962 amendments essentially stated that premarket notification was not sufficient. The amendments put in force a premarket approval system, giving the FDA authority to review the safety as well as the effectiveness of a new drug before it could be marketed. Its consumer protection role now enabled the FDA to prevent harm before it occurred. The new rule, however, was criticized for slowing down the introduction of new drugs and, consequently, denying patients the early benefit of the latest treatments.

In the late 1980s, pressure on the FDA from those wanting rapid access to new drugs for the treatment of HIV infection called for a reconsideration of the drug review process (Rakich et al., 1992, p. 186). Also, the Orphan Drug Act of 1983 and subsequent amendments were passed to provide incentives for pharmaceutical firms to develop new drugs for rare diseases and conditions. Incentives such as grant funding were made available because a relatively small number of people are afflicted by these rare conditions, creating a relatively small market. As a result of the Orphan Drug Act, certain new drug therapies have become available for conditions that affect fewer than 200,000 people in the United States.

In 1992, Congress passed the Prescription Drug User Fee Act, which authorized the FDA to collect fees from pharmaceutical companies to review their drug applications. According to the U.S. General Accounting Office, the fees have allowed the FDA to make new drugs available more quickly by shortening the time it takes for approvals. On the flip side, there has been a rise in the percentage of drugs that have had to be withdrawn from the market after approval because of safety-related concerns (New Leadership for the FDA, 2002). There is clearly a tradeoff between accelerating the review process and potential safety risks.

On November 21, 1997, Congress passed the Food and Drug Administration Modernization Act. The law provides for increased patient access to experimental drugs and medical devices. It provides for "fast-track" approvals when the potential benefits of new drugs for serious or life-threatening conditions are considered significantly greater than those for currently available therapies.

Legislation to Regulate Devices

The FDA was first given jurisdiction over medical devices under the Federal Food, Drug, and Cosmetic Act of 1938. Initially, such jurisdiction was confined to the sale of products that were believed to be unsafe or that made misleading claims of effectiveness (Merrill, 1994). In the 1970s, several deaths and miscarriages were attributed to the Dalkon Shield, which had been marketed as a safe and effective contraceptive device (Flannery, 1986). The Medical Devices Amendments of 1976 extended the FDA's authority to include premarket review of medical devices divided into three classes.

- Class I: Devices subject to general controls regarding misbranding, that is, fraudulent claims regarding the therapeutic effects of certain devices.
- Class II: Devices subject to certain performance standards.
- Class III: Devices that come under the most stringent requirements of premarket approval regarding safety and effectiveness. Devices in this class support life, prevent health impairment, or prevent an unreasonable risk of illness or injury (Rakich et al., 1992).

The Safe Medical Devices Act of 1990 has particular relevance for health care providers who are required by law to report to the manufacturer and, in some cases to the FDA as well, all injuries and deaths caused by medical devices. Requirements under this Act serve as an early warning system for any serious device-related problems that could potentially become widespread.

Although the FDA's protocols for evaluating the safety and effectiveness of therapeutic products are relatively well established, at present no such capability exists for the assessment of medical and surgical procedures (Rettig, 1994).

Research on Technology

The Agency for Healthcare Research and Quality (AHRQ), originally named the Agency for Health Care Policy and Research, was established in 1989 under the Omnibus Budget Reconciliation Act of 1989. A division of the DHHS, the AHRQ is the lead federal agency charged with supporting research to improve the quality of health care, reduce health care costs, and improve access to essential services. The agency's reports on technology assessment are made available to medical practitioners, consumers, and other health care purchasers.

The federal government is also a major provider of financial support to private and public institutions for biomedical research. The AHRQ and the National Institutes of Health (NIH) support both basic and applied biomedical research in the United States.

IMPACT OF MEDICAL TECHNOLOGY

The effects of advances in scientific knowledge and medical technology have been far-reaching and pervasive. The effects often overlap, making it difficult to pinpoint accurately the impact of technology on the delivery of health care.

Impact on Quality of Care

For most Americans, high-technology medicine is synonymous with high-quality care although such an association is not always accurate. Quality is enhanced only when new procedures can prevent or delay the onset of serious disease, provide better diagnosis, make quicker and more complete cures possible, increase safety of medical treatment, minimize undesirable side effects, promote faster recovery from surgery, increase life expectancy, and add to quality of life (**Exhibit 5.4**). Improvements in diagnostic capabilities increase the likelihood that timely and more appropriate treatments will be provided. Technology can provide new remedies where none existed before. Technology also offers improved remedies that are more effective, less invasive, or safer. The outcomes can be increased longevity and decreased morbidity, both of which are indicators of better quality of health care.

Exhibit 5.4 Criteria for Quality of Care

- Prevent or delay disease onset
- More accurate diagnosis than currently available
- Quicker cure
- More complete cure
- Increase safety of treatment
- Minimize side effects
- Faster recovery from surgery
- Increase life expectancy
- Add to quality of life

Numerous examples illustrate the role of technology in enhancing the quality of care. Tiny cardiac pacemakers and implantable cardioverter defibrillators (ICDs) can be implanted in the human body to prevent sudden cardiac death. New imaging technologies such as positron emission tomography (PET) and single-photon emission computed tomography (SPECT) are available as advanced diagnostic tools to study brain function and locate both physical and mental disorders. Laser technology permits surgery with less trauma, better precision, and quicker postsurgical recovery. Advanced lasers are now available for high precision eye surgery. New blood screening methods, such as nucleic acid testing, have made the nation's blood supply far safer than it was a few years ago. Molecular and cell biology are being employed to screen for genetic disorders and provide gene therapy. Major pharmaceutical breakthroughs now enable Americans suffering from heart disease, cancer, AIDS, and preterm birth to have much longer life expectancies and improved health status (Kleinke, 2001).

Amid all the enthusiasm that emerging technologies might garner, some degree of caution must prevail. Past experience shows that greater proliferation of technology may not necessarily equate to higher quality. Unless the effect of each individual technology is appropriately assessed, some innovations may actually be wasteful, and others may possibly be harmful.

Impact on Quality of Life

Quality of life indicates a patient's overall satisfaction with life during and after medical treatment. For example, quality of life is enhanced when technology enables people to live normal lives despite disabling conditions affecting speech, hearing, vision, and movement. Major technological advances have furnished the clinical ability to help patients cope with diabetes, heart disease, end-stage renal disease, and HIV/AIDS. Thanks to modern treatments, HIV/AIDS has become a chronic disease, not a death sentence (Komaroff, 2005). New categories of drugs are also instrumental in relieving pain and suffering. For example, for cancer pain management, new opioids have been developed for transdermal, nasal, and nebulized administration that allow needleless means of controlling pain (Davis, 2006). Finally, minimally invasive surgical procedures, such as lithotripsy, which crushes kidney and bile stones by using shock waves, have improved quality of life by reducing pain and suffering and allowing a quicker return to normal life. Procedures such as coronary artery bypass graft (CABG) surgery—an open-heart surgical procedure to correct blockage of coronary arteries—has made it possible for people with severe heart disease to return to normal activity within a few weeks after surgery. Previously, such patients would have required lifelong medication and suffered prolonged disability (Nitzkin, 1996).

Impact on Health Care Costs

Measurement of the impact of technology on health care costs is rather imprecise, but technology proliferation has unquestionably contributed to rising health care expenditures (Littell & Strongin, 1996). According to some experts, technology diffusion may be the single most important factor in medical cost inflation (Cassell, 1993). Unlike other industries in which new technology often reduces labor force and production costs, the addition of new technology in health care usually increases both labor and capital costs (Iglehart, 1982). Exhibit 5.5 summarizes the main reasons behind technology-driven cost escalation. First, there is the cost of acquiring the new technology and equipment. Second, specially trained physicians and technicians are often needed to operate the equipment and to analyze the results, which often leads to increases in labor costs. Third, new technology may also require special housing and setting requirements, resulting in facilities costs (McGregor, 1989). Finally, the utilization of new technology is assured when it is covered by insurance.

High R & D costs invested in developing new technology and precision manufacturing necessitate a high price tag. From a systems perspective, however, total purchase price represents only a small fraction of the total annual U.S. health care expenditures. Costs associated with utilization of technology after it becomes available are more important.

Exhibit 5.5 Cost Increases Associated with New Medical Technology

- Capital costs: Acquisition costs are often high because of R & D and precision manufacturing
- Training or hiring of technicians with special skills
- Facilities may require refurbishing or expansion to accommodate new technology
- Utilization when covered by insurance (moral hazard and provider-induced demand)

Although it is true that many new technologies increase costs, others actually reduce costs when they replace treatments that are more expensive. **Exhibit 5.6** shows the three main areas in which technology has saved health care costs. Cost-saving technologies include peripheral vascular angioplasty, lithotripsy, endoscopic lasers, valvuloplasty, and automated clinical chemistry analyzers (Stripp, 1989). Minimally invasive technologies have reduced costs indirectly by eliminating the need for overnight hospital stays. Technology should also be credited for an overall reduction in the need for hospitalization. For example, antiretroviral therapies have been largely credited with the dramatic reduction in the hospitalization of AIDS patients (CDC, 1999). Breakthroughs in antidepressants and antipsychotics have been instrumental in reducing admissions for inpatient psychiatric care.

Impact on Access

Geographic access can be improved for many people by providing mobile equipment or by using new communications technologies that allow remote access to centralized equipment and specialized personnel. Mobile equipment can be transported to rural and remote sites, making it accessible to those populations. Mobile cardiac catheterization laboratories, for example, can provide high technology in rural settings.

Exhibit 5.6 Cost-Saving Medical Technology

- Replacement of earlier, more expensive procedures
- Minimally invasive procedures that eliminate the need for overnight hospital stays
- Technologies that shorten hospital stays

Impact on the Structure and Processes of Health Care Delivery

Medical technology has transformed large urban hospitals into medical centers where the latest diagnostic and therapeutic remedies are offered, but technology also takes modern medicine to alternative locations such as patients' own homes. The notable growth in outpatient and home care has been made possible by new technology, and at the same time, costs have been reduced because previously similar technology was available only in hospitals. Without technological innovations, extensive adaptations of modern treatments to these alternative sites would not have been possible. For example, monitoring devices can permit cardiac implants to transmit vital information over telephone lines, respirators maintain breathing in the home, and kidney dialyzers are commonly used at home. Common outpatient surgical procedures now include hernia repair, surgery for kidney and gallbladder stones, cataract removal, tonsillectomy, carpal tunnel release, left heart catheterization, knee arthroscopy, and much gynecological surgery. Numerous diagnostic procedures are also performed in outpatient settings.

Managed care has been instrumental in transforming the way in which health services are delivered in the United States. Simpson (1994) observed that without technology, managed care would not be possible because it is based on managing information, and managing information requires technology. For example, information management is the backbone for the monitoring of cost-effectiveness and quality of delivered services and for the tracking of referrals to specialized services.

Impact on Global Medical Practice

The United States leads the world in medical technology, producing more than half of the $175 billion in health care technology products purchased worldwide each year (AdvaMed, 2004). Many nations wait for the United States to develop new technologies that can then be introduced into their systems in a more controlled and manageable fashion. This process gives them access to high-tech medical care with less national investment because they forego the high R & D costs. If technology development was slowed by a modest amount in the United States, it would likely have serious health consequences globally (Massaro, 1990). Telemedicine has also made clinical care, distance education, and medical research possible in parts of the world traditionally unexposed to such advancements (Umar, 2003).

Impact on Bioethics

Increasingly, technological change is raising serious ethical and moral issues. Gene mapping of humans, genetic cloning, stem cell research, genetic engineering, genetic testing, and so forth may hold potential benefits, but they also present serious ethical dilemmas. For example, research on embryonic stem cells may lead one day to the discovery of treatments and cures for diseases and other long-term degenerative illnesses such as cardiac failure, Parkinson's disease, spinal cord injury, and diabetes. However, the use of human embryos for research is highly controversial. Life support technology also raises serious ethical issues in medical decisions, whether life support should continue when a patient may only exist in a permanent vegetative state or whether life support should be discontinued, and if so, at what point.

ASSESSMENT OF MEDICAL TECHNOLOGY

Technology assessment refers to the evaluation of medical technology to determine its efficacy, safety, and cost-effectiveness. Assessment can go beyond examining the direct effects of technology and can include its social, economic, and ethical consequences (Institute of Medicine, 1985). The objective of technology assessment is to establish the appropriateness of medical technology for widespread use. Hence, technology assessment should govern decisions to adopt and disseminate new technology.

Efficacy and safety are the basic starting points in evaluating the overall usefulness of medical technology. Cost-effectiveness goes a step further in evaluating the safety and efficacy in relation to the cost of using technology. Efficacy and safety are evaluated through clinical trials. A clinical trial is a carefully designed research study in which human subjects participate under controlled observations. Cost-effectiveness is determined by using economic models that compare the benefits of a treatment in relation to its costs.

In the United States, it is primarily the private sector that conducts technology assessment, unlike nations such as Sweden, the Netherlands, and Canada, which have centralized technology assessment agencies (Neumann & Sandberg, 1998). Hence, much of the talent needed to assess medical technology is also located, organized, and financed in the private sector.

Efficacy

Efficacy may be defined simply as the health benefit to be derived from the use of technology or how effective a given technology is in diagnosing or treating a condition. If a product or service actually produces some health benefits, it can be considered *efficacious* or *effective*. Decisions about efficacy require that the right questions be asked. For example, is the current diagnosis satisfactory? What is the likelihood that a different procedure would result in a better diagnosis? If the problem is more accurately diagnosed, what is the likelihood of a better cure? Apart from evaluating the effects on mortality and morbidity, psychosocial and functional factors are also recognized as important outcomes, even though they may be difficult to measure.

Safety

Safety considerations are designed to protect patients against unnecessary harm from the use of technology. As a primary benchmark, benefits must outweigh any negative consequences. Clinical trials are used to evaluate both efficacy and safety. After safety has been experimentally determined, the outcomes from the wider use of a certain technology are closely monitored over time to identify any problems.

Cost-Effectiveness

Cost-effectiveness, or cost-efficiency, is a step beyond the determination of efficacy and safety. It weighs benefits against costs. When a medical treatment is first introduced in caring for a patient, the benefits generally exceed the costs, and the use of technology is regarded as cost-effective. Additional treatments begin to lower the benefits in relation to rising costs. At some point along a time line, continued medical interventions yield benefits that roughly equal the additional costs. Optimal cost-effectiveness is achieved when additional benefits equal the additional cost of treatment. From that point on, additional interventions either deliver no further benefits or the cost of providing additional care begins to exceed the benefits. In these cases, additional care becomes wasteful. In cost-effectiveness analysis, potential risk from medical treatment can also be incorporated as a type of cost, recognizing that most medical procedures are associated with varying degrees of risk or potential harm.

Experts believe that much of the medical care delivered in America is wasteful because, after a certain point, additional care adds little or no health benefits while the costs continue to accumulate. One of the problems is that little is known about the cost-effectiveness of even well-established health care technologies. As the overall health care cost burden continues to mount, technology assessment will play a considerable role in future health care planning, policy, financing, and delivery. Establishing the cost-effectiveness of various treatments can potentially relieve physicians and insurers from the responsibility of making certain treatment decisions that otherwise become controversial and lead to conflict and legal battles.

BENEFITS OF TECHNOLOGY ASSESSMENT

From the previous section, some of the main benefits of technology assessment become obvious. For example, the safety and efficacy of new technology are essential to prevent potential harm to patients. Other beneficial effects discussed earlier, such as improved quality of care, better quality of life, better access, and control of costs, are all based on the use of technologies that pass rigorous examination of their safety, efficacy, and cost-effectiveness.

Delivering Value

Possibilities regarding what technology can achieve are potentially limitless as the rapid rate of technological development continues to advance. However, health services decision making is increasingly being governed by asking the question "what is appropriate?" rather than "what is possible?" (Abele, 1995). The concept of *value*—improved benefits at lower costs—is becoming important to those who finance health care, including private employers, the government, and managed care organizations. Value can be increased by improving quality, reducing cost, or doing both. The problem is that insured patients often want to use all available medical resources regardless of how little health benefit is received in relation to cost. Physicians often find themselves in a precarious situation when they are required to withhold treatment because of its cost-inefficiency. Payers generally get blamed as uncaring profit mongers when they intervene in the delivery of medical care based on costs. Eventually the government may find itself in a central position for issuing practice guidelines based on cost-efficiency.

Cost-Containment

Simply pointing to technology as the culprit for cost escalations and putting arbitrary restraints on technology development and dissemination would be a misdirected strategy. As stated earlier, technology has the potential to not only enhance health benefits but also reduce costs. Demands for reducing costs without sacrificing quality must influence technological change. Also, a greater emphasis should be placed on developing technology specifically for reducing costs.

Standardized Practice Protocols

Medical practice guidelines (or clinical practice guidelines) are systematically developed protocols to assist practitioners in delivering appropriate health care for specific clinical circumstances (Field & Lohr, 1990). Technology assessment plays a significant role in the development of clinical protocols. Practice guidelines result from an evaluation of medical procedures regarding their effectiveness, appropriateness, and safety, and the integration of these assessments into clinical practice. Unlike some other countries, however, cost-effectiveness has not taken central stage in health care delivery in the United States. Rising health care costs and excessive spending in the United States are of growing concern to most Americans.

CONCLUSION

Medical technology includes drugs, devices, procedures, facilities, information systems, and organizational systems. Thanks to American beliefs and values, the use of all available medical technology has been firmly entrenched in the American health care system. The United States is foremost in both the production and use of medical technology. Other countries adopt the technology developed in the United States and save on the high R & D costs. Other nations also use supply-side rationing to contain the diffusion and use of technology. Such an approach has been unacceptable to most Americans. Consequently, medical technology has been one of the primary factors in the growth of health care expenditures in the United States.

The FDA regulates the introduction of new drugs and devices based on efficacy and safety. The notion of cost-effectiveness is used in other countries, but Americans thus far have been unwilling to accept denial of medical care on that premise. Experts believe that much of the medical care delivered in America is actually wasteful, but at this point, no one is quite sure how to contain Americans' insatiable demand for the almost indiscriminate use of technology.

REFERENCES

Abele, J. 1995. Health reform and technology—What does it mean for us? *Biomedical Instrumentation and Technology* 29 (6):476–478.

AdvaMed (Advanced Medical Technology Association). 2004. *Industry profile—Medical technology*. Retrieved July 2008 from http://www.advamed.org/MemberPortal/About/NewsRoom/MediaKits/industryprofilemedical technology.htm.

Anderson, G., and P. S. Hussey. 2001. Comparing health system performance in OECD countries. *Health Affairs* 20 (3):219–232.

Blumenthal, D. 2002. Doctors in a wired world: Can professionalism survive connectivity? *Milbank Quarterly* 80 (3):525–546.

Bronzino, J. D., et al. 1990. *Medical Technology and Society: An Interdisciplinary Perspective*. Cambridge, MA: MIT Press.

Cassell, E. J. 1993. The sorcerer's broom: Medicine's rampant technology. *Hastings Center Report* 23 (6):32–39.

CDC (Centers for Disease Control and Prevention). 1999. *New Data Show AIDS Patients Less Likely to Be Hospitalized*. Retrieved July 2008 from http://www.cdc.gov/od/oc/media/pressrel/r990608.htm/.

Clayton, P. D. 2001. Confidentiality and medical information. *Annals of Emergency Medicine* 38 (3):312–316.

Davis, M.P. 2006. Management of cancer pain: Focus on new opioid analgesic formulations. *American Journal of Cancer* 5 (3):171–182.

Evans, M. 2008. Primary-care worries. *Modern Healthcare* 38 (7):8–9.

Field, M. J., and J. Grigsby. 2002. Telemedicine and remote patient monitoring. *Journal of the American Medical Association* 288:423–425.

Field, M. J., and K. N. Lohr (eds.). 1990. *Clinical Practice Guidelines: Directions for a New Agency*. Washington, DC: National Academy Press.

Flannery, E. J. 1986. Should it be easier or harder to use unapproved drugs and devices? *Hastings Center Report* 16 (1):17–23.

Gelijns, A., and N. Rosenberg. 1994. The dynamics of technological change in medicine. *Health Affairs* 13 (3):28–46.

Hamilton, M., et al. 2005. Financial anatomy of biomedical research. *Journal of the American Medical Association* 294 (11):1333–1342.

Hay, J. W. 2006. Where's the value in health care? *Value in Health* 9 (3):141–143.

Iglehart, J. K. 1982. The cost and regulation of medical technology: Future policy directions. In J. B. McKinlay (ed.). *Technology and the Future of Health Care* (pp. 69–103). Cambridge, MA: MIT Press.

Institute of Medicine. 1985. *Assessing Medical Technologies*. Washington, DC: National Academy Press.

Institute of Medicine. 2003. *Key Capabilities of an Electronic Health Records System*. Washington, DC: National Academy Press.

Kim, M., et al. 2001. How interested are Americans in new medical technologies? A multicountry comparison. *Health Affairs* 20 (5):194–201.

Kleinke, J. D. 2001. The price of progress: Prescription drugs in the health care market. *Health Affairs* 20 (5):43–60.

Komaroff, A. L. 2005, December 12. Beyond the horizon. *Newsweek* 146:82–84.

Littell, C. L., and R. J. Strongin. 1996. The truth about technology and health care costs. *IEEE Technology and Society Magazine* 15 (3):10–14.

Maheu, M.M. et al. 2001. *E-Health, Telehealth, and Telemedicine: A Guide to Start-Up and Success*. San Francisco: Jossey-Bass.

Massaro, T.A. 1990. Impact of new technologies on health care costs and on the nation's health. *Clinical Chemistry* 36 (8B):1612–1616.

McClellan, M., and D. Kessler. 1999. A global analysis of technological change in health care: The case of heart attacks. *Health Affairs* 18 (3):250–257.

McGregor, M. 1989. Technology and the allocation of resources. *New England Journal of Medicine* 320 (2):118–120.

Merrill, R. A. 1994. Regulation of drugs and devices: An evolution. *Health Affairs* 13 (3):47–69.

Morrissey, J. 2002. Hospitals offer remote control. *Modern Healthcare* 32 (51):32–35.

Mullan, F., and G. Lundberg. 2000. Looking back, looking forward: Straight talk about U.S. medicine. *Health Affairs* 19 (1):117–123.

Neumann, P. J., and E. A. Sandberg. 1998. Trends in health care R & D and technology innovation. *Health Affairs* 17:111–119.

New Leadership for the FDA. 2002. *Lancet* 360 (9341):1183.

Nitzkin, J. L. 1996. Technology and health care: Driving costs up, not down. *IEEE Technology and Society Magazine* 15 (3):40–45.

Rakich, J. S., et al. 1992. *Managing Health Services Organizations*. Baltimore, MD: Health Professions Press.

Rettig, R. A. 1994. Medical innovation duels cost containment. *Health Affairs* 13 (3):7–27.

Robeznieks, A. 2007. Don't LOL at virtual visits. *Modern Healthcare* 37 (41): 6–7, 16.

Simpson, R. L. 1994. The role of technology in a managed care environment. *Nursing Management* 25 (2):26–28.

Stripp, D. 1989, November 11. A two-edged sword. *Wall Street Journal*, R21–R23.

Tan, J. K. H. 1995. *Health Management Information Systems: Theories, Methods, and Applications*. Gaithersburg, MD: Aspen Publishers.

Umar, K. Office of Minority Health Resource Center. 2003. Telemedicine works: Quality, access, and cost impacts cited. *Closing the Gap* (January–February 2003). Washington, DC: Department of Health and Human Services.

Walker, M. 1999, March 5. Canadians with medical needs follow their doctors south. *Wall Street Journal*, A15.

Chapter 6

Financing and Reimbursement Methods

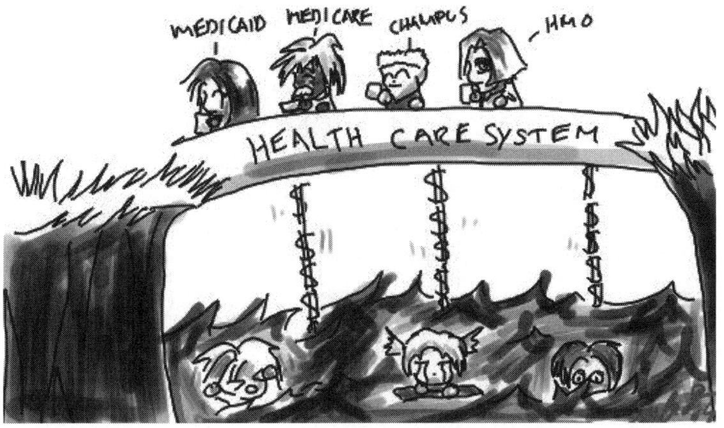

INTRODUCTION

Financing refers to any mechanism that gives people the ability to pay for health care services. In most cases, financing is necessary in order to access health care. Some uncompensated or charity care, mainly through free clinics, community health centers, and hospital emergency departments, is delivered to those who have little or no means to finance their health care. For most Americans, however, health insurance is the most common avenue for receiving health care. Most health insurance in the United States is privately financed. Also, certain categories of people are eligible for public insurance programs, such as Medicare, Medicaid, or State Children's Health Insurance Program. Financing also includes the various methods of paying providers in exchange for the health care they deliver. Hence, the two functions encompassed in financing are purchase of health insurance and payment for delivery of services.

The complexity of financing is one of the primary characteristics of medical care delivery in the United States. A multitude of programs and health plans exist to provide health insurance coverage. In 2006, 59% of Americans had private health insurance, most of which was job based; 14% were covered under Medicare; 12% had coverage under Medicaid and various other public programs; and 16% were uninsured (Henry J. Kaiser Family Foundation, 2007a).

The actual payment to providers of care is also handled in numerous ways. In most cases, patients directly pay a relatively small portion of the total cost of the services they receive. Various private and government insurance plans pay the bulk of the cost of health care, and they use several different types of payment mechanisms. The financing of health care through the various private and public sources ultimately aggregates into national health care expenditures, which measure the total amount of money a nation spends on health care delivery and other health-related activities. **Figure 6.1** illustrates the relationships between financing, insurance, access, payment, and total expenditures.

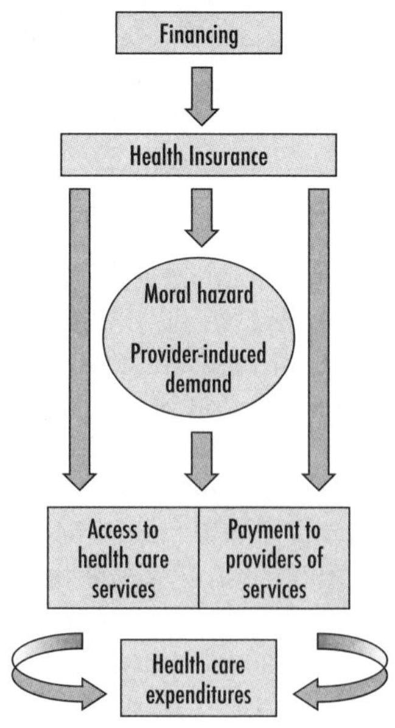

Figure 6.1 Relationships Between Financing, Insurance, Access, Payment, and Expenditures

Employers and the government are the primary financiers of health care in the United States. From an economic perspective, one could argue that Americans, through employment and taxes, finance their own health care and subsidize health care for those who cannot afford it. For instance, employer-paid health insurance actually represents an exchange for salary. Working Americans also have Medicare tax deducted from their paychecks, which amounts to prepayment of Medicare benefits they can expect to receive at the age of 65 years. General taxes collected from working Americans subsidize health care for the poor. Uninsured Americans receive catastrophic health care (medical services received when they are sick or injured) that is financed by insured Americans through cost shifting and through tax subsidies.

EFFECTS OF HEALTH CARE FINANCING AND INSURANCE

Health care financing produces effects that go beyond merely providing access and paying the providers (**Exhibit 6.1**). It also produces some undesirable effects.

Financing and insurance are instrumental in creating the demand for health care services. In a free market, demand is determined by the prices of goods and services on the one hand and people's ability to pay for them on the other. Health insurance lends people the ability to pay, but it also desensitizes both consumers and providers to the price of services. First, it creates excessive demand from consumers who want to use their health insurance benefits. When services are covered under insurance, consumers are driven to utilize more of them than if they had to pay the entire price out

Exhibit 6.1 Health Care Financing and Its Effects

- Financing of private and public health insurance—hence, a means of access to health care
- Payment to providers
- Moral hazard
- Provider-induced demand
- Services with liberal reimbursement proliferate
- Total health care expenditures are greater than if the same services were to be paid by the patients
- Growth of medical technology

of their own pockets. Consumer behavior that leads to a higher utilization of health care services when the services are covered by insurance is referred to as *moral hazard* (Feldstein, 1993, p. 125).

Financing also exerts powerful influences on supply-side factors, such as how much health care is delivered. Services with more liberal reimbursement proliferate rapidly. When reimbursement is constrained, the supply of services is curtailed accordingly. Health insurance also desensitizes the providers against the price of services, with the result that providers deliver additional and more expensive services. Again, if consumers had to pay for these services out of their own pockets, many of them would not be used. The providers' ability to create demand is referred to as *provider-induced demand*. As explained in Chapter 5, these additional services often provide little or no additional health benefits. Thus, financing indirectly affects the growth of medical technology.

Financing eventually affects the total health care expenditures (also referred to as health care costs or health care spending) incurred by a health care delivery system. Both moral hazard and provider-induced demand waste health care resources and add to the rising cost of health care. It is because of both moral hazard and provider-induced demand that countries with national health insurance have to implement rationing measures by restricting the supply of services. This *supply-side rationing* is accomplished through central health planning, which focuses on restricting the availability of expensive medical technology. Otherwise, the health care expenditures in these countries would be astronomical. The United States accomplishes similar results by not extending health insurance to all residents. This is called *demand-side rationing*. Without insurance, people face barriers to obtaining health care that they would have the desire to use if they were insured. On the flip side, the extension of health insurance to the uninsured, without other restrictions, would increase total health care expenditures. Such increases for 1994, when a national health care program was last proposed by President Clinton, have been estimated to range between $16.3 and $24.8 billion (Short et al., 1997). Even though these estimates represent only about 2% to 3% of total health care spending, moral hazard and provider-induced demand could substantially raise the estimated costs. Various types of supply-side approaches to the rationing of health care would have to be employed to restrain cost escalations, as shown by the experiences of other nations that have national health care programs.

INSURANCE: ITS NATURE AND PURPOSE

Basic Insurance Concepts

Insurance is a mechanism for protection against risk. In the context of insurance, *risk* refers to the possibility of a substantial financial loss from some event. In health care, illnesses requiring expensive treatments and hospitalization pose substantial financial risk to most people. Similarly, the cost of most surgeries and subsequent treatment would be beyond the means of many people to pay out of pocket. Insurance, in a general sense, is primarily designed to protect people against such eventualities. Health care providers are also subject to substantial risk when they are required to treat the sick and injured who cannot pay.

An individual who is protected by insurance against the possible risk of financial loss is called the *insured*. The insured is also referred to as the *enrollee* or the *beneficiary*. The insuring agency that assumes risk is called the insurer or underwriter. *Underwriting* is a systematic technique for evaluating, selecting (or rejecting), classifying, and rating risks. Four fundamental principles underlie the concept of insurance (Health Insurance Institute, 1969, p. 9; Vaughn & Elliott, 1987, p. 17).

- Risk is unpredictable for the individual insured.
- Risk can be predicted with a reasonable degree of accuracy for a group or a population.
- Insurance provides a mechanism for transferring or shifting risk from the individual to the group through the pooling of resources.
- Actual losses are shared on some equitable basis by all members of the insured group.

Based on underwriting, the insurer determines a fair price to insure against specified risks. The amount charged for insurance coverage is called a *premium*, which is usually paid every month. The average monthly cost of health insurance premiums in 2008 was $392 for a single plan and $1,057 for a family plan (Claxton et al., 2008).

Cost Sharing

Insurance requires some type of *cost sharing* so that the insured assumes at least part of the risk. The purpose of cost sharing is to reduce the misuse of insurance benefits. There are three main types of cost sharing in private health insurance: premium cost sharing, deductibles, and copayments.

In employer-sponsored health insurance, the employee is generally required to share in the total cost of the premium. Of the premium costs given previously, insured workers paid 15.3% of the cost for single plans and 26.5% of the cost for family plans (Claxton et al., 2008). In addition to paying a share of the cost of premiums through payroll deductions, insured individuals also generally pay a portion of the actual cost of medical services out of their own pockets. These out-of-pocket expenses are in the form of deductibles and copayments and are incurred if and when medical care is used.

A *deductible* is the amount the insured must first pay before any benefits by the plan are payable. A deductible commonly must be paid on an annual basis. For example, suppose a plan requires the insured to pay a $250 deductible. When the insured receives medical care, the plan starts paying only after the cost of medical services received by the insured has exceeded $250 in a given year. The insured must pay the first $250. In many managed care plans, preventive care is exempt from the deductible. However, separate deductibles often apply for hospitalization and outpatient surgery.

Another type of shared cost is the *copayment*. It is the amount that the insured has to pay out of pocket each time health services are received after the deductible amount has been paid. Suppose a plan requires a $250 deductible and offers 80:20 coinsurance. After the deductible requirement has been met, the plan starts paying 80% of all covered medical expenditures; the insured pays the remaining 20% as copayment. The 80:20 ratio of cost sharing between the insurance plan and the insured is referred to as *coinsurance*. The dollar amount paid is the copayment. Most plans include a *stop-loss* provision, which is the maximum out-of-pocket liability an insured would incur in a given year. In case of a catastrophic illness or injury, the copayment amount can add up to a substantial sum. The purpose of the stop-loss provision is to limit the total out-of-pocket costs to a certain amount, for example, $1,500. This means that after the deductible and copayments have totaled $1,500 in a given year, no further copayments are required and the plan pays 100% of any additional expenses. Some plans have set lifetime limits on benefits of $1 to $2 million; others have no such limits.

The rationale for cost sharing is to control the utilization of health care services. Because insurance creates moral hazard by insulating the insured against the cost of health care, making the insured pay part of the cost promotes more responsible behavior in health care utilization. A comprehensive study employing a controlled experimental design conducted in the 1970s, commonly referred to as the Rand Health Insurance Experiment, demonstrated that cost sharing had a material impact on lowering utilization without any significant negative health consequences.

PRIVATE INSURANCE

Private health insurance is also referred to as voluntary health insurance because it is not mandatory. The origins and rise of private health insurance in America were discussed in Chapter 3. The modern health insurance industry is pluralistic. Private insurance includes many different types of health plan providers, such as commercial insurance companies (e.g., Aetna, Cigna, Metropolitan Life, Prudential), Blue Cross/Blue Shield, self-insured employers, and managed care organizations (MCOs). The nonprofit Blue Cross and Blue Shield Associations function much like private health insurance companies.

Private insurance is generally available in the form of single or family plans. A family plan covers the spouse and children of the subscriber, along with the subscriber. In contrast, government programs such as Medicare and Medicaid do not offer family plans; each individual is an independent beneficiary. There are five main types of private insurance: group insurance, self-insurance, individual private insurance, managed care plans, and high-deductible health plans (HDHPs).

Group Insurance

Group insurance can be obtained through an entity such as an employer, a union, or a professional organization. A group insurance program anticipates that a substantial number of people in the group will participate in purchasing insurance through its sponsor. Risk and often the cost of insurance are distributed equally among the insured.

Earlier health insurance plans were designed to protect against financial hardships that could occur because of the high cost of hospitalization, extended illness, and expensive surgery. These plans were referred to as "major medical plans." Since the 1970s, health insurance plans have commonly combined major medical coverage with all-inclusive comprehensive coverage, which includes basic and routine physician office visits and diagnostic services.

Self-Insurance

Large employers often have workforces that are big enough and sufficiently well diversified in terms of risk so that they can self-insure. Rather than pay insurers a dividend to bear the risk, large employers can simply assume the risk by budgeting a certain amount to pay medical claims incurred by their employees. Being self-insured also gives such employers a greater degree of control. Self-insured employers can protect themselves against any potential risk of high losses by purchasing *reinsurance* from a private insurance company. Many of these employers found managed care to be a more economical alternative. Consequently, the number of self-insured plans declined during the 1990s.

Individual Private Insurance

Although most Americans obtain health insurance coverage through employer-sponsored group plans or government programs, individually purchased private health insurance is an important source of coverage for many Americans. In 2006, approximately 5% of Americans were covered under private nongroup plans (Henry J. Kaiser Family Foundation, 2007a). The family farmer, the early retiree, the employee of a business that does not offer health insurance, and the self-employed make up the bulk of the people who rely on private nonemployer-related health insurance. Unlike group insurance in which risk is spread over the entire group, individual private insurance determines premium price and eligibility based on the risk indicated by each individual's health status and demographics (U.S. General Accounting Office, 1996). Consequently, high-risk individuals are often unable to obtain privately purchased health insurance.

Managed Care Plans

MCOs, such as health maintenance organizations (HMOs) and preferred provider organizations (PPOs), emerged in response to the rapid escalation of health care costs during the 1970s and 1980s. Managed care plans are a type of health insurance because they assume risk in exchange for an insurance premium. Unlike traditional insurance companies, however, MCOs also assume the responsibility for delivering health care to their enrollees by contracting with a network of providers. Patients are expected to obtain services from in-network providers at nominal out-of-pocket costs. Some MCOs allow patients to go out of network, but in doing so, patients incur a higher out-of-pocket expense. MCOs also use a variety of mechanisms to monitor utilization and a variety of methods to reimburse providers for the services rendered. A detailed discussion on managed care is presented in Chapter 9.

High-Deductible Health Plans

HDHPs are an emerging type of health insurance that is expected to grow in popularity because of their low premium costs. For example, in 2008, single plans cost 17% less and family plans cost 20% less than managed care plans, mainly because of the high-deductible feature of HDHPs. In 2008, among employers that offered health insurance to workers, 13% offered an HDHP, up from 4% in 2005, and covered approximately 5.5 million workers (Claxton et al., 2008).

Generally, health plans that carry at least $1,000 deductible for single coverage or $2,000 for family coverage are considered HDHPs. There are two types of HDHP arrangements. Both link a personal savings account to HDHP insurance. The savings accounts give consumers greater control over how to use the funds. Hence, these plans are also referred to as *consumer-driven health plans*.

The first type includes a health reimbursement arrangement (HRA) (HDHP/HRA). The HRA is funded by the employer; employees are prohibited from contributing. The funds are used to reimburse the insured for qualified medical expenses, which include payment for HDHP premiums and premiums for long-term care insurance. Employees do not pay taxes on the payments made to them from HRAs. Although participants in an HRA are not required to have an HDHP, the arrangement commonly includes both.

The second type of arrangement combines a health savings account (HSA) with an HDHP (HDHP/HSA) that meets federal standards. For example, federal regulations require reasonable caps on out-of-pocket expenses. Also, the HDHP deductible amounts are indexed annually (e.g., $1,100 and $2,200 for single and family plans, respectively, in 2008). HSAs were authorized under the Medicare Prescription Drug,

Improvement, and Modernization Act, 2003. Under the law, HSA holders must have an HDHP. Employers may contribute, but are not required to do so. A little less than half of the employers currently make contributions to HSAs. Funds belong to the account holder and can accumulate without limit. HSAs have significant tax advantages. Contributions are tax-deductible. Withdrawals used to pay for medical expenses are exempt from federal income taxes. Account earnings are also tax-exempt.

PUBLIC INSURANCE

A significant portion of health services delivered in the United States is supported through public programs. In 2005, government financing accounted for 45.4% of total U.S. health care expenditures (Figure 6.2). The most notable shift from the private share of national health expenditures to the government's share occurred soon after the Medicare and Medicaid programs were created in 1965. Since then, the government has continued to liberalize benefits and has added new programs in a piecemeal fashion, most recently, the addition of prescription drug benefit to the Medicare program. This will further shift the burden of national health care spending to taxpayers.

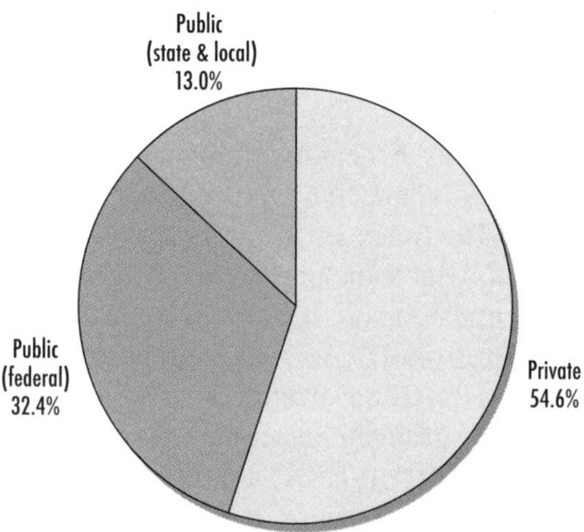

Figure 6.2 Private and Public Health Care Expenditures: 2005. Data from NCHS. *Health, United States, 2007*, p. 375. Hyattsville, MD: US DHHS.

The creation of Medicare and Medicaid programs under the Social Security Amendments of 1965 was discussed in Chapter 3. This section discusses the financing, eligibility requirements, and covered services for the major public health insurance programs.

Public financing supports *categorical programs*, each designed to provide benefits to a certain category of people who meet the eligibility criteria to become beneficiaries. The United States does not have publicly financed health insurance specifically for the unemployed. Even though public insurance is financed by the government, for the most part, services are purchased from providers in the private sector. One notable exception is the Department of Veterans Affairs (VA), which runs its own health care system to provide most of the services to its beneficiaries.

Medicare

The Medicare program, also referred to as Title 18 of the Social Security Act, finances medical care for three categories of people:

- Persons 65 years and older
- Disabled individuals of any age who are entitled to Social Security benefits
- People of any age who have permanent kidney failure (end-stage renal disease)

Medicare is a federal program administered by the Centers for Medicare and Medicaid Services (CMS), an agency under the U.S. Department of Health and Human Services (DHHS). In 1966, shortly after the program was created, it had 19.1 million enrollees. According to the 2008 annual report of the Medicare's boards of trustees, in 2007, there were 44.1 million Medicare enrollees (36.9 million elderly and 7.2 million nonelderly) in all U.S. states, territories, and the District of Columbia. Although the program was initially created for the elderly, over 16% of the enrollees are younger than 65 years of age who qualify on the basis of their disability. With the aging of the population, the program is expected to grow to 61 million enrollees by the year 2020. Medicare poses the single greatest future challenge to taxpayers of all government programs.

Deductibles, copayments, and noncovered services can leave Medicare beneficiaries with substantial out-of-pocket costs. It is estimated that the elderly spend an average of 22% of their annual income for out-of-pocket health care expenditures (Caplan & Brangan, 2004). Roughly 20% of the Medicare beneficiaries also qualify for Medicaid, which then picks up the expenses not covered by Medicare. Roughly 25% of Medicare participants privately purchase supplemental insurance policies from insurance companies. These policies are referred to as *Medigap* policies, which cover all or a portion of Medicare deductibles and copayments and may pay for services not covered by Medicare. Hence, private Medigap insurance plays an important role in meeting the medical needs of the elderly.

For almost 30 years after its inception, Medicare had a dual structure comprising two separate insurance programs referred to as Part A and Part B. Now Medicare has a four-part structure.

Hospital Insurance (Part A)

Part A, the hospital insurance (HI) portion of Medicare, is financed by special payroll taxes collected for Social Security. These mandatory taxes are paid by all working individuals, including those who are self-employed. All earnings are subject to the Medicare tax. The employer and employee share equally in financing the HI Trust Fund. Part A is designed to cover hospitalization, short-term convalescence and rehabilitation in a skilled nursing facility (SNF), and home health care. For terminally ill patients, Medicare pays for care provided by a Medicare-certified hospice. **Figure 6.3** shows the distribution of Part A payments for various services. As of the year 2003, hospice payments have exceeded payments for home health services. (Note the managed care expenditures are for Medicare Advantage, which is discussed later.)

The structure of Part A benefits is rather complex. For hospital and nursing home stays, the timing of benefits is determined by what is referred to as a *benefit period*. It begins on the day a beneficiary is hospitalized. It ends when the beneficiary has not been in a hospital or an SNF for 60 consecutive days. If after 60 days the beneficiary is hospitalized again, a new benefit period begins. The number of benefit periods a beneficiary can have over his or her lifetime is unlimited. The following is a brief description of acute care, postacute skilled nursing care, home health, and hospice benefits under Part A.

With regard to acute care, all covered hospital services are fully paid for the first 60 days in a benefit period after a deductible ($1,068 in 2009) has been met. Part A deductible applies to each benefit period. If ongoing

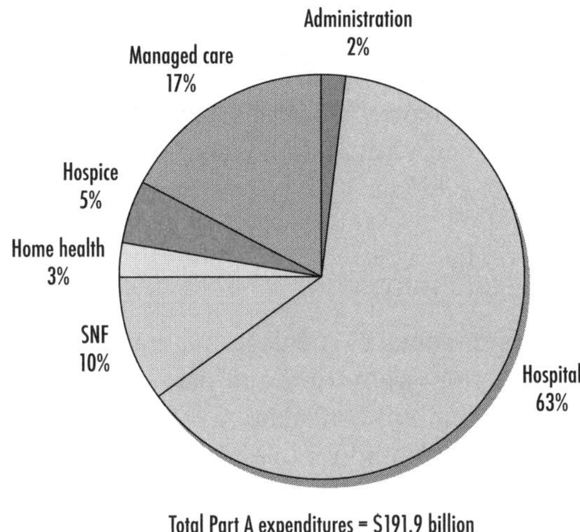

Figure 6.3 Part A Expenditures: 2006 (estimates). Data from NCHS. *Health, United States, 2007*, p. 408. Hyattsville, MD: US DHHS.

hospitalization beyond 60 days is necessary, a copayment ($267 per day in 2009) must be paid from days 61 through 90, and a higher copayment ($534 per day in 2009) applies beyond 90 days. A benefit period has 90 days of maximum coverage. Beyond the 90 days, there is a lifetime reserve of 60 additional hospital inpatient days. Benefits for medical care in a psychiatric hospital are limited to 190 days in the beneficiary's lifetime. Private funds, Medigap insurance benefits, or Medicaid (if a person qualifies) must be used if the need for hospitalization exceeds the limits specified by Medicare.

For postacute care, Medicare pays for up to 100 days in a Medicare-certified SNF subsequent to inpatient hospitalization for at least 3 consecutive days, not including the day of discharge. Admission to the SNF must occur within 30 days of hospital discharge, and it must be related to the same condition for which the beneficiary was hospitalized. All covered services are fully paid for the first 20 days. Beyond that, a copayment ($133.50 per day in 2009) must be paid from days 21 through 100.

Medicare pays for home health care when a person is homebound and requires intermittent or part-time skilled nursing care or rehabilitation care determined to be "reasonable and necessary." Part A home care benefits cover up to 100 home health visits following a hospital stay. Durable medical equipment (DME), such as wheelchairs, hospital beds, walkers, and medical supplies, are also covered. Home health visits do not have a deductible, but a 20% coinsurance applies to DME.

For terminally ill patients, Medicare pays for care provided by a Medicare-certified hospice. A small copayment of up to $5 applies for prescription drugs for these patients.

Supplementary Medical Insurance (Part B)

Part B, the supplementary medical insurance (SMI) portion of Medicare, is a voluntary program, financed partly by general tax revenues and partly by required premium contributions. Almost 95% of people entitled to hospital insurance also choose to enroll in SMI because they cannot get similar coverage at that price from private insurers. Coverage includes physician, ambulance, outpatient rehabilitation, and limited preventive services; hospital outpatient services such as outpatient surgery, diagnostic tests, radiology, and pathology; emergency department visits; renal dialysis; prostheses; and medical equipment and supplies. Part B also covers limited home health services beyond what Part A covers.

Participation in Part B requires the beneficiaries to pay a monthly premium. Effective 2007, the premium became income-based. The standard premium for 2009 is $96.40 per month. For those earning more than $85,000 and filing individual tax returns (or earning more than $170,000 and filing joint tax returns), 2009 premiums range between $134.90 and $308.30 depending on income. Part B also carries an annual deductible ($135 in 2009), and an 80:20 coinsurance applies to most services.

Medicare Advantage (Part C)

In reality, Part C is not a special program that offers specifically defined medical services. The program was formerly called Medicare+Choice, which took effect on January 1, 1998 and was mandated by the Balanced Budget Act of 1997. The law expanded the role of private managed care health plans such as HMO and PPO plans. The beneficiaries, however, do have the choice to remain in the original Medicare fee-for-service program.

Under the Medicare Advantage program, Medicare pays a set amount of money each month to the participating private health plans on behalf of each beneficiary. In turn, the plan manages Medicare benefits for its members. To attract Medicare enrollees, private companies may offer extra benefits that may lower the beneficiaries' out-of-pocket costs. Hence, Part C is generally a good option for low-income beneficiaries because it may eliminate the need for Medigap coverage.

Prescription Drug Coverage (Part D)

Part D was added to the existing Medicare program under the Medicare Prescription Drug, Improvement, and Modernization Act (MMA) of 2003 and was fully implemented in January 2006. The program is available to anyone, regardless of income, who has coverage under Part A or Part B. Coverage is offered through two types of private plans approved by Medicare: (a) Stand-alone prescription drug plans (PDPs) that offer only drug coverage are available to those who want to stay in the original Medicare fee-for-service program. (b) Medicare advantage prescription drug plans (MA-PDs) are available to those who want to obtain all health care services through MCOs participating in Part C.

Like Part B, the program is voluntary because it requires payment of a monthly premium that varies from plan to plan. For 2008, the average was estimated to be $25 per month for a basic plan. More generous plans can cost over $100 per month. After an annual deductible ($295 in 2009), benefits are paid according to three layers of personal out-of-pocket spending on prescription drugs (see **Table 6.1**). Clearly, the program is designed to help everyone at a basic threshold level of spending and, beyond that, those

Table 6.1 Part D Standard Benefits and Individual Out-of-Pocket Costs for 2009

	Drug Costs	Medicare Pays	Beneficiary Pays
Deductible	$295	None	$295
Initial coverage	$296–2,700	75% up to $1,803.75	25% up to $601.25
Gap or "doughnut hole"	$2,701–6,153.75	None	100% up to $3,453.75
Catastrophic coverage	Over $6153.75	Approximately 95%	Approximately 5%

Note: The beneficiary must pay a total of $4,350 before catastrophic coverage begins.

who have excessive needs for prescription drugs. For example, in 2009, the program pays 95% of the cost of prescription drugs after a beneficiary incurs $4,350 in out-of-pocket costs.

Services Not Covered Under Medicare

Neither Part A nor Part B offers comprehensive coverage. Services such as vision care, eyeglasses, dentures, hearing aids, routine physical exams, and many preventive services are not covered by either plan. Exceptions are screening Pap smears, mammography, screening for colorectal and prostate cancer, glaucoma screening, flu shots, and vaccinations against pneumonia. These are covered for Part B enrollees.

Medicaid

Medicaid, also referred to as Title 19 of the Social Security Act, finances health care services for the indigent; however, Medicaid does not provide medical assistance for all poor persons. Each state has established its own criteria for determining eligibility according to income and other resources such as bank accounts, real property, and other assets. Although a person does not need to be on welfare to be eligible for Medicaid, federal law requires that certain low-income people be covered. Examples include many of the elderly, the blind, and the disabled receiving Supplemental Security Income (SSI), and some pregnant women. Medicaid is instrumental in providing health insurance to children in low-income families (**Figure 6.4**). In addition, most states, at their discretion, have defined other "medically needy" categories. Most important among these are individuals who are institutionalized in nursing or psychiatric facilities and individuals who are receiving community-based services but would otherwise be eligible for Medicaid if institutionalized. All of these people have to qualify based on assets and income, which must be below the threshold levels established by each state. Hence, Medicaid is a *means-tested program.*

The program is jointly financed by the federal and state governments. The federal government provides matching funds to the states based on the per capita income in each state. Wealthier states have a smaller share of their costs reimbursed by the federal government.

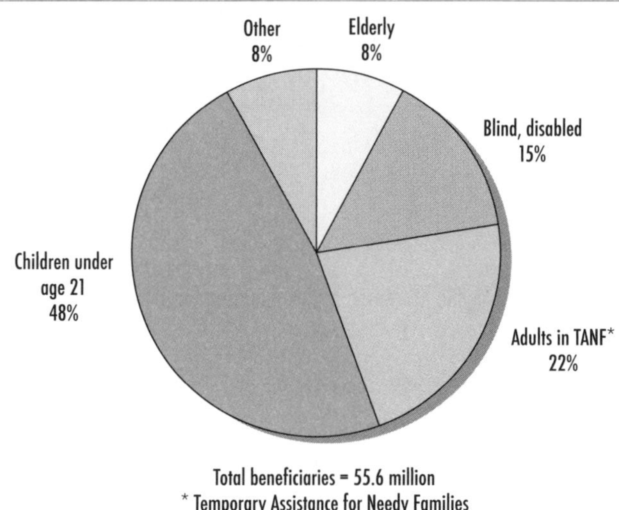

Figure 6.4 Medicaid Recipient Categories: 2004. Data from NCHS. *Health, United States, 2007*, p. 413. Hyattsville, MD: US DHHS.

Each state administers its own Medicaid program. Hence, eligibility criteria, covered services, and payments to providers vary considerably from state to state. However, for a state to receive federal matching funds, the state must provide some specific health services (see Table 6.2).

State Children's Health Insurance Program

The State Children's Health Insurance Program (SCHIP), codified as Title 21 of the Social Security Act, was enacted under the Balanced Budget Act of 1997. Initially created for 10 years, federal funding for SCHIP was extended through March 2009 under the Medicare, Medicaid, and SCHIP Extension Act of 2007.

When the program was initiated, nearly one quarter of the children in low-income families were uninsured. The program offers additional federal matching funds to states to expand Medicaid eligibility to enroll children under 19 years of age who otherwise would not qualify for coverage

Table 6.2 Federally Mandated Services for State Medicaid Programs

Hospital inpatient care

Hospital outpatient services

Physician services

Laboratory and x-ray services

Nursing facility services

Home health services for those eligible for care in a skilled nursing facility

Prenatal care

Family planning services and supplies

Rural health clinic services

Preventive, diagnostic, and treatment services (including vaccinations) for dependent children under the age of 21 years

Nurse-midwife services

Certain federally qualified ambulatory and health center services

Pediatric and family nurse–practitioner services

Data from Health Care Financing Review, Statistical Supplement, 2001: 14.

because their families' incomes exceed the Medicaid threshold levels. Certain adults, such as pregnant women, parents, and caretaker relatives, may also be covered under SCHIP.

In most states, SCHIP is available to families with incomes up to 200% of the federal poverty level, or about $42,400 (higher in Alaska and Hawaii) for a family of four in 2008–2009, and if they are not covered under a private insurance plan. SCHIP offers participating states three options: (1) expansion of Medicaid, (2) establishment of a special child-health assistance program, or (3) a combination of the two approaches. States are required to screen applicants for Medicaid eligibility and to enroll eligible children in Medicaid rather than in the SCHIP program. In 2005, 6.1 million children were enrolled in SCHIP, and another 28.3 million were in Medicaid, up from 3.4 million and 21.8 million, respectively, in the year 2000 (Henry J. Kaiser Family Foundation, 2007b).

REIMBURSEMENT METHODS

Insurance companies, MCOs, Blue Cross/Blue Shield, and the government (for Medicare and Medicaid) are referred to as *third-party payers*, the other two parties being the patient and the provider (Wilson & Neuhauser, 1985, p. 118). Payment made by third-party payers to the providers of services is called *reimbursement*.

Various methods are in use for determining how much providers should be paid. Traditionally, providers have preferred the fee-for-service method, which has fallen into disfavor with payers because of cost escalations. Private payers as well as the government have devised various methods aimed at limiting the amount of reimbursement.

Fee for Service

Fee-for-service reimbursement is based on the assumption that services are provided in a set of identifiable and individually distinct units of services. For example, physician services may include units such as an examination, x-ray, urinalysis, and a tetanus shot. For surgery, individual services may include an admission kit, numerous medical supplies (each accounted for separately), surgeon's fees, anesthesia, anesthesiologist's fees, recovery room charges, and so forth. Each of these services is separately billed.

Initially, fee-for-service charges were set by providers, and insurers passively paid the claims. Later, insurers started to limit reimbursement to a "usual, customary, and reasonable" (UCR) amount that was determined by each payer. In this case, providers would *balance bill*, that is, ask the patients to pay the difference between the actual charges and the payments received from insurers.

The main problem under fee-for-service arrangements is that providers have an incentive to induce demand and deliver additional services that are nonessential. Hence, this method of reimbursement has been gradually replaced by other methods and is now rarely used. On the other hand, some providers such as dentists and optometrists still get paid under the fee-for-service method.

Package Pricing

In package pricing, also referred to as *bundled charges*, a number of related services are included in one price. For example, normal vaginal delivery may have one set fee that includes predelivery and postdelivery care (Williams, 1995, p. 114). Optometrists sometimes advertise package prices that include the charges for eye exams, frames for eyeglasses, and corrective lenses.

Resource-Based Relative Value Scale

Under the Omnibus Budget Reconciliation Act of 1989, Medicare developed a method to reimburse physicians according to a "relative value" assigned to each physician service. Relative values are based on the time, skill, and intensity it takes to provide a service, and the actual reimbursement is derived using a complex formula. Each year, Medicare publishes the Medicare Fee Schedule, which gives the reimbursement amount for each of the services and procedures under a current procedural terminology (CPT) code. The reimbursement amounts are adjusted for the geographic area in which the practice is located.

Reimbursement Under Managed Care

Three distinct approaches are used by MCOs. PPOs use a variation of the fee-for-service method. The PPO establishes fee schedules based on discounts negotiated with providers participating in its network. HMOs sometimes have physicians on their staff who are paid a salary. Capitation is another mechanism used by HMOs. Under *capitation*, a provider is paid a set monthly fee per enrollee (sometimes referred to as per member per month or PMPM rate), regardless of whether an enrollee sees the provider or not, and regardless of how often an enrollee sees the provider. Capitation removes the incentive for provider-induced demand. It makes providers prudent and encourages them to provide only necessary services.

From Retrospective to Prospective Reimbursement

Traditionally, Medicare and Medicaid established *per diem* (daily) rates for reimbursing hospitals, nursing homes, and other inpatient facilities. The per diem rates were based on the actual costs the providers had incurred during the previous year. Because rates were set after evaluating the costs retrospectively, the method was referred to as *retrospective reimbursement*. Home health was also reimbursed on the basis of cost.

Because the retrospective method was based on costs that were directly related to length of stay, services rendered, and the cost of providing the services, providers had no incentive to control costs. Services were rendered indiscriminately because health care institutions could increase their profits by increasing costs. Because of the perverse financial incentives inherent in retrospective cost-based reimbursement, it has been largely replaced by prospective methods of reimbursement.

In contrast to retrospective reimbursement, where historical costs are used to determine the amount to be paid, *prospective reimbursement* uses certain pre-established criteria to determine in advance the amount of reimbursement. Medicare has been using the prospective payment system (PPS) to reimburse inpatient hospital acute care services under Medicare Part A since 1983.

The Balanced Budget Act of 1997 mandated implementation of a PPS for hospital outpatient services and postacute care providers such as SNFs, home health agencies, and inpatient rehabilitation facilities. Depending on the type of service setting, the four main prospective reimbursement methods currently in use are based on diagnosis-related groups (DRGs), ambulatory payment classifications (APCs), resource utilization groups (RUGs), and home health resource groups (HHRGs).

DRGs

This method is used to pay for hospital inpatient services. Medicare has established approximately 500 DRGs corresponding to the most prevalent diagnoses among patients using inpatient services. Instead of a per diem rate, the reimbursement method based on DRGs prospectively sets a bundled price according to the principal diagnosis at the time of admission. The hospital receives the predetermined fixed rate for that particular DRG classification.

The primary factor governing the amount of reimbursement is the main clinical diagnosis, but additional factors can create differences in reimbursement for the same DRG. Such factors include differences in wage levels in various geographic areas, an urban versus a rural hospital location, whether the institution is a teaching hospital (i.e., it has residency programs for medical graduates; adjustments in reimbursement are based on the intensity of teaching), and an adjustment related to treating a disproportionately large share of low-income patients (HCFA, 1996).

The DRG-based prospective reimbursement has forced hospitals to control their costs. By keeping the actual cost of services below the fixed reimbursement amount, a hospital gets to keep the difference as profit. A hospital loses money when its costs exceed the prospective reimbursement rate.

APCs

This prospective payment method, implemented in August 2000, is associated with Medicare's Outpatient Prospective Payment System for services provided by hospital outpatient departments. Outpatient clinics not associated with hospitals are currently exempt. The APC divides all outpatient services into more than 300 procedural groups. Reimbursement rates are associated with each APC group. The rates are also adjusted for geographic variations in wages. APC reimbursement includes services such as anesthesia, certain drugs, supplies, and recovery room charges in a package price established by Medicare.

RUGs

Medicare pays SNFs on the basis of RUGs, but the method differs from the way in which DRG-based payments are used for hospitals. Whereas a fixed amount of reimbursement is associated with each DRG, RUG categories are used for determining an SNF's overall intensity of health conditions requiring medical and nursing intervention. The overall acuity level in a facility, as determined by the severity of the patients' condition, is referred to as its *case mix*. It is determined by first evaluating each patient's medical and nursing care needs. Based on this evaluation, each patient is classified into one of 44 RUGs. The case-mix composite of an institution is then used to determine a fixed per diem amount associated with the case mix. The higher the case mix score, the higher the reimbursement.

Adjustments to the PPS rate are made for differences in wages prevailing in various geographic areas and for facility location in urban as opposed to rural areas.

HHRGs

Implemented in October 2000, the PPS for home health care pays a fixed, predetermined rate for each 60-day episode of care, regardless of the specific services delivered. Thus, all services provided by a home health agency are bundled under one payment made on a per patient basis. An assessment instrument called Outcomes and Assessment Information Set (OASIS) is used to rate each patient's functional status and clinical severity level. The assessment measures translate into "points." The points are totaled to determine the patient's HHRG. Payment is based on the patient's specific HHRG category. Beginning in 2008, the HHRG classification uses 153 distinct groups (previously there were 80) in which patients can be classified according to clinical severity, functional status, and the need for rehabilitation therapies.

NATIONAL HEALTH EXPENDITURES

National health expenditures (also called national health spending or national health care costs) are an estimate of the amount spent for all health services and supplies and health-related research and construction activities in the United States during a calendar year (NCHS, 1996, p. 303). In 2006, national health expenditures in the United States amounted to $2.105 trillion. To put some meaning into such large expenditures, it is common to compare the total health care expenditures to the total economic consumption. The *gross domestic product* (GDP) measures the total value of goods and services produced and consumed. In 2006, the GDP was $13.195 trillion. Hence, 16% of the total economic output in 2006 was consumed by health care. Another way to look at health care expenditures is in terms of the average per capita spending, which controls for changes in the size of the population. In 2006, the average per capita spending for health care amounted to $7,026 for each American. National health expenditures from 1960 to 2006 are presented in Table 6.3.

Table 6.3 National Health Expenditures, Selected Years

Year	Amount (in billions of $)	Percentage of Gross Domestic Product	Amount per Capita
1960	27.5	5.2	$148
1970	74.9	7.2	356
1980	253.9	9.1	1,102
1990	714.0	12.3	2,813
2000	1353.3	13.8	4,790
2006	2105.5	16.0	7,026

Data from NCHS. *Health, United States, 2007*, pp. 375, 378; and Catlin, A. et al., 2008. National Health Spending in 2006: A Year of Change for Prescription Drugs. *Health Affairs* 27 (1):14–29.

Figure 6.5 shows the breakdown of how 2006 national health dollars were used. Approximately 84% of total national health expenditures were used for personal health services and products, which include hospital care, physician and clinical services, dental care, other professional services, nursing home care, home health care, prescription drugs, medical supplies, durable medical equipment (DME), vision care, and other personal health care products and services. The remaining 16% of national expenditures are accounted for by public health services, research, investment in structures and equipment, costs related to administration of government programs, and administrative costs of private insurance.

The annual growth in health care spending, or health care cost inflation, is a matter of concern for almost all nations. Cost inflation in health care is evaluated by comparing it to the growth of the GDP and also to the *consumer price index* (CPI), which measures inflation in the general economy. As Table 6.4 shows, health care cost inflation has exceeded the growth in the GDP and CPI. The reasons for cost inflation are discussed in Chapter 12.

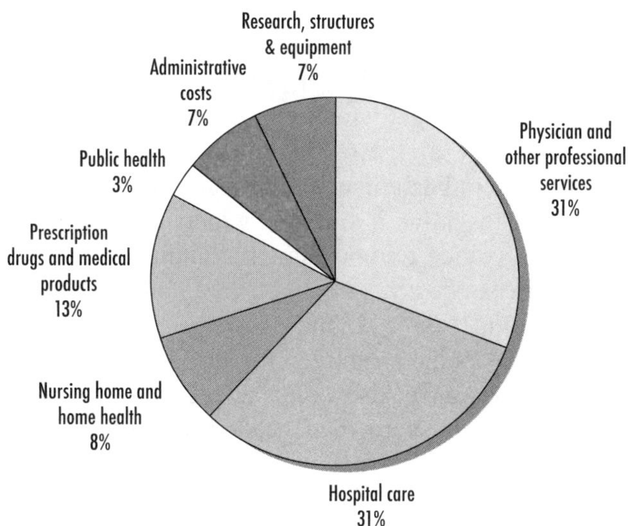

Figure 6.5 Breakdown of National Health Expenditures, 2006. Data from Catlin, A., et al., 2008. National Health Spending in 2006: A Year of Change for Prescription Drugs. *Health Affairs* 27 (1): 14–29.

Table 6.4 Growth Comparisons of National Health Expenditures to the GDP and CPI: 1990–2005

	1990	**2005**
National health expenditures	$714.0 billion	$1987.7 billion
Average annual increase		7.1%
GDP	$5803.0 billion	$12,456.0 billion
Average annual increase		5.2%
CPI	130.7	195.3
Average annual increase		2.7%

Data from NCHS. *Health, United States, 2007*, pp. 375, 376, 378.

CONCLUSION

Financing plays a critical role in health care delivery. For consumers, it pays for insurance coverage, which enables them to obtain health care services. For providers, it reimburses them for the services they provide.

The methods of reimbursement were changed from retrospective to prospective mechanisms after it became widely known that cost-based methods and fee-for-service reimbursement contained perverse incentives for providers to increase the costs of health care delivery. Prospective payment methods, now widely in use, and capitation, used by health maintenance organizations, contain incentives for the delivery of cost-effective health care. Health insurance also contains perverse incentives for consumers to use more health care than needed, a phenomenon known as moral hazard. Deductibles and copayments were instituted after it became known that these methods of cost sharing reduce the excessive use of health care.

The financing of health care is shared between private and public sources. Contrary to what many people might think, the government incurs a sizable proportion of total health care expenditures, estimated to be over 45% of all health care expenditures in the United States. Hence, at least from a financing standpoint, the United States has a quasi-national health care system. The share of public expenditures in the future is expected to grow with the recent expansion of Medicare and a growing elderly population.

REFERENCES

Caplan, C., and N. Brangan. 2004. Out-of-Pocket Spending on Health Care by Medicare Beneficiaries Age 65 and Older in 2003. Research Report, AARP Public Policy Institute (September 2004). Retrieved October 2008 from http://www.aarp.org/research/medicare/outofpocket/aresearch-import-912-DD101.html.

Claxton, G., et al. 2008. *The Kaiser Family Foundation and Health Research and Educational Trust Employer Health Benefits 2008 Annual Survey*. Menlo Park, CA: Henry J. Kaiser Family Foundation and Chicago, IL: Health Research and Educational Trust.

Feldstein, P. J. 1993. *Health Care Economics*, 4th ed. New York: Delmar Publishers.

Health Care Financing Administration (HCFA). 1996. *Medicare and Medicaid Statistical Supplement, 1996*. Pub. No. 03386. Baltimore, MD: U.S. Department of Health and Human Services.

Health Insurance Institute. 1969. *Modern Health Insurance*. New York: Health Insurance Institute.

Henry J. Kaiser Family Foundation. 2007a. *Health Insurance Coverage in the U.S., 2006*. Retrieved July 2008 from http://facts.kff.org/?CFID=33558548&CFTOKEN=27078486.

Henry J. Kaiser Family Foundation. 2007b. *Medicaid and SCHIP Enrollment of Children, 1998-2005*. Retrieved July 2008 from http://facts.kff.org/chart.aspx?ch=469.

National Center for Health Statistics (NCHS). 1996. *Health, United States 1995*. Hyattsville, MD: U.S. Department of Health and Human Services.

Short, P. F., et al. 1997. The effect of universal coverage on health expenditures for the uninsured. *Medical Care* 35 (2):95–113.

U.S. General Accounting Office. 1996. *Private Health Insurance: Millions Relying on Individual Market Coverage Face Cost and Coverage Trade-Offs*. Washington, DC: U.S. General Accounting Office.

Vaughn, E. J., and C. M. Elliott. 1987. *Fundamentals of Risk and Insurance*. New York: John Wiley & Sons.

Williams, S. J. 1995. *Essentials of Health Services*. Albany, NY: Delmar Publishers.

Wilson, F. A., and D. Neuhauser. 1985. *Health Services in the United States*, 2nd ed. Cambridge, MA: Ballinger Publishing.

Chapter 7

Outpatient Services and Primary Care

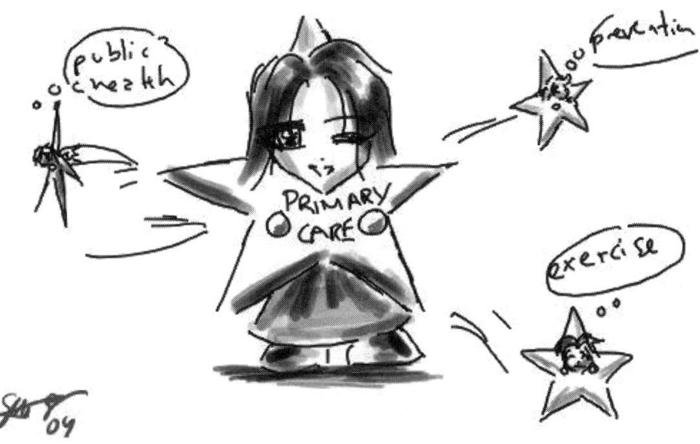

INTRODUCTION

Historically, outpatient care has been independent of services provided in health care institutions. In earlier days, physicians saw patients in their clinics, and most physicians also made home visits to treat patients. Given the limitations of medical science in those days, physicians generally provided the full spectrum of medical services, including diagnosis, treatment, surgery, and dispensing of medications. With the advancements in medical science, the locus of health care delivery became concentrated around the institutional core of community hospitals. As the range of services that could be provided on an outpatient basis continued to expand, hospitals gradually became the dominant players in providing the vast majority of outpatient care, with the exception of cognitive and basic diagnostic care provided in physicians' offices (Barr & Breindel, 1995). In recent years, the process of health care delivery has increasingly shifted away from expensive stays in acute-care hospitals, and many intensive procedures are increasingly performed on an outpatient basis. Unlike hospitals, independent providers face capital constraints and competitive pressures in the health care marketplace, with most solo practitioners consolidating into group practices.

State and local government agencies have also actively sponsored limited outpatient services to meet the needs of underserved populations, mainly indigent patients who lack personal resources to obtain health care in the private sector. Community health centers, which primarily depend on federal and state funds, serve a number of rural and inner-city areas, providing a wide array of outpatient services.

WHAT IS OUTPATIENT CARE?

The terms "outpatient" and "ambulatory" are used interchangeably, although the term outpatient is more comprehensive. Strictly speaking, ambulatory care consists of diagnostic and therapeutic services and treatments provided to the "walking" (ambulatory) patient. Hence, in a restricted sense, ambulatory care refers to care rendered to patients who come to physicians' offices, outpatient departments of hospitals, and health centers to receive care; however, patients do not always ambulate to the service centers to receive ambulatory care. For example, in a hospital emergency department (ED), patients may arrive by land or air ambulance. In other instances, such as in mobile diagnostic units and home health care, services are transported to the patient instead of the patient coming to receive the services. Hence, the terms "outpatient" and "inpatient" are more precise, and the term *outpatient services* refers to any health care services that do not require an overnight stay in an institution of health care delivery, such as a hospital or long-term care facility. Some outpatient services may be offered by a hospital or nursing home. For instance, besides EDs, many hospitals have other outpatient service centers such as outpatient surgery, rehabilitation, and specialized clinics.

In recent years, there has been extraordinary growth in the volume of outpatient services and the emergence of new types of settings where outpatient services are delivered. The most basic outpatient services, such as physical exams and minor treatments, are still delivered in a physician's office. Advanced outpatient care has traditionally been provided in hospital-based facilities, generally in various building complexes surrounding the main hospital. Also, in recent years, there has been an explosive growth in the type and ownership of nonhospital-based facilities offering ambulatory care (see **Exhibit 7.1**).

In 2004, Americans made approximately 910.9 million visits, or more than 3 visits per person, to office-based physicians. Physicians in general and family practice accounted for the largest share of these visits (22.8%), followed by physicians in internal medicine (18.1%), pediatrics (12.8%), and obstetrics and gynecology (7.2%). Doctors of osteopathy accounted for 7.2% of the visits. The South led the nation in physician visits (38.8%), followed by the Midwest (21.7%), the West (20.8%), and the Northeast (18.7%). Ambulatory visits per person were the highest in the South (3.4 visits) and lowest in the West (2.9 visits). Most physician office visits (86.8%) took place in metropolitan areas. Visits per person were also higher in metropolitan areas (3.3) than in rural areas (2.7), reflecting poorer access to primary care in rural areas of the United States.

SCOPE OF OUTPATIENT SERVICES

Outpatient care now includes much more than primary care services. For example, most surgeries are now performed in outpatient settings. Previously, many of these same procedures could be performed only in hospitals. The shift to outpatient care is expected to endure. As hospital occupancy rates have declined over the past decade, hospital executives have increasingly viewed

Exhibit 7.1 Outpatient Settings and Services

- Private practice
- Hospitals
- Freestanding surgical facilities
- Mobile facilities for medical, diagnostic, and and screening services
- Patient's home
  - Telephone triage
  - Home health services
  - Hospice care
- Outpatient long-term care services
- Public health services
- Community health centers and free clinics
- Alternative medicine clinics

outpatient care as an essential portion of their health care business (Barr & Breindel, 1995). Establishing a firm position in the outpatient care market has become critical to continued hospital survival, as has expanding into services previously not considered part of their core business.

The growth of nonhospital-based outpatient services has intensified competition for outpatient medical services between hospitals and community-based providers. Examples of such competition include home health care, ambulatory clinics for routine and urgent care, and outpatient surgery. On the other hand, several other services, such as dental care and optometric services, continue to be office based. Financing is the main reason that dental and optometric services have not been integrated with other outpatient medical services. Traditionally, medical insurance plans have been separate from dental and vision care plans. Philosophical and technical differences account for other variations. Chiropractic care, for instance, is generally covered by most health plans but remains isolated from the mainstream practice of medicine. Other services, such as alternative therapies and self-care, are not covered by insurance yet have experienced remarkable growth in recent years.

Several key changes have been instrumental in shifting the balance between inpatient and outpatient services. These factors can be broadly classified as reimbursement, technologic factors, utilization control factors, and social factors.

Reimbursement

Today, both private and public payers have a clear preference for outpatient treatment because it costs less than inpatient care. Quicker discharge of patients from hospital beds under prospective and capitated reimbursement methods created a substantial market for outpatient services. In response to the changes in financial incentives to reimburse for outpatient care, hospitals aggressively developed outpatient services to offset declining inpatient income. The financial factors, for instance, have provided a major impetus for the unprecedented growth of home health care.

Technologic Factors

The development of new diagnostic and treatment procedures and less invasive surgical methods has made it possible to provide services in outpatient settings that previously had required inpatient stays in hospitals. Shorter acting anesthetics and the proliferation of minimally invasive technologies have made many surgical procedures less traumatic and recovery time much shorter. Many office-based physicians have expanded their capacity to perform outpatient diagnostic, treatment, and surgical services because the acquisition of technology has become more feasible and cost-effective.

Utilization Control Factors

Inpatient hospital stays have been strongly discouraged by various payers. Prior authorization for inpatient admission and close monitoring during hospitalization have been actively pursued with the objective of minimizing the length of stay. Utilization control methods are discussed in Chapter 9.

Social Factors

In addition to the financial, technologic, and utilization control factors just mentioned, social factors have contributed to the growth of outpatient services. Patients generally have a strong preference for receiving health care in home and community-based settings. Unless absolutely necessary, most patients do not want to be institutionalized. Staying in their own homes gives people a strong sense of independence and control over their lives, elements considered important for quality of life.

OUTPATIENT CARE SETTINGS AND METHODS OF DELIVERY

The myriad outpatient care and community-based services now in existence sometimes make it difficult to differentiate adequately among the structural settings in which these services are provided (see Exhibit 7.1). For example, agencies providing home health services can be freestanding, hospital based, or nursing home based; physician group practices, in many instances, are merging with hospitals, and hospitals and freestanding surgical clinics often compete against each other for various types of surgical procedures. Therefore, the classifications used in this section are only illustrative because there are many exceptions to the arrangements presented here. Also, in this constantly evolving system, new settings and methods are likely to emerge. The various settings for outpatient services found in the U.S. health care delivery system can be grouped as follows.

Private Practice

Physicians, as office-based practitioners, form the backbone of ambulatory care and constitute the vast majority of primary care services. Most visits entail relatively limited examination and testing, and encounters with the physician are generally of a relatively short duration. The waiting time in the office is typically longer than the actual time spent with the physician.

In the past, the solo practice of medicine and small partnership arrangements attracted the most practitioners. Self-employment offered a degree of independence not generally available in large organizational settings. During the past few years, group practice and institutional affiliations, such as employment by a managed care organization (MCO), have expanded dramatically. Few graduates of residency programs are entering solo practice. Several factors account for this shift: uncertainties created by rapid changes in the health care delivery system, contracting by MCOs with consolidated rather than solo entities, competition from large health care delivery organizations, the high cost of establishing a new practice, complexity of billings and collections in a multiple-payer system, and increased external controls over the private practice of medicine. Group practice and other organizational arrangements offer the benefits of a patient referral network, negotiating leverage with MCOs, sharing of overhead expenses, ease of obtaining coverage from colleagues for personal time off, and in a growing number of instances, attractive starting salaries along with benefits and profit-sharing plans. Most young physicians find that these advantages far outweigh the allure of being an independent solo practitioner.

Hospitals

Many hospital outpatient clinics, particularly those in inner-city areas, function as the community's safety net, providing primary care to the medically indigent and uninsured populations. Outpatient services now constitute a key source of profits for hospitals. Consequently, hospitals have expanded their outpatient departments, and utilization has grown. This trend is the result of fierce competition in the health care industry, in which MCOs emphasizing preventive and outpatient care have waged a relentless drive to cut costs. As hospitals have seen inpatient revenues steadily erode, they have begun sprucing up and expanding outpatient services. A hospital providing both inpatient and outpatient services can enhance its revenues by referring postsurgical cases to its affiliated units for rehabilitation and home care follow-up. Patients receiving various types of hospital-affiliated outpatient services become an important source of referrals back to the hospitals for inpatient care. A hospital can thus expand its patient base.

Hospital-based outpatient services can be broadly classified into five main types: clinical (typically for the uninsured or those in research studies), surgical (patient is discharged on the day of surgery), home health care (postacute care and rehabilitation), women's health, and traditional emergency care.

Freestanding Facilities

Various types of proprietary, community-based, freestanding medical facilities have opened across the country. They are known as walk-in clinics, urgent care centers, and surgical centers. *Walk-in clinics* provide outpatient services ranging from basic primary care to urgent care, but they are generally used on a nonroutine, episodic basis. *Urgent care centers* accept patients without appointments and generally offer a wide range of routine services for basic and acute conditions on a first-come first-served basis. The main advantages of walk-in clinics and urgent care centers are convenience of location, evening and weekend hours, and availability of services on a walk-in, no-appointment basis. *Surgicenters* are freestanding outpatient surgery centers independent of hospitals. They usually provide a full range of services for the types of surgery that can be performed on an outpatient basis and do not require overnight hospitalization. Other types of outpatient facilities include outpatient rehabilitation centers, optometric centers, and dental clinics.

Mobile Facilities for Medical, Diagnostic, and Screening Services

Mobile health care services are transported to patients and constitute an efficient and convenient means for providing certain types of routine health services. Mobile diagnostic services include mammography and magnetic resonance imaging. Such mobile units take advanced diagnostic services to small towns and rural communities. Screening vans, staffed by volunteers who are trained professionals, are generally operated by various nonprofit organizations and are often seen at malls and fairgrounds. Various types of health education and health promotion services and screening checks such as blood pressure and cholesterol screening are commonly performed for anyone who walks in.

Telephone Triage

Telephone access, referred to as telephone triage, is a means of bringing expert opinion and advice to the patient, especially during the hours when physicians' offices are generally closed. The system is staffed by specially trained nurses who have access to patient medical records and provide guidance with the use of standardized protocols. They can consult with primary care physicians when necessary or refer patients to an urgent care facility or ED (Appleby, 1995).

Home Health Care

In home health care, services are brought to patients in their own homes. Without home services, the only alternative for such patients would be institutionalization in a hospital or nursing home. Home health care is consistent with the philosophy of maintaining people in the least restrictive environment possible. Most people express a strong preference for receiving health services at home. Home health services typically include nursing care, such as changing dressings, monitoring medications, and providing help with bathing; short-term rehabilitation, such as physical therapy, occupational therapy, and speech therapy; homemaker services, such as meal preparation, shopping, transportation, and some specific household chores; and certain medical supplies and equipment, such as ostomy supplies, hospital beds, oxygen tanks, walkers, and wheelchairs (the latter are referred to as durable medical equipment).

Hospice Services

The term "hospice" refers to a cluster of comprehensive services for the terminally ill who have a life expectancy of six months or less. Hospice programs provide services that address the special needs of dying persons and their families. Hospice is a method of care, not a location, and services are taken to patients and their families wherever they happen to be located. Hospice services include medical, psychologic, and social services provided in a holistic context. The two primary areas of emphasis in hospice care are (1) pain and symptom management, which is referred to as *palliative care*, and (2) psychosocial and spiritual support.

Outpatient Long-Term Care Services

Long-term care (LTC) has typically been associated with care provided in nursing homes, but during the past several years, a number of alternative settings, forming a continuum, have emerged. Two types of ambulatory LTC services are case management and adult day care. Case management provides coordination and referral among a variety of health care services. The objective is to find the most appropriate setting to meet a patient's health care needs. Adult day care complements informal care provided at home by family members with professional services available in adult day care centers during the day. Both of these services are discussed in more detail in Chapter 10.

Public Health Services

Public health services in the United States are typically provided by local health departments, and the range of services offered varies greatly by locality. Generally, public health programs are limited in scope. They include well-baby care, venereal disease clinics, family planning services, screening and treatment for tuberculosis, and outpatient mental health care. States vary in the range and extent of public health services offered.

Community Health Centers and Free Clinics

The creation of community health centers was authorized during the 1960s, primarily to reach the medically underserved regions of the United States. Community health centers operate under the auspices of the Bureau of Primary Health Care (BPHC), which is part of the U.S. Department of Health and Human Services (DHHS). Community health centers are required by law to be located in medically underserved areas and provide services to anyone seeking care, regardless of insurance status or ability to pay (McAlearney, 2002). The "medically underserved" designation is determined by the federal government. Community health centers provide family-oriented preventive care, primary care, and dental care and serve as a primary care safety net.

Other community health centers developed through federal funding are migrant health centers, serving transient farm workers in agricultural communities, and rural health centers in isolated, underserved rural areas. The

Community Mental Health Center program was established to provide outpatient mental health services in underserved areas.

Modeled after the 19th century dispensary (see Chapter 3), a related category of provider, the free clinic, is a general ambulatory care center serving primarily the poor, the homeless, and the uninsured. Free clinics have three main characteristics: (1) services are provided at no charge or at a very nominal charge, (2) the clinics are not directly supported or operated by a government agency or health department, and (3) services are delivered mainly by trained volunteer staff.

The combination of free clinics, community health centers, public health services, and some hospitals now form a significant safety net of providers for individuals who lack private or public health insurance.

Alternative Medicine Clinics

Alternative medicine, or complementary and alternative medicine (CAM), refers to the broad domain of all health care resources, other than those intrinsic to biomedicine, to which people have recourse (CAM Research Methodology Conference, 1997). Alternative therapies are regarded as nontraditional and include a wide range of treatments such as homeopathy, herbal remedies, natural products used as preventive and treatment agents, acupuncture, meditation, yoga exercises, biofeedback, and spiritual guidance or prayer. Chiropractic is also largely regarded as a complementary treatment. Alternative medicine is not yet a system of healing endorsed by conventional Western medicine, although the traditional medical establishment has shown growing interest in the efficacy of these treatments.

No particular settings of health care delivery are involved in alternative treatments. Many of the therapies are self-administered or at least require active patient participation.

PRIMARY CARE

Primary care is the conceptual foundation for outpatient services, but not all outpatient care is primary care. For example, hospital ED services are not intended to be primary in nature. On the other hand, services other than primary health care have now become an integral part of outpatient services. Thanks to the technologic advancements in medicine, many secondary and tertiary treatments are now provided in ambulatory care settings.

What Is Primary Care?

Primary care plays a central role in a health care delivery system. Other essential levels of care include secondary and tertiary care. Secondary- and tertiary-care services are more complex and specialized than primary care. Primary care is distinguished from secondary and tertiary care according to its duration, frequency, and level of intensity. *Secondary care* is usually short term, involving sporadic consultation from a specialist to provide expert opinions and/or surgical or other advanced interventions that primary care physicians are not equipped to perform. Secondary care thus includes hospitalization, routine surgery, specialty consultation, and rehabilitation. *Tertiary care* is the most complex level of care and is needed for conditions that are relatively uncommon. Typically, tertiary care is institution based, highly specialized, and technology driven. Much of tertiary care is rendered in large teaching hospitals, especially university hospitals. Examples include trauma care, burn treatment, neonatal intensive care, tissue transplants, and open-heart surgery. In some instances, tertiary treatment may be long-term in nature, and the tertiary-care physician may assume long-term responsibility for the bulk of the patient's care.

In defining primary care, the focus is often on the type or level of services, such as prevention, diagnostic and therapeutic services, health education and counseling, and minor surgery. Although primary care specifically emphasizes these services, many specialists also provide the same spectrum of services; therefore, primary care should be more appropriately viewed as an approach to providing health care rather than as a set of specific services (Starfield, 1994). The World Health Organization (WHO) and the Institute of Medicine (IOM) offer useful definitions of primary care which differentiate primary health care and primary care. Although primary health care focuses on its function as the point of entry into a health service system and coordinating the delivery of health services, primary care is more involved in the integration of health care services and the accountability of clinicians and patients to the health care system.

WHO Definition

According to the WHO, primary health care is essential health care that is based on practical, scientifically sound, and socially acceptable methods and technology. Such care is universally accessible to individuals and families in the community by means acceptable to them and at a cost that the community and the country can afford to maintain at every stage of their development in a spirit of self-reliance and self-determination. Primary health care serves as the foundation of ambulatory services, characterized by the first level of contact between individuals, the family, and the community on one hand and the health care delivery system on the other hand, bringing health care as close as possible to where people live and work. It constitutes the first element of a continuing health care process (WHO, 1978, p. 25).

IOM Definition

The IOM Committee on the Future of Primary Care recommended that *primary care* be the usual and preferred route of entry, although not the only route of entry, into the health care system. The IOM defined primary care as follows (Vanselow et al., 1995, p. 192):

> The provision of integrated, accessible health care services by clinicians who are accountable for addressing a large majority of personal health care needs, developing a sustained partnership with patients, and practicing in the context of family and community.

Domains of Primary Care

These definitions highlight several important domains, which are critical to understanding primary care. Three elements in the WHO and two elements in the IOM definitions are particularly noteworthy for an understanding of primary care, as summarized in **Exhibit 7.2**.

Exhibit 7.2 Domains of Primary Care

- Point of entry
- Coordination of care
- Essential care
- Integrated care
- Accountability

Point of Entry

Primary care is the point of entry into a health services system in which health care delivery is organized around primary care (Starfield, 1992, p. vii). Primary care is the first contact a patient makes with the health care delivery system. This first contact feature is closely associated with the gatekeeper role of the primary care practitioner. *Gatekeeping* implies that patients do not visit specialists and are not admitted to a hospital without being referred by their primary care physicians. On the surface, gatekeeping may appear to be a controlling mechanism for denying needed care. In most cases, however, primary care protects patients from unnecessary procedures and overtreatment (Franks et al., 1992) because specialists use medical tests and procedures to a much greater extent than do primary care providers, and such interventions carry a definite risk of iatrogenic (caused by the process of health care) complications (Starfield, 1994).

One of the goals of primary care is to bring health care as close as possible to where people live and work. In other words, true primary care is community based. It represents convenience and easy accessibility. To make such services widely available to communities in urban, suburban, and rural areas, the nature of primary care services must remain basic, routine, and inexpensive. Yet appropriate technology must be incorporated into the delivery of primary care so that costly referrals to other components of the health delivery system are made only when necessary.

Coordination of Care

One of the main functions of primary care is to coordinate the delivery of health services between the patient and the myriad components of the system. Hence, in addition to providing basic services, primary care professionals serve as patient advisors and advocates. In this coordinating role, the provider refers patients to sources of specialized care, gives advice regarding various diagnoses and therapies, discusses treatment options, and provides continuing care for chronic conditions (Williams, 1993). Coordination of an individual's total health care needs is meant to ensure continuity and comprehensiveness. These desirable goals of primary care are best achieved when the patient and provider have formed a close mutual relationship over time. Primary care can be regarded as the hub of the health care delivery system wheel. The various components of the health care delivery system are located around the rim, and the spokes signify the coordination of continuous and comprehensive care (see **Figure 7.1**).

Countries whose health systems are oriented more toward primary care achieve better health levels, higher satisfaction with health services among their populations, and lower expenditures in the overall delivery of health care (Starfield, 1994). Countries with weak primary care infrastructures incur poorer health outcomes and higher health care costs. Even in the United States, those states with higher ratios of primary care physicians show better health outcomes associated with the availability of better primary care (Shi, 1992, 1994). Higher ratios of family and general practice physicians in the population are also associated with lower hospitalization rates for conditions treatable with good primary care (Parchman & Culler, 1994). Adults who have primary care physicians as their regular source of care subsequently experience lower death rates and incur lower health care costs (Franks & Fiscella, 1998).

An ideal system of health care delivery is based on primary care but is closely interlinked to adequate and timely specialized services. Continuous and coordinated care requires that secondary and tertiary services be integrated with primary care through appropriate interaction and consultation among physicians. Coordination of health care has certain definite advan-

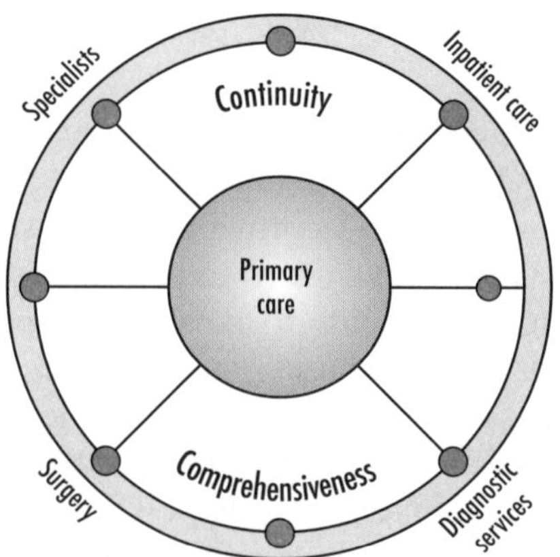

Figure 7.1 Coordination Role of Primary Care in Health Delivery

tages. Studies have shown that both the appropriateness and the outcomes of health care interventions are better when primary care physicians refer patients to specialists than they are when patients self-refer (Bakwin, 1945; Roos, 1979).

Essential Care

Primary health care is regarded as essential health care. As such, the goal of the health care delivery system is to optimize population health, not just the health of individuals who have the means to access health services. Achievement of this goal requires that disparities across population subgroups be minimized to ensure equal access. Because financing of health care is a key element in determining access, the goal of optimizing population health is better achieved under a national health care program. For this reason, the lack of access to primary care for countless millions remains a nagging concern in the United States.

In the United States, the mixture of public and private financing has created a fragmented system in which primary care does not form the organizing hub for continuous and coordinated health services. Although the primary care model has gained increased popularity under the managed care system, its current role appears to be limited to low-cost general medicine and gatekeeping, controlling access to the rest of the health care system. In reality, primary care is much more than that.

Integrated

The term "integrated" embodies the concepts of comprehensive, coordinated, and continuous services that provide a seamless process of care. Primary care is comprehensive because it addresses any health problem at any given stage of a patient's life cycle. The coordinating function ensures the provision of a combination of health services to best meet the patient's needs. Continuity refers to care over time by a single provider or a team of health care professionals. The IOM definition goes further to emphasize accessibility and accountability as key characteristics of primary care. Accessibility refers to the ease with which a patient can initiate an interaction with a clinician for any health problem. It includes efforts to eliminate barriers such as those posed by geography, financing, culture, race, and language.

Accountability

The IOM Committee recognizes that both clinicians and patients have accountability. The clinical system is accountable for providing quality care, producing patient satisfaction, using resources efficiently, and behaving in an ethical manner. On the other hand, patients are responsible for their own health to the extent that they are capable of influencing it. Patients also have the responsibility to be judicious in their use of resources when they need health care. Partnership between a patient and a clinician does not necessarily imply an equal role for each party. The role played by each party will vary, both over time and from case to case. Mutual trust, respect, and responsibility are the hallmarks of this partnership. The IOM Committee has proposed that primary care clinicians must possess the knowledge and skills necessary to manage most of the physical, mental, social, and emotional concerns that affect the functioning of patients. Primary care clinicians must use their best judgment to involve other practitioners in diagnosis, treatment, or both when it is appropriate to do so (Vanselow et al., 1995).

Community-Oriented Primary Care

The 1978 International Conference on Primary Health Care (Alma Ata, USSR, under the auspices of WHO) concluded that people throughout the world had very little control over their own health care and that emphasis should be placed on attaining health through a response from the community to their health problems (WHO, 1978). More positive outcomes occur when people have a greater sense of ownership of health programs that address their needs. It requires a partnership between health care providers and the communities in which they serve. It has been suggested that collective action by a community may enhance the competence of communities in mitigating risk factors and thereby reduce their vulnerability to social problems and disease (Minkler, 1992).

Community-oriented primary care incorporates the elements of good primary care delivery and adds a population-based approach to identifying and addressing community health problems. Current thoughts about primary care delivery have extended beyond the traditional biomedical paradigm, which focuses on medical care for the individual in an encounter-based system. The broader biopsychosocial paradigm emphasizes the health of the population, as well as that of the individual (Lee, 1994).

Primary Care Effectiveness

Although preventive interventions might be better performed by specialists if the interventions are in the specialists' area of expertise, it is in primary care that preventive interventions not related to any one disease or organ system are best carried out. For example, rates of cholesterol testing might be highest among cardiologists, who are more likely to follow patients with cardiovascular disease; however, immunizations and the encouragement of healthy personal behavior are best carried out by primary care physicians, given their focus on the entire person rather than a particular body system or disease and their reach to a broader cross-section of the population.

U.S. states with higher ratios of primary care physicians to population have lower smoking rates, less obesity, and higher seatbelt use than states with lower primary care physician-to-population ratios (Shi, 1994; Shi & Starfield, 2000). Continuity of care with a single provider was positively associated with primary preventive care, including smoking cessation and influenza immunization, in a large ongoing 60-community study in the United States (Saver, 2002). Studies have shown that an increase of one primary care physician per 10,000 population is linked to a reduction of 1.44 deaths per 10,000 population, 2.5% reduction in infant mortality, and a 3.2% reduction of low birth weight on average (Thesis Proposal 19). Population subgroups with a good primary care source have better birthweight distributions than comparable populations without good primary care. In 2000, it was shown that in white and black populations in both urban and rural areas of the United States birth weights were higher when the source of care was a community health center designed to provide good primary care than they were in the comparable population as a whole (Politzer et al., 2001). The likelihood of preventive visits among disadvantaged children is much greater when their source of care is a good primary care practitioner (Gadomski et al., 1998). Early detection of breast cancer is also enhanced when the supply of primary care physicians (at least relative to specialists) is adequate while a one-third increase in the supply of family physicians correlates to a 20% decrease in the mortality rates of cervical cancer (Ferrante et al., 2000; Macinko et al., 2005). Additionally, studies have suggested that as many as 127,617 deaths in the United States can be prevented annually with an increase of one primary care physician per 10,000 population (Macinko et al., 2005).

Secondary Prevention

To the extent that most secondary preventive activities are disease focused, better quality for primary care (compared with specialty care) would not necessarily be expected; however, the evidence suggests otherwise for those conditions that are common and, hence, are in the province primarily of primary care. For example, several studies have demonstrated positive associations among the cardinal features of primary care and improved access to care and health outcomes (Bertakis et al., 1998; Bindman et al., 1996; Flocke et al., 1998; Greenfield et al., 1992).

Disease Management

Following the line of reasoning just established, it might be expected that specialists would perform better than generalists and achieve better outcomes for those conditions within their purview. Even when considering care for many specific common diseases, primary care physicians do at least as well as specialists. For uncommon conditions, appropriate specialist care is undoubtedly better because primary care physicians would not see the patients frequently enough to maintain competence in managing them (Bartter & Pratter, 1996; Donohoe, 1998; Grumbach et al., 1999; Harrold et al., 1999; Hirth et al., 1996; Kaag et al., 1996; Starfield et al., 2003).

Hospitalizations and Use of Emergency Care

The literature is strong in showing that lower rates of hospitalization for ambulatory care-sensitive conditions (hospitalizations that could be prevented with good primary care) are strongly associated with receiving primary care. Children receiving their care from a good primary care source have lower hospitalization rates for these conditions as well as lower hospitalization rates overall; these findings are associated with the better receipt of preventive care from primary care providers (Gadomski et al., 1998). Rates of hospital admission are lower in U.S. communities in which primary care physicians are more involved in the care of children both before and during hospitalization (Perrin et al., 1996). Adolescents with the same regular source of care for preventive and illness care (i.e., a source of primary care) are much more likely to receive indicated preventive care and less likely to seek care in emergency rooms (Ryan et al., 2001). Thus, there is strong and consistent evidence that hospitalizations, and especially hospitalizations for ambulatory care-sensitive conditions, are less frequent when primary care is strong.

The geographic distribution of primary care physicians has also been found to be an important factor. Parchman and Culler (1994, p. 45), for instance, demonstrated that geographic areas with more family and general care physicians per population had lower hospitalization rates for conditions that could be preventable with good primary care (including diabetes mellitus or pneumonia in children and congestive heart failure, hypertension, pneumonia, and diabetes mellitus in adults). Another study found that poor primary care resources were independently associated with higher rates of hospitalization for conditions preventable by adequate primary care.

Cost of Care

Areas in which primary care is stronger, as measured by primary care physician-to-population ratios, have much lower total health care costs than other areas. This has been demonstrated to be the case among the elderly in the United States who live in metropolitan areas, both for total costs (inpatient and outpatient) (Mark et al., 1996; Welch et al., 1993) and for the total population in the United States (Franks & Fiscella, 1998), as well as in an international comparison of industrialized countries (Starfield & Shi, 2002). Care for illnesses common in the population (e.g., community-acquired pneumonia) is more expensive if provided by specialists than if provided by generalists, with no difference in outcomes (Rosser, 1996; Whittle et al., 1998).

Morbidity

Primary care physician supply has been associated with lower rates of self-reported poor health in 60 representative U.S. communities, after controlling for a wide range of sociodemographic and socioeconomic characteristics (Shi & Starfield, 2000). Data from this same survey confirmed the positive impact of primary care by showing that those who actually experienced better primary care reported better health (Shi et al., 2002). Birth weight and infant mortality were also associated with primary care physician supply in U.S. states. Higher primary care physician supply has been associated with lower low-birth-weight percentages and lower infant mortality, even after controlling for educational levels, unemployment, racial/ethnic composition, income inequality, and urban–rural differences (Shi et al., 2003).

One population-based study (Roetzheim et al., 1999) in an entire U.S. state found that detection of colorectal cancer at earlier stages was better in areas that had a greater supply of primary care physicians. Conversely, diagnosis tended to be later in areas with more specialist physicians. The nature of the findings led the authors to conclude that a lower supply of specialists enhances the likelihood that primary care physicians screen for such cancers.

Several studies have shown the importance of primary care as an entrance point to the health care system for a majority of conditions. For example, one study demonstrated that entry-level access is associated with better outcomes for 16 common conditions in children and youth (Starfield, 1985). Although only conducted among men, another study showed that men who lack a primary care provider were at greater risk for severe uncontrolled hypertension than those who lacked medical insurance or had alcohol-related problems (Shea et al., 1992).

Mortality

Perhaps the most frequent demonstration of the benefits of primary care has been with regard to mortality (death rates). One line of evidence comes from ecological studies of the relationship between primary care personnel-to-population ratios and various types of health outcomes in the United States. Two separate studies found better health outcomes in states with higher primary care physician-to-population ratios after controlling for sociodemographic measures (percentage of elderly, percentage of urban, percentage of minority, education, income, unemployment, pollution) and lifestyle factors (seatbelt use, obesity, and smoking) (Shi, 1992, 1994). The supply of primary care physicians has also been shown to exert a strong and significant direct influence on life expectancy, stroke, and postnatal and total mortality (Shi et al., 1999).

Studies using multiple years of data also show a relationship between primary care physician supply and mortality outcomes, where increases in the supply of primary care physicians are associated with decreases in overall and cause-specific population mortality rates (Shi et al., 2003; Villalbi et al., 1999). There is a significant positive association between life expectancy and higher numbers of primary care physicians. The greater the ratio of physicians per population, the greater is the life expectancy (Shi et al., 1999).

CONCLUSION

Outpatient services now transcend basic and routine primary care services. Many general medical and surgical interventions are provided in ambulatory care settings. In response to the changing economic incentives in the health care delivery system, numerous types of ambulatory services have emerged, and a variety of settings for the delivery of services have developed. In most settings, patients go to the delivery sites to receive services. In other cases, services are brought to the patients.

Primary care is the point of entry into a health services system in which health care delivery is organized around primary care. It is regarded as essential health care. One of the main functions of primary care is to coordinate the delivery of health services between the patient and the myriad delivery components of the system to maintain long-term health for patients. Continuity of care over a period of time is essential, not just for individuals, but also for an entire community. Primary care is comprehensive because it addresses any health problem at any given stage of a patient's life cycle. Primary care plays a central role in a health care delivery system because it is linked to both improved patient health status and cost-effectiveness.

REFERENCES

Appleby, C. 1995. Boxed in? *Hospitals and Health Networks* 69 (18):28–34.

Bakwin, H. 1945. *Pseudodoxia pediatrica. New England Journal of Medicine* 232:691–697.

Barr, K. W., and C. L. Breindel. 1995. Ambulatory care. In L. F. Wolper (ed.). *Health Care Administration: Principles, Practices, Structure, and Delivery*, 2nd ed. (pp. 547–573). Gaithersburg, MD: Aspen Publishers.

Bartter, T., and M. R. Pratter. 1996. Asthma: Better outcome at lower cost? The role of the expert in the care system. *Chest* 110 (6):1589–1596.

Bertakis, K. D., E. J. Callahan, L. J. Helms, R. Azari, J. A. Robbins, and J. Miller 1998. Physician practice styles and patient outcomes: Differences between family practice and general internal medicine. *Medical Care* 36 (6):879–891.

Bindman, A. B., K. Grumbach, D. Osmond, K. Vranizan, and A. L. Stewart. 1996. Primary care and receipt of preventive services. *Journal of General Internal Medicine* 11 (5):269–276.

Complementary and Alternative Medicine Research Methodology Conference. 1997. Defining and describing complementary and alternative medicine. *Alternative Therapies* 3(2):49–56.

Donohoe, M. T. 1998. Comparing generalist and specialty care: Discrepancies, deficiencies, and excesses. *Archives of Internal Medicine* 158 (15):1596–1608.

Ferrante, J. M., E. C. Gonzalez, N. Pal, and R. G. Roetzheim. 2000. Effects of physician supply on early detection of breast cancer. *Journal of the American Board of Family Practice* 13 (6):408–414.

Flocke, S. A., K. C. Stange, and S. J. Zyzanski. 1998. The association of attributes of primary care with the delivery of clinical preventive services. *Medical Care* 36(8 Suppl):AS21–AS30.

Franks, P., and K. Fiscella. 1998. Primary care physicians and specialists as personal physicians. Health care expenditures and mortality experience. *Journal of Family Practice* 47 (2):105–109.

Franks, P., et al. 1992. Gatekeeping revisited: Protecting patients from overtreatment. *New England Journal of Medicine* 327 (4):424–429.

Gadomski, A., P. Jenkins, and M. Nichols. 1998. Impact of a Medicaid primary care provider and preventive care on pediatric hospitalization. *Pediatrics* 101 (3):E1. http://www.pediatrics.org/cgi/content/full/101/3/e1.

Greenfield, S., et al. 1992. Variations in resource utilization among medical specialties and systems of care. Results from the medical outcomes study. *Journal of the American Medical Association* 267 (12):1624–1630.

Grumbach, K., J. V. Selby, J. A. Schmittdiel, and C. P. Quesenberry, Jr. 1999. Quality of primary care practice in a large HMO according to physician specialty. *Health Services Research* 34 (2):485–502.

Harrold, L. R., T. S. Field, and J. H. Gurwitz. 1999. Knowledge, patterns of care, and outcomes of care for generalists and specialists. *Journal of General Internal Medicine* 14 (8):499–511.

Hirth, R. A., A. M. Fendrick, and M. E. Chernew. 1996. Specialist and generalist physicians' adoption of antibiotic therapy to eradicate *Helicobacter pylori* infection. *Medical Care* 34 (12):1199–1204.

Kaag, M. E, D. Wijkel, and D. de Jong. 1996. Primary health care replacing hospital care: The effect on quality of care. *Int J Qual Health Care* 8 (4):367–373.

Lee, P. R. 1994. Models of excellence. *Lancet* 344 (8935):1484–1486.

Mark, D. H., M. S. Gottlieb, B. B. Zellner, V. K. Chetty, and J. E. Midtling. 1996. Medicare costs in urban areas and the supply of primary care physicians. *Journal of Family Practice* 43 (1):33–39.

McAlearney, J. S. 2002. The financial performance of community health centers, 1996–1999. *Health Affairs* 21 (2):219–225.

Minkler, M. 1992. Community organizing among the elderly poor in the United States. *International Journal of Health Services* 22 (2):303–316.

Parchman, M. L., and S. Culler. 1994. Primary care physicians and avoidable hospitalizations. *Journal of Family Practice* 39 (2):123–128.

Perrin, J. M., et al. 1996. Primary care involvement among hospitalized children. *Archives of Pediatric and Adolescent Medicine* 150 (5):479–486.

Politzer, R.M., J. Yoon, L. Shi, R. G. Hughes, J. Regan, and M. H. Gaston. 2001. Inequality in America: The contribution of health centers in reducing and eliminating disparities in access to care. *Medical Care Research and Review* 58 (2):234–248.

Roetzheim, R. G., et al. 1999. The effects of physician supply on the early detection of colorectal cancer. *Journal of Family Practice* 48 (11):850–858.

Roos, N. 1979. Who should do the surgery? Tonsillectomy and adenoidectomy in one Canadian province. *Inquiry* 16 (1):73–83.

Rosser, W. W. 1996. Approach to diagnosis by primary care clinicians and specialists: Is there a difference? *Journal of Family Practice* 42 (2):139–144.

Ryan, S., A. Riley, M. Kang, and B. Starfield. 2001. The effects of regular source of care and health need on medical care use among rural adolescents. *Archives of Pediatric and Adolescent Medicine* 155 (2):184–190.

Saver, B. 2002. Financing and organization findings brief. *Academy for Research and Health Care Policy* 5 (1):1–2.

Shea, S., D. Misra, M. H. Ehrlich, L. Field, and C. K. Francis. 1992. Predisposing factors for severe, uncontrolled hypertension in an inner-city minority population. *New England Journal of Medicine* 327 (11):776–781.

Shi, L. 1992. The relation between primary care and life chances. *Journal of Health Care for the Poor and Underserved* 3:321–335.

Shi, L. 1994. Primary care, specialty care, and life chances. *International Journal of Health Services* 24 (3):431–458.

Shi, L., and B. Starfield. 2000. Primary care, income inequality, and self-rated health in the United States: A mixed-level analysis. *International Journal of Health Services* 30:541–555.

Shi, L., et al. 1999. Income inequality, primary care, and health indicators. *Journal of Family Practice* 48:275–284.

Shi, L., et al. 2002. Primary care, self-rated health, and reductions in social disparities in health. *Health Services Research* 37:529–550.

Shi, L., J. Macinko, B. Starfield, J. Regan, R. Politzer, and J. Wulu. 2004. Primary care, infant mortality, and low birthweight in US states. *Journal of Epidemiology and Community Health*. 58 (5):374–380.

Starfield, B. 1985. Motherhood and apple pie: The effectiveness of medical care for children. *Milbank Memorial Fund Quarterly. Health and Society* 63 (3):523–546.

Starfield, B. 1992. *Primary Care: Concept, Evaluation, and Policy*. New York: Oxford University Press.

Starfield, B. 1994. Is primary care essential? *Lancet* 344 (8930):1129–1133.

Starfield, B., and L. Shi. 2002. Policy relevant determinants of health: An international perspective. *Health Policy* 60:201–218.

Starfield, B., K. W. Lemke, T. Bernhard, S. S. Foldes, C. B. Forrest, and J. P. Weiner. 2003. Comorbidity: Implications for the importance of primary care in 'case' management. *Annals of Family Medicine* 1:8–14.

Vanselow, N. A., et al. 1995. From the Institute of Medicine. *Journal of the American Medical Association* 273 (3):192.

Villalbi, J. R., et al. 1999. An evaluation of the impact of primary care reform on health. *Aten Primaria* 24 (8):468–474.

Welch, W. P., M. E. Miller, H. G. Welch, E. S. Fisher, and J. E. Wennberg. 1993. Geographic variation in expenditures for physicians' services in the United States. *New England Journal of Medicine* 328 (9):621–627.

Whittle, J. C., et al. 1998. Relationship of provider characteristics to outcomes, process, and costs of care for community-acquired pneumonia. *Medical Care* 36 (7):977–987.

Williams, S. J. 1993. Ambulatory health care services. In S. J. Williams and P. R. Torrens (eds.). *Introduction to Health Services*, 4th ed. Albany, NY: Delmar Publishers.

World Health Organization. 1978. *Primary Health Care*. Geneva: Author.

Chapter 8

Hospitals

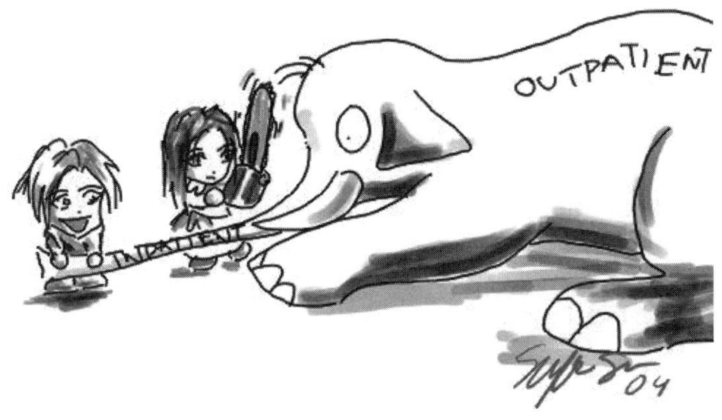

INTRODUCTION

The term *inpatient* refers to a patient staying overnight in a health care facility, such as a hospital or a nursing care facility. Outpatient, as discussed in Chapter 7, refers to services provided while the patient is not lodged in the hospital or some other health care institution. This chapter describes what a hospital is, its evolution, and its current role in health care delivery.

The American Hospital Association (AHA) defines a hospital as an institution with at least six beds whose primary function is "to deliver patient services, diagnostic and therapeutic, for particular or general medical conditions" (AHA, 1994). In addition, a hospital must be licensed, must have an organized physician staff, and must provide continuous nursing services under the supervision of registered nurses (RNs). A hospital must have a designated governing body or board that is legally responsible for the conduct of the hospital and a full-time chief executive officer (CEO) who is responsible for the hospital's operations. The hospital must also maintain medical records on each patient, have pharmacy services available within the institution, and provide food services to meet the nutritional and therapeutic requirements of the patients (Health Forum, 2001). The construction and operation of the modern hospital are governed by federal laws, state health regulations, city ordinances, standards of the Joint Commission on Accreditation of Healthcare Organizations, and national codes for building, fire protection, and sanitation.

In the past 200 years or so, hospitals have gradually evolved from ordinary institutions of refuge for the homeless and poor to ultramodern facilities providing the latest medical services to the critically ill and injured. The term *medical center* is used by some hospitals, reflecting their high level of specialization and wide scope of services. Medical centers often engage in teaching and research. Since the 1980s, many hospitals have expanded their scope of services to include outpatient care.

EVOLUTION OF THE HOSPITAL IN THE UNITED STATES

The major stages of hospital evolution in the United States are listed in **Exhibit 8.1**. As discussed in Chapter 3, before 1850 or so, only a few hospitals existed, and these were confined to major U.S. cities. The main health care institutions were the almshouses (also called poorhouses). Their services were more akin to social welfare than to medicine, consisting

Exhibit 8.1 Major Stages of Hospital Evolution

- Almshouses as primarily institutions of social welfare
- Community-owned private hospitals as charitable institutions supported by affluent donors
- Institutions of medical practice and training serving the needs of all members of society; able to make a profit
- Emergence of a relatively small number of physician-owned proprietary hospitals
- University-based centers of medical research
- Emergence of medical systems providing a large array of health services

mainly of providing food and shelter to the destitute and some nursing care to the sick. At that time, however, medicine and nursing as the professions we know today had not emerged. People generally stayed in these institutions for months rather than days.

During the latter half of the 1800s, hospitals evolved from the almshouses and pesthouses (places for those with contagious diseases), but they continued to serve mainly the poor. At this point, hospitals also began to transition from being primarily government-run institutions to community institutions supported mainly through private charitable donations. Influential donors also exercised control over the hospital as members of the board of trustees. Since then, private nonprofit rather than government-owned hospitals have continued to dominate the hospital landscape in America.

Medical discoveries during the latter half of the 1800s (summarized in Exhibit 3.4) were instrumental in transforming hospitals into true institutions of medical practice. Discoveries that had a profound impact on hospitals included anesthesia, which aided significantly in advancing new surgical techniques, and the development of the germ theory of disease, which led to the subsequent discovery of antiseptic and sterilization techniques (Haglund & Dowling, 1993). From around 1850 onward, technological progress led to the development of advanced equipment, facilities, and personnel training, which became centered in the hospital. Hospitals established laboratories and x-ray units so that physicians could have convenient access to diagnostic technology. These advances made it necessary for physicians to treat acute illness in hospitals, which also became centers where physicians received their practical training. From this point on, hospitals came to be regarded as a necessity because the superior medical services and surgical procedures offered there could not be obtained at home. Thus, hospitals began to attract well-to-do patients who could afford to pay privately. Gradually, hospitals no longer had to depend totally on charitable contributions. They could now generate a profit. At this stage, some physicians started opening their own small hospitals, thus laying the foundation of *proprietary* (for-profit) hospitals in the United States.

Today, many hospitals affiliate with university-based medical schools and have become centers of medical research where new discoveries are made. They disseminate their findings through publications in medical journals to advance new medical knowledge throughout the world.

Today's hospitals are complex organizations. The field of hospital administration is a discipline in its own right. To manage hospitals, administrators need expertise in financial management and good organizational and human relations skills. Also, departments such as food service, pharmacy, x-ray, and the laboratory require well-trained professional staff to manage the delivery of services.

In recent years, local market pressures have prompted many hospitals to merge or enter into formal affiliations with other hospitals. In urban areas, *medical systems* have formed. These health systems may include more than one hospital to serve a large geographical area. They also are increasingly providing a full array of health care services. These services include outpatient clinics, same-day surgery, outpatient imaging services, outpatient rehabilitation therapies, nursing home care, and home health services. Many health systems have also opened special women's centers and fitness centers. Increasingly, community services such as health education, promotion of healthy lifestyles, and prevention of disease have become an important part of a hospital's mission.

EXPANSION AND DOWNSIZING OF HOSPITALS IN THE UNITED STATES

The number of hospital beds in the United States grew from 35,604 in 1872 to 907,133 in 1929 (Haglund & Dowling, 1993). This phenomenal growth started after hospitals became institutions of medical practice, serving the needs of all members of society and making a profit. The factors contributing to the growth of hospitals from the preindustrial era to around 1980 are listed in **Exhibit 8.2**. Technological advances led to a growth in the volume of surgical work, which at that time could be done only in hospitals. As new beds were built, they were quickly filled by patients needing

Exhibit 8.2 Factors Contributing to the Growth of Hospitals

- Broad appeal, once hospitals evolved into institutions of medical practice as a result of technological advances and professional training of health care professionals
- Private health insurance
- Hill-Burton Act
- Medicaid and Medicare

acute treatment or surgery. Advances in medical science, as well as professional training of nurses and other health care professionals, played an important role in creating a demand for more beds.

After 1930, it was the increased availability of private health insurance that enabled more and more people to pay for hospital services, which became increasingly more costly and unaffordable. Once people had health insurance, that in itself generated new demand. Early insurance plans provided generous coverage for inpatient care, and there were few restrictions on the use of hospital services.

In the 1940s, the U.S. government recognized a severe shortage of hospitals. In response, Congress passed the Hospital Survey and Construction Act of 1946, which is more commonly known as the Hill-Burton Act. It provided federal grants to the states for the construction of new hospital beds. The objective of Hill-Burton was to ensure 4.5 beds per 1,000 population (Teisberg et al., 1991). The Hill-Burton program has been regarded as the greatest single factor in increasing the nation's bed supply. The program made it possible for even small remote communities to have their own hospitals (Wolfson & Hopes, 1994).

The creation of Medicaid and Medicare in 1965 made public health insurance available to a large segment of the U.S. population. Hospital demand continued to grow. Between 1965 and 1980, the number of community hospitals in the United States increased from 5,736 (741,000 beds) to 5,830 (988,000 beds) (AHA, 1990). By 1980, the United States had also reached its goal of 4.5 community hospital beds per 1,000 civilian population (National Center for Health Statistics, 2002).

In 1983, the U.S. government decided to contain the exploding cost of hospital care, mostly because of its impact on the rising cost of Medicare (see **Figure 8.1** for the rise in costs between 1970 and 1980). The goal of cost containment was achieved by enacting the Social Security Amendments of 1983. The law required Medicare to stop paying hospitals per diem rates established on the basis of their costs of operation (retrospective reimbursement). Instead, a prospective payment system (PPS) was established to reimburse hospitals on the basis of diagnosis-related groups (DRGs). Under this method, hospitals received a pre-established fixed rate per admission, as explained in Chapter 6. In order not to lose money, they had to cut their costs of operation. They also had to discharge patients quicker than before because keeping patients in the hospital longer than necessary cut into the hospital's profits. Many hospitals had to close

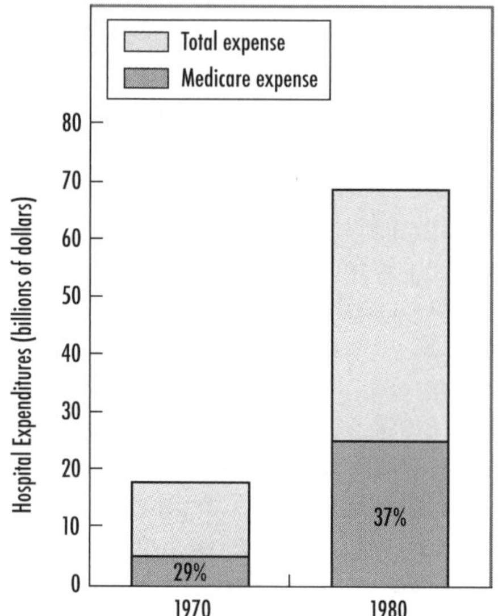

Figure 8.1 Medicare's Share of Hospital Expenses

because they had difficulty coping with the new method of reimbursement. Other hospitals continued to operate but had to take unused beds out of service. PPS triggered the downsizing phase in the U.S. hospital industry.

During the 1990s, the growth of managed care played a significant role in curtailing inpatient utilization even further. Managed care has emphasized cost containment and efficient delivery of care. Because inpatient care in hospitals is costly, managed care has emphasized early discharge from hospitals and, if necessary, continuing the delivery of care through home health agencies and skilled-care nursing homes. In other instances, the emphasis has been on using outpatient services whenever appropriate instead of admitting patients to hospitals.

The three main factors just discussed (and summarized in **Exhibit 8.3**) were largely successful in reducing the growth of national spending on hospital care. **Figure 8.2** illustrates the growth of spending in hospital inpatient care compared with the growth of national health expenditures. Notice the slower rates of growth after the implementation of the PPS between

Exhibit 8.3 Factors Contributing to the Downsizing of Hospitals

- Change in Medicare reimbursement to hospitals from a retrospective to a prospective method, leading to shorter hospital stays
- Hospital closings
- Managed care's emphasis on cost-containment and use of services such as outpatient, home health, and skilled nursing care

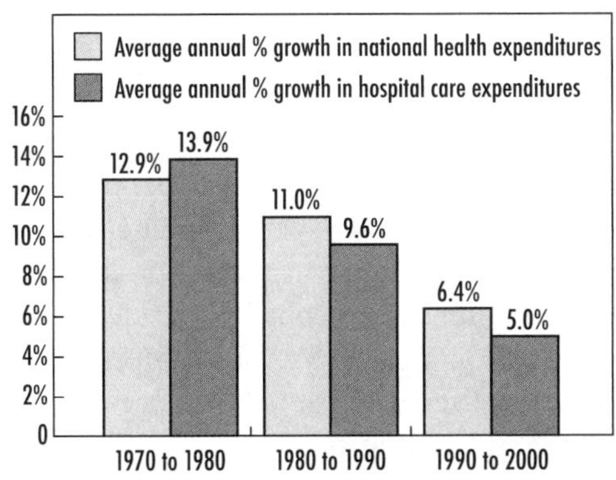

Figure 8.2 Comparison of Growths in Hospital and National Health Expenditures

1980 and 1990 and a further slowdown between 1990 and 2000 resulting from managed care.

ACCESS AND UTILIZATION BY THE U.S. POPULATION

Access

The total number of patient discharges per 1,000 population is an indicator of access to hospital inpatient services. Because newborn infants are not included in admissions, discharges provide a more accurate measure of the number of people served by a hospital. *Discharges* refer to the total number of patients released from a hospital's acute care beds during a given period also including deaths.

Utilization

An *inpatient day* (also referred to as a patient day or a hospital day) is a night spent in the hospital by a patient. The average number of days a patient spends in the hospital is called the *average length of stay* (ALOS). The total number of inpatient days incurred by a population over a given period of time is referred to as *days of care*. Mathematically,

$$\text{days of care} = \text{number of discharges} \times \text{ALOS}$$

National data on days of care per 1,000 population show that the elderly spend more time in hospitals than do younger people. Even after adjusting for childbearing among women 18 years of age and older, women are admitted to hospitals more often than men, but men incur longer stays. Hospital utilization is higher among blacks than whites and is also higher among the poor than the nonpoor. Various factors (education, socioeconomic status, behaviors, lifestyles, heredity, access to primary care, etc. discussed in Chapter 2) interact to produce differences in health status and onset of acute conditions between the different population groups. Hence, some groups incur more frequent hospitalizations and also longer stays once admitted. From this information, it can also be concluded that overall hospital utilization is higher among Medicare and Medicaid recipients than in the rest of the population.

Since 2003, the ALOS for community hospitals in the United States has been 4.8 days, the lowest ever recorded. First, the PPS had a marked influence on the decline in the ALOS. This was followed by the influence of managed care during the 1990s. The sharp decline in ALOS during the 1990s became possible with the growth of alternative services, such as home health and subacute long-term care, which enabled people to be discharged earlier than was previously possible. Thanks to the development of these substitute sites of care and better technology, there has been no evidence that quicker discharges of patients from hospitals under the PPS or managed care payment systems has resulted in medical harm to patients.

UTILIZATION OF HOSPITAL CAPACITY

Capacity refers to the number of beds set up, staffed, and made available by a hospital for inpatient use. Eighty-four percent of all community hospitals in the United States have fewer than 300 beds. Nationally, a typical rural hospital has 65 beds, and an urban hospital has 231 beds (Anonymous, 2002).

The term *census* refers to the number of patients in a hospital on a given day. The cumulative census is called *patient days*. The average census over a given period of time is called the *average daily census* (see Table 8.1). Mathematically,

$$\text{average daily census} = \text{patient days over a defined period} \div \text{number of days in the period}$$

The average daily census in a hospital represents the average number of beds occupied per day.

Occupancy rate is the percentage of capacity used during a defined period of time. It is derived by dividing the average daily census for that

Table 8.1 Relationship Between the Various Measures of Capacity Utilization

Day Number	Census	Patient Days
1	100	100
2	104	204
3	101	305
4	99	404
5	98	502
6	102	604
7	103	707

Patient days for this week: 707. Average daily census: 707 ÷ 7 = 101. If hospital capacity is 153, the occupancy rate is 66% [(101 ÷ 153) × 100].

period by the capacity (see Table 8.1). The fraction is expressed as a percentage (% beds occupied). An individual hospital's performance in capacity utilization can be meaningfully compared with local and national composite occupancy rates. In 2005, the occupancy rate for all U.S. community hospitals was 67.3%.

HOSPITAL EMPLOYMENT

The U.S. health care sector employs approximately 14.4 million civilians. Of these, 5.7 million, or approximately 40%, are employed in hospitals. Hospital employment accounts for roughly 4% of the employed (full- and part-time) civilian population. Hospitals have been hiring an increasing number of personnel. Between 2000 and 2006, hospital employment grew by 1.6% per year (National Center for Health Statistics, 2007, p. 354). The average annual rate of increase in hospital employment between 2004 and 2014 is expected to be 1.5% (U.S. Census Bureau, 2008, p. 395).

Among all health services sites, average hourly earnings are the highest in hospitals. In 2006, the average hourly earnings of nonmanagement workers in hospitals amounted to $22.19 (U.S. Census Bureau, 2008, p. 406).

TYPES OF HOSPITALS

The United States has a variety of institutional forms, with both private and government-owned institutions under independent management. A hospital can be classified under more than one category.

Community Hospitals

Approximately 85% of all U.S. hospitals are classified as community hospitals. The identifying characteristics of these hospitals are listed in **Exhibit 8.4**. By definition, a *community hospital* is a nonfederal, short-stay hospital whose services are available to the general public. This excludes federal hospitals, such as those in the Department of Veterans Affairs (VA) and military systems, and hospital units of institutions, such as prisons and infirmaries in colleges and universities because their services are not available to the general public. However, hospitals operated by local and state

Exhibit 8.4 Characteristics of a Community Hospital

- Nonfederal: hospitals operated by local and state governments can be community hospitals
- Short stay: ALOS must be ≤ 30 days
- Open to the general public
- Private for-profit or nonprofit; general or specialty

governments are generally community hospitals. Also excluded from the definition of a community hospital are long-stay hospitals, such as psychiatric facilities, tuberculosis hospitals, and other chronic disease hospitals. In long-stay hospitals, the ALOS is more than 30 days.

Public Hospitals

In health care, the word "public" connotes government ownership. *Public hospitals*, therefore, are hospitals owned by agencies of federal, state, or local governments. Approximately 19% of the U.S. hospital bed capacity is in the public sector (**Figure 8.3**).

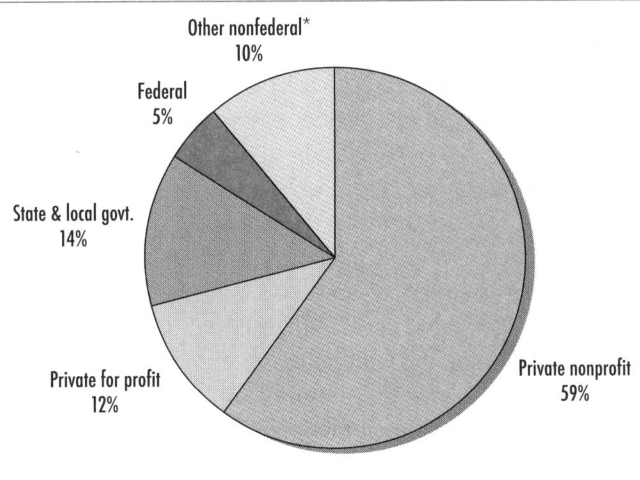

Figure 8.3 Proportion of Hospital Beds by Type of Hospital, 2005.

A public hospital is not necessarily a hospital that is open to the general public. For example, being government owned, federal hospitals are classified as public hospitals, but they are not community hospitals because they do not serve the general public. Federal hospitals are maintained primarily for special groups of federal beneficiaries such as Native Americans, military personnel, and veterans. VA hospitals constitute the largest group among federal hospitals. The VA system operates approximately 170 medical centers across the country.

State governments have generally limited themselves to the operation of mental and tuberculosis hospitals, reflecting the government's early role in protecting communities by isolating the mentally ill and persons with contagious diseases.

On the other hand, most hospitals operated by local governments, such as counties and cities, are public hospitals because they are government owned, but they are also classified as community hospitals because people from the community can utilize them. Government-owned community hospitals are often located in large urban areas where they serve mainly the inner-city indigent and disadvantaged populations. Because of the poor health status of these populations and inner-city violence, these hospitals incur higher utilization than hospitals located in suburban areas. Most of these hospitals are of small to moderate size (the average size is 115 beds). Some large public hospitals are affiliated with medical schools, and they play a significant role in training physicians and other health care professionals. Medicare, Medicaid, and state and local tax dollars pay for almost 80% of the services these hospitals provide (Safety Net in Shreds, 2002). These hospitals provide a substantial amount of charity care and often suffer financial losses that are covered by funneling tax dollars into the operations. Because of increasing financial pressures, many public hospitals have had to privatize or close. Consequently, the number of state and local government-owned community hospitals declined by 23% between 1990 and 2005. During this same period, the number of federal hospitals, which are not community hospitals, declined by almost 33%. In contrast, the number of private nonprofit hospitals declined by only 7%, and for-profit hospitals actually increased by 16% during the same period (National Center for Health Statistics, 2007, p. 364).

Private Nonprofit Hospitals

Private nonprofit hospitals are also called *voluntary hospitals*. The majority of these hospitals are operated by community associations, but other nongovernment organizations, such as philanthropic foundations and fraternal orders and societies, also operate a few. Church-owned hospitals also play a significant role in delivering hospital services in the United States. For example, Catholic and various Protestant denominations operate some of the multihospital chains. Hospitals are also established by Jewish philanthropic organizations. These hospitals were first established so that Jewish patients could observe their dietary laws more faithfully and so that Jewish physicians could find sites for training and work opportunities (Raffel, 1980, p. 241). Now, almost all church-affiliated hospitals are community hospitals. These hospitals are not discriminatory in terms of access to care; however, they are generally sensitive to the special spiritual or dietary needs of the sponsoring denomination (Raffel & Raffel, 1994, p. 131–132).

Almost 60% of the hospital beds in the United States are under private nonprofit ownership (Figure 8.3). The primary mission of these hospitals is to benefit the communities in which they are located. The operating expenses are covered from patient fees, third-party reimbursement, donations, and endowments.

Lay people make a common assumption that nonprofit (sometimes referred to as not-for-profit) organizations do not make a profit. The fact is that every corporation, regardless of whether it is for profit or nonprofit, has to make a profit (a surplus of revenues over expenses) to survive over the long term. No business can survive for long if it continually spends more than it takes in. This is as true for nonprofit organizations as it is for the for-profit sector (Nudelman & Andrews, 1996). The Internal Revenue Code, Section 501(c)(3), grants tax-exempt status to nonprofit organizations. As such, these institutions are exempt from federal, state, and local taxes such as income, sales, and property taxes. In general, these organizations must (1) provide some defined public good, such as service, education, or community welfare and (2) not distribute any of the profits to any individual. The rationale behind tax exemption is that these facilities provide an essential community benefit, principally for charitable, training, or research purposes. Discussions in the U.S. Congress over the years have suggested that benefits received by a community should at least be equal to the benefit of tax exemption enjoyed by the organization (Wolfson & Hopes, 1994).

The fact, however, is that nonprofit hospitals, in many instances, compete head-on with for-profit hospitals. Competition commonly occurs in the same communities, for the same patients, with revenues coming from the same public and private third-party sources, and often the same physician providers have admitting privileges at more than one hospital.

Moreover, many nonprofit hospitals engage in the same kinds of aggressive marketplace behaviors that for-profit hospitals pursue. In general, for-profit and nonprofit hospitals provide similar levels of charity and uncompensated care. Hence, whether nonprofit hospitals are indeed charitable institutions remains controversial. Many nonprofit entities must redefine their missions in order to differentiate themselves and provide tangible evidence of the benefits to the community in exchange for the tax benefits they receive.

Private For-Profit Hospitals

Private for-profit or *proprietary hospitals*, also referred to as investor-owned hospitals, are owned by individuals, partnerships, or corporations. They are operated for the financial benefit of the entity that owns the institution, that is, the stockholders. At the beginning of the 20th century, more than half of the nation's hospitals were proprietary. Most of these hospitals were small and were established by physicians who wanted a place to hospitalize their own patients (Stewart, 1973). Later, most of these institutions were closed or acquired by community organizations or hospital corporations because of population shifts, increased costs, and the necessities of modern clinical practice (Raffel & Raffel, 1994, p. 133).

For-profit corporations operate some of the largest multihospital chains in the United States. One of the most significant trends over the past few years has been the building or acquisition of a substantial number of hospitals by large investor-owned corporations. Still, most multihospital health care systems today are operated by nonprofit corporations. Although a major goal for a for-profit organization is to provide a return on investment to its shareholders, it achieves this goal primarily by excelling at accomplishing its basic mission. The basic mission of any health services provider is to deliver the highest quality of care possible at the most reasonable price possible.

General Hospitals

A *general hospital* provides diagnostic, treatment, and surgical services for patients with a variety of acute medical conditions. Services may include general and specialized medicine, general and specialized surgery, and obstetrics. Most hospitals in the United States are general hospitals, but they are not all community hospitals because most federal hospitals are general hospitals too.

The term "general hospital" does not imply that these hospitals are less specialized or that their care is inferior to that of specialty hospitals. The difference lies in the nature of services, not the quality. General hospitals provide a broader range of services for a larger variety of conditions, whereas specialty hospitals provide a narrow range of services for specific medical conditions or patient populations.

Specialty Hospitals

Specialty hospitals admit only certain types of patients or those with specified illnesses or conditions (Rakich et al., 1992, p. 261). Specialty hospitals have traditionally included tuberculosis, psychiatric, rehabilitation, and children's hospitals. With increasing competition, other types of specialty hospitals have emerged to provide treatments that are also available in many general hospitals. Examples include hospitals specializing in orthopedic surgery and cardiology. Specialty hospitals forge a distinct service niche in a given market. These hospitals are community hospitals as long as they meet the criteria discussed in that section.

In the entire nation, only a handful of tuberculosis hospitals are now left. Brief discussions of the other three categories of specialty hospitals follow.

Psychiatric Hospitals

The primary function of a psychiatric hospital is to provide diagnostic and treatment services for patients who have psychiatric illnesses. Specifically, such an institution must have facilities to provide psychiatric, psychological, and social work services. A psychiatric hospital must also have a written agreement with a general hospital for the transfer of patients who may require medical, obstetric, or surgical care (Health Forum, 2001, p. A3). Historically, state governments have taken the primary responsibility for establishing facilities to care for the mentally ill, but as new therapies have become available to treat mental illness, most mental health services are now delivered in private psychiatric facilities and outpatient treatment centers.

Rehabilitation Hospitals

Rehabilitation hospitals specialize in therapeutic services to restore the maximum level of functioning in patients who have suffered recent disability due to illness or accident. These hospitals serve patients who generally cannot be cured but whose functioning can be improved. These patients include amputees, patients who have sustained spinal cord or sports injuries, stroke victims, and others (Raffel & Raffel, 1989, p. 160). Patients often transfer to such facilities after orthopedic surgery in a general hospital. Facilities and staff are available to provide physical, occupational, and speech and language therapy.

Children's Hospitals

Children's hospitals are community hospitals that typically have special facilities and trained staff to deal with the unique medical problems of children, particularly those with complex and rare conditions. Roughly three-fourths of the inpatients in children's hospitals are treated for chronic or congenital conditions. The remaining require intensive care for a variety of needs, such as cancer treatment, treatment of cystic fibrosis, and tissue transplants. Children's hospitals account for less than 4% of all U.S. hospitals, but they provide the vast majority of the highly specialized care that many children require.

These hospitals have equipment and furnishings that are specially designed for children—from newborn babies requiring intensive care to teens with chronic illnesses. These hospitals also maintain a nurse staffing ratio that is higher than in general hospitals because children require more nursing care than adults.

Rural Hospitals

A *rural hospital* is one that is located in a county that is not part of a metropolitan statistical area (MSA). The U.S. Bureau of the Census has defined an MSA as a geographical area that includes at least (1) one city with a population of 50,000 or more or (2) an urbanized area of at least 50,000 inhabitants and a total MSA population of at least 100,000. Compared with other hospitals, rural hospitals generally treat a larger percentage of poor and elderly patients. Such hospitals often find themselves in financial trouble and sometimes face closure.

Teaching Hospitals

A *teaching hospital* offers one or more graduate residency programs approved by the American Medical Association (AMA). Hence, the primary role of a teaching hospital is to train physicians. Although these hospitals may also be actively involved in training nurses and other health professionals, such as therapists and dietitians, unless they train physicians, they cannot be called teaching hospitals.

Depending on the type and number of residency programs offered, a hospital is either a major or a minor teaching institution. To be a full teaching hospital, it should offer, at a minimum, residencies in general medicine, surgery, obstetrics and gynecology, and pediatrics. Many teaching hospitals offer residencies in every subspecialty of medicine and surgery in addition to pathology, anesthesiology, family practice, and other programs (Wolper & Peña, 1995). Most major teaching hospitals are affiliated with medical schools of large universities. In addition to a substantial teaching and research mission, they also deliver specialized care for a variety of complex medical problems. These hospitals often operate several intensive care units, possess the latest medical technologies, and attract a diverse group of physicians representing most specialties and many subspecialties. Major teaching hospitals also offer many unique tertiary care services not generally found in other institutions, such as burn care, trauma care, and organ transplantation.

Osteopathic Hospitals

For all practical purposes, osteopathic hospitals are community, general hospitals. In 1970, osteopathic hospitals became eligible to apply for registration with the AHA (AHA, 1994). There are approximately 200 osteopathic hospitals in the United States. Osteopathic medicine represents an approach to medical practice that employs all the methods traditionally associated with allopathic medicine, such as pharmaceuticals, laboratory tests, x-ray diagnostics, and surgery. Osteopathic medicine, however, takes a holistic approach and goes a step further in advocating treatment that involves correction of the position of the joints or tissues and in emphasizing diet and environment as factors that might influence natural resistance. For many years after osteopathy was established as a separate branch of medicine in 1874, osteopaths had to develop their own hospitals because of antagonism from the established allopathic medical practitioners. Both groups have now inspected each other's medical schools and satisfied themselves that each is worth associating with and that each could serve on the other's faculties and practice side by side in the same hospitals (Raffel & Raffel, 1994, p. 45).

LICENSURE, CERTIFICATION, AND ACCREDITATION

State governments oversee the *licensure* of health care facilities, and each state sets its own standards for licensure. All facilities must be licensed to operate, but as a general rule, they are not required to be certified or accredited. The licensure function is usually carried out by each state's department of health. State licensure standards strongly emphasize compliance with building codes, fire safety, climate control, space allocations, and sanitation. States have also established minimum standards for equipment and personnel that health care organizations must meet in order to be licensed.

Certification gives a hospital the authority to participate in the Medicare and Medicaid programs. Legislation in 1972 mandated federal oversight of hospitals that wanted to participate in the Medicare and Medicaid programs. The U.S. Department of Health and Human Services (DHHS) developed standards referred to as *conditions of participation*. The DHHS generally contracts with each state's department of health to carry out inspections to verify whether facilities meet the conditions of participation. Facilities meeting these conditions are certified.

The Joint Commission on Accreditation of Hospitals, a private nonprofit body, was formed in 1951 with the approval of the various medical and hospital organizations. The organization changed its name in 1987 to the Joint Commission on Accreditation of Healthcare Organizations (Joint Commission or JCAHO), which more accurately describes the variety of health facilities it accredits. The JCAHO sets standards and accredits most of the nation's general hospitals, as well as many of the long-term care facilities, psychiatric hospitals, substance abuse programs, outpatient surgery centers, urgent care clinics, group practices, community health centers, hospices, and home health agencies. Different sets of standards apply to each category of health care organization. Seeking accreditation is voluntary, but the passage of Medicare in 1965 specified that accredited facilities were eligible for Medicare reimbursement. Medicare regulations confer *deemed status* on hospitals accredited by JCAHO. Deemed status means an accredited hospital is deemed to have met the conditions of participation for Medicare and Medicaid certification. Over the years, the JCAHO has refined its accreditation standards and process of verifying compliance to put greater emphasis on quality of care.

HOSPITAL ORGANIZATION

Hospitals are complex organizations. A hospital is generally responsible to numerous stakeholders, such as the community, the government, insurers, managed care organizations, and accreditation agencies. Internally, hospital governance involves three major sources of power, whose motivations are sometimes at odds. The organizational structure of a hospital also differs substantially from that of other large organizations. The CEO receives delegated authority from the governing body (board) and is responsible for managing the organization with the help of senior executives. In large hospitals, these senior executives often carry the title of senior vice president or vice president responsible for various key service areas, such as nursing services, rehabilitation services, human resources, and finance. Most physicians belong to a separate organizational structure parallel to the administrative structure (Figure 8.4). Such a dual structure is rarely seen in other types of businesses and presents numerous opportunities for conflict to arise between the CEO and the medical staff. Sometimes matters can be further complicated because most physicians are not employed by the hospital, yet they must be closely involved in its operations. Also, the nursing

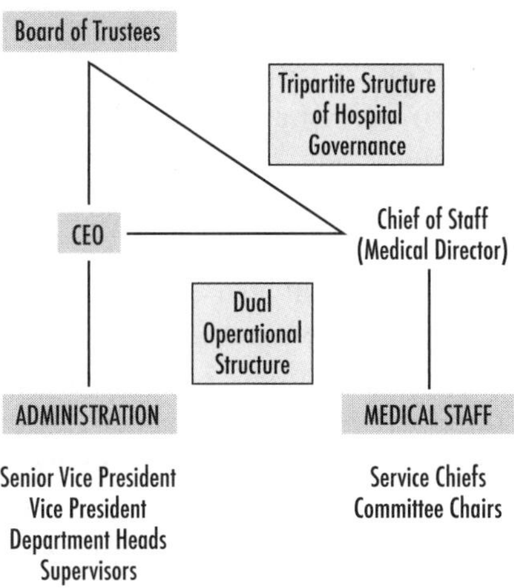

Figure 8.4 Hospital Governance and Operational Structures

staff, pharmacists, diagnostic technicians, dietitians, and others are administratively accountable to the CEO but professionally accountable to the medical staff (Raffel & Raffel, 1994, p. 139). One main exception to the medical staff organization described here is employment of physicians on salary in organizations such as veterans hospitals.

ETHICS AND PUBLIC TRUST

Ethical issues arise in all types of health services organizations, but the most significant ones occur in acute-care hospitals. Increasing levels of technology create situations requiring decision making under complex circumstances. Constraints on reimbursement often make it essential to cut costs or eliminate unprofitable services, which also can raise ethical concerns.

Ethical Challenges

Physicians and other caregivers have moral responsibilities when delivering clinical care. These professionals are guided by the principles of beneficence and nonmaleficence. *Beneficence* means that a health services organization has an ethical obligation to do all it can to alleviate suffering caused by ill health and injury. This obligation includes providing essential services, such as emergency care, to needy individuals who do not have the ability to pay. Closely related to beneficence, *nonmaleficence* means that care providers have a moral obligation not to harm the patients. Nevertheless, many physicians encounter issues such as legalized abortion, physician-assisted suicide, artificial prolongation of life, and experimentation.

No less challenging is the ethical issue surrounding the definition of extraordinary or heroic measures to sustain a person's life. Medical and legal experts differ on the controversial issue of withdrawing nutrition and other means of life support for dying patients (Bresnohan & Drane, 1986). Such issues do not have easy answers, and most of the time physicians must follow their own consciences and apply personal ethical values. Other legal and ethical standards in medical treatment require the patient's consent before treatment is rendered, a discussion of the various treatment alternatives, and patient's participation in decision making and the selection of treatment options. Health care providers are duty bound to hold all patient information in strict confidence. Fairness, equality, and nondiscrimination are also essential in the delivery of health care.

Addressing Ethical Issues

Many health care organizations, especially large acute care hospitals, now have ethics committees. The ethics committee is charged with the responsibility of developing guidelines and standards for ethical decision making in the provision of health care (Paris, 1995). Ethics committees are also responsible for resolving issues related to medical ethics. Such committees are interdisciplinary, involving physicians, nurses, clergy, social workers, legal experts, ethicists, and administrators.

Certain legal mechanisms are also available to help deal with difficult decisions about life and death. The Patient Self-Determination Act of 1990 applies to all health care facilities participating in Medicare or Medicaid. The law requires hospitals and other facilities to provide all patients, on admission, with information on patients' rights.

Informed consent is a basic patient right. The patient has the right to make an informed choice regarding medical treatment, including the right to refuse treatment. For a patient who is mentally capable, physicians must provide all the information the patient asks for or should have to make a properly informed decision.

Patients also have the right to formulate *advance directives*. It means that the patient can express in advance his or her wishes regarding continuation or withdrawal of treatment in the event that he or she becomes incompetent. When advance directives are not available, the burden of ethical decision making falls squarely on the shoulders of those responsible for providing health care services. In actual practice, however, discussions between physicians and patients about the prognosis at the end of life are infrequent and limited in scope (Bradley et al., 2001). Hence, relatively few people use advance directives. Physicians can play an important role by engaging in discussions about patients' preferences regarding end-of-life decisions.

Public Trust

Communities must place a high degree of trust in their hospitals, but occasionally, behavior of some hospitals has called this trust into question. Hospital administrators have a fiduciary responsibility. They are responsible for acting prudently in managing the affairs of the organization. Because a hospital's mission is to benefit the community, the hospital should be viewed as a community asset regardless of whether it is investor owned or nonprofit. When such a viewpoint is lost and a hospital's board and its executives start placing other priorities ahead of their main responsibility to serve the community, a breach of public trust can occur. As business enterprises, hospitals must respond to changes in the health care delivery system. Hospitals must also maintain their financial and operational integrity. The real danger is when these concerns are put above a genuine concern for the welfare of the patients and the community. Because hospitals form the institutional hub of health care delivery, their integrity within the system is crucial.

There have been instances where a relentless pursuit of profits may have blinded the management to the primary mission of their institutions. For example, in a survey of 23,768 patients who had been discharged from hospitals in 12 states, concerns were expressed regarding reduced access to care, higher expenses, a sense that medical decisions were not made in the patients' best interests, and a feeling that caregivers were uncaring and impersonal (Lagnado, 1997). Other public-opinion surveys have shown eroding public trust in hospitals, along with a widespread belief that fraud is rampant in health care. Several hospitals and multihospital systems have been under investigation for Medicare fraud and abuse. In some instances, fines and jail sentences have resulted for hospital executives indicted for fraud. Although most hospital executives are honest, the wide negative publicity such reports generate does influence the public's perception of hospitals in general. Hospital boards and administrators have a responsibility to take aggressive steps to prevent the erosion of public trust. Rebuilding lost trust in the face of scandals and negative press can squander resources that are actually meant for serving the public.

Hospitals are increasingly being held accountable for enhancing the health status of the communities they are supposed to serve. A growing emphasis on wellness and health promotion is part of this mandate.

CONCLUSION

Any facility that treats patients on the basis of an overnight stay is called an inpatient facility. The most common types of inpatient facilities are hospitals and nursing homes. Both of these institutions trace their beginnings to the almshouses of the 18th and 19th centuries, but as medical science advanced, hospitals emerged as institutions specializing in acute care and surgical services. Today, along with physician offices, hospitals are primary settings for health care delivery. By entering into other types of services such as long-term care and outpatient services, hospitals in many parts of the country have been transformed into integrated delivery systems that deliver a full range of health care services.

REFERENCES

American Hospital Association. 1990. *Hospital Statistics 1990–1991 Edition.* Chicago: American Hospital Association.

American Hospital Association. 1994. *AHA Guide to the Health Care Field 1994 Edition.* Chicago: American Hospital Association.

Anonymous. 2002. Nearly half of U.S. public hospitals had negative margins in 2000. *Healthcare Financial Management* 56 (9):22–23.

Bradley, E. H., et al. 2001. Documentation of discussions about prognosis with terminally ill patients. *American Journal of Medicine* 111 (3):218–223.

Bresnohan, J. F., and J. F. Drane. 1986. A challenge to examine the meaning of living and dying. *Health Progress* 67:32–37, 98.

Haglund, C. L., and W. L. Dowling. 1993. The hospital. In S. J. Williams and P. R. Torrens (eds.). *Introduction to Health Services*, 4th ed. (pp. 135–176). Albany, NY: Delmar Publishers.

Health Forum. 2001. *AHA Guide to the Health Care Field. 2001–2002 Edition.* Chicago: Health Forum.

Lagnado, L. 1997, January 28. Patients give hospitals poor score card. *Wall Street Journal*, B1.

National Center for Health Statistics. 2002. *Health, United States, 2002.* Hyattsville, MD: Department of Health and Human Services.

National Center for Health Statistics. 2007. *Health, United States, 2007.* Hyattsville, MD: US Department of Health and Human Services.

Nudelman, P. M., and L. M. Andrews. 1996. The "value added" or not-for-profit health plans. *New England Journal of Medicine* 334 (16):1057–1059.

Paris, M. 1995. The medical staff. In L. F. Wolper (ed.). *Health Care Administration: Principles, Practices, Structure, and Delivery*, 2nd ed. (pp. 32–46). Gaithersburg, MD: Aspen Publishers.

Raffel, M. W. 1980. *The U.S. Health System: Origins and Functions*. New York: John Wiley and Sons.

Raffel, M. W., and N. K. Raffel. 1989. *The U.S. Health System: Origins and Functions*, 3rd ed. Albany, NY: Delmar Publishers.

Raffel, M. W., and N. K. Raffel. 1994. *The U.S. Health System: Origins and Functions*, 4th ed. Albany, NY: Delmar Publishers.

Rakich, J. S., et al. 1992. *Managing Health Services Organizations*, 3rd ed. Baltimore, MD: Health Professions Press.

Safety Net in Shreds. 2002. *Trustee* 55:3.

Stewart, D. A. 1973. The history and status of proprietary hospitals. *Blue Cross Reports—Research Series 9*. Chicago: Blue Cross Association.

Teisberg, E. D., et al. 1991. *The Hospital Sector in 1992*. Boston: Harvard Business School.

U.S. Census Bureau. 2008. *Statistical Abstract of the United States, 2008*. Washington, DC: U.S. Census Bureau.

Wolfson, J., and S. L. Hopes. 1994. What makes tax-exempt hospitals special? *Healthcare Financial Management* July:56–60.

Wolper, L. F., and J. J. Peña. 1995. History of hospitals. In L. F. Wolper (ed.). *Health Care Administration: Principles, Practices, Structure, and Delivery*, 2nd ed. (pp. 3–15). Gaithersburg, MD: Aspen Publishers.

Chapter 9

Managed Care and Integrated Systems

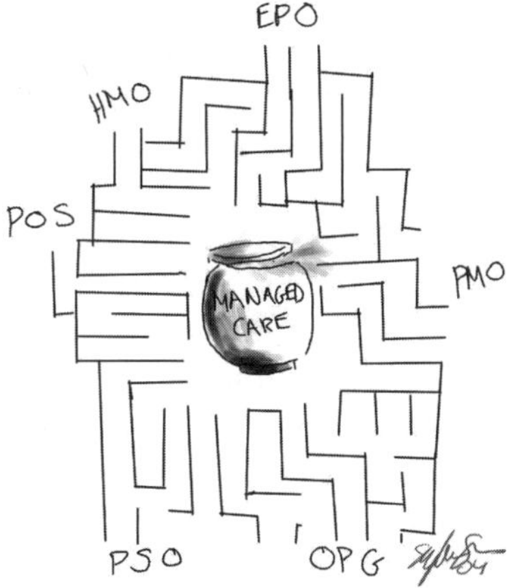

INTRODUCTION

Since around 1990, managed care has been the single most dominant force in the fundamental transformation of health care delivery in the United States. At first, some observers viewed the managed care phenomenon as an aberration. However, as private employers began to realize cost savings and public policy makers and administrators saw the opportunity to slow down the growing expense of providing health care through the Medicare and Medicaid programs, they increasingly turned to managed care. For now, managed care has become firmly entrenched in the United States, and some other countries have adopted its features to reform their own traditional mechanisms of health care delivery.

Shortly after the birth of health insurance in the United States, Blue Cross/Blue Shield and then other commercial insurance companies started to dominate the health insurance market. Health insurance became employer based, but neither the employers nor the insurance companies had any incentive to manage the delivery of services or payments made to providers. Providers showed a strong preference to be paid on a fee-for-service basis. Thus, both the delivery of health care and payment got out of control. Managed care was designed to control both the quantity of health care delivered and the amount of reimbursement to providers.

Managed care has experienced unprecedented success. For example, only 27% of the employees insured through employer-sponsored health insurance were enrolled in managed care plans in 1988. By 2002, 95% were enrolled in managed care. This growth occurred despite attacks on managed care from physicians and consumers. In 2007, only 3% of workers were enrolled in employer-sponsored conventional health insurance plans (Claxton et al., 2007). Many conventional insurance companies and Blue Cross/Blue Shield have been offering managed care plans.

By enrolling a large segment of the insured U.S. population and taking responsibility to procure cost-effective health care for the enrollees, managed care organizations (MCOs) garnered enormous buying power. To a large extent, consolidation by providers was in response to this growing power of MCOs. These changes have given rise to new organizational arrangements. The freestanding hospital and the solo practitioner continue to be replaced with hospital systems and group practices of physicians as they integrate their services (Johnson, 1994). In many instances, physicians and hospitals have been forming partnerships. These organizational alliances and networks are referred to as integrated delivery systems or health networks.

WHAT IS MANAGED CARE?

Managed care is a mechanism of providing health care services in which a single organization takes on the management of financing, insurance, delivery, and payment. (1) Financing: Premiums are usually negotiated between employers and the MCO. Generally, a fixed premium per enrollee includes all health care services provided for in a contract. (2) Insurance: The MCO collects premiums for insuring groups of enrollees. It then functions like an insurance company by assuming all risk. In other words, it takes financial responsibility if the total cost of services provided exceeds the revenue from fixed premiums. MCOs retain approximately 15%

to 20% of the premium dollar to manage risk and to cover their own administrative expenses. The rest is spent on health care services. (3) Delivery: Unlike conventional insurance, the MCO arranges to provide health care to its enrollees. To do so, most MCOs establish contracts with physicians, clinics, and hospitals. These providers operate independently but are linked to the MCO through legal contracts. Some very large MCOs have their own physicians on salary and operate their own clinics, and in some instances, MCOs even operate their own hospitals. To keep costs under control, MCOs use various methods to manage the utilization of health care services. (4) Payment: The most common methods used for reimbursing providers are capitation and discounted fees. Under *capitation*, the provider is paid a fixed monthly sum per enrollee, often called a per member per month (PMPM) payment. The provider receives the capitated fee per enrollee regardless of whether the enrollee uses health care services and regardless of the quantity of services used. The provider is responsible for providing all needed health care services determined to be medically necessary. Thus, under capitation, a portion of the risk is shifted from the MCO to the provider. When providers have to bear some of the risk, they become prudent in providing services cost-effectively. They can lose money if they deliver services indiscriminately. The discounted fee arrangement uses a modified form of fee for service. After services have been delivered, the provider can bill the MCO for each service separately but is paid according to a schedule of fees. The fee schedule is prenegotiated and is based on discounts off the regular fees the provider would otherwise charge. Providers agree to discount their regular fees in exchange for the volume of patients the MCO brings them. (See **Exhibit 9.1**.)

Exhibit 9.1 Main Characteristics of Managed Care

MCOs manage financing, insurance, delivery, and payment for providing health care:

- Premiums are usually negotiated between MCOs and employers.
- MCOs function like an insurance company and assume risk.
- MCOs arrange to provide health care, mainly through contracts with providers.
- MCOs manage the utilization of health care services.
- Common payment methods are capitation and discounted fees.

Since 1991, MCOs have been accredited by the National Committee for Quality Assurance (NCQA). Accreditation is voluntary. The NCQA has also designed a set of standardized performance measures for MCOs. Commonly referred to as managed care report cards, the national standards and performance reports on individual MCOs are contained in the Health Plan Employer Data and Information Set (HEDIS). The report cards are voluntary efforts and were begun out of concerns that controlling health care utilization could adversely affect the quality of care. HEDIS data include a number of different measures on cost and quality. Although there is no federal legislation requiring that MCOs comply with HEDIS standards, compliance is required in some states.

EVOLUTION AND GROWTH OF MANAGED CARE

In the early 1900s, certain railroad, mining, and lumber companies located in isolated areas employed salaried physicians to provide medical care to workers. In other instances, such companies contracted with physicians and hospitals at a flat fee per worker. Such arrangements can be viewed as prototypes of today's managed care. The first known private health insurance plan started at the Baylor University Hospital in Dallas, Texas, in 1929 was also a prepaid plan. For a predetermined fixed fee per month, Baylor, and subsequently other hospitals, provided inpatient services. Thus, the financing of the first health insurance plan was based on capitation. Later, during the 1940s, some large health plans emerged in New York, California, Washington state, and St. Louis. These also provided comprehensive health care to enrolled populations for a capitated fee. For example, the well-known Kaiser Permanente plan started in California in 1942 when the industrialist Henry J. Kaiser was faced with the problem of providing health care to his 30,000 workers. In 1945, the Permanente Health Plan was made available to the general public. Even today, the Kaiser Foundation Health Plan, operated by Kaiser Permanente, is the largest health maintenance organization (HMO) in the United States. In the rest of the country, however, delivery of health care was predominantly under the fee-for-service system. Commercial insurance companies were the dominant players in the private health insurance market.

The Health Maintenance Organization Act of 1973 was passed out of concern for escalating health care expenditures. Subsequent to the creation of Medicare and Medicaid, national health expenditures rose at more than double the rate of growth in the consumer price index during the 5-year period from 1966 to 1971 (**Figure 9.1**). The law was designed to provide an alternative to the traditional fee-for-service practice of medicine. It was aimed at stimulating the growth of HMOs by providing federal funds to establish new HMOs (Wilson & Neuhauser, 1985, p. 206). The reasoning behind promoting HMO growth was that medical care delivery under capitation would stimulate competition among health plans, increase efficiency, and slow the rate of growth in health care expenditures. The law's objective was to create 1,700 HMOs to serve 40 million members by 1976 (Iglehart, 1994). By the end of the 1970s, however, enrollment in HMOs was still below 10 million.

During the 1980s, managed care experienced relatively slow growth, but in states such as California and Minnesota, growth was faster than in most parts of the United States. However, health care costs continued to rise uncontrollably (**Figure 9.2**). Private businesses were increasingly

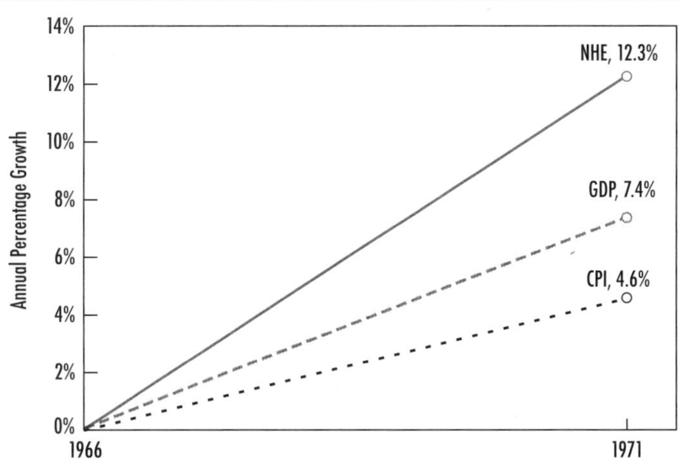

Figure 9.1 Average Annual Rates of Increase in National Health Expenditures (NHE), Gross Domestic Product (GDP), and Consumer Price Index (CPI) Between 1966 and 1971.

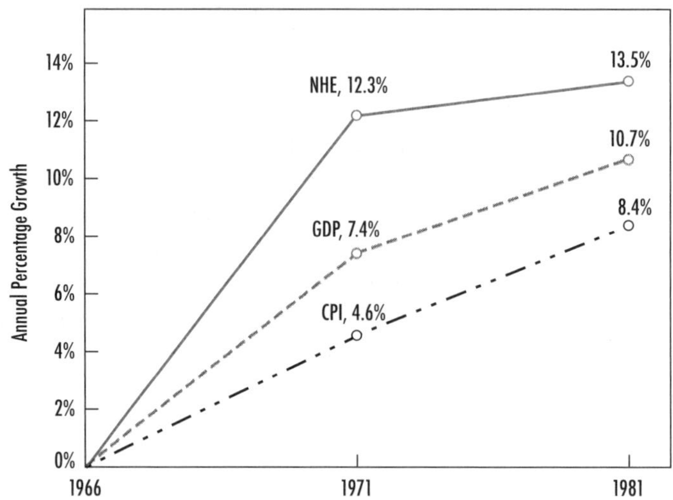

Figure 9.2 Average Annual Rates of Increase in NHE, GDP, and CPI Between 1966 and 1971 and Between 1971 and 1981.

threatened by the erosion of profits resulting from double-digit increases in the cost of health care premiums. As health insurance became less and less affordable, employers started switching from traditional health insurance to managed care plans during the 1980s, but it was not until the early 1990s that a veritable managed care revolution got under way as private employers experienced a total increase of 217% (12.2% average annual increase) in the cost of health insurance between 1980 and 1990. **Figure 9.3** illustrates the growth of enrollment in managed care plans.

As managed care grew, competition among MCOs gave rise to new forms of managed care plans. To differentiate among themselves, some new organizations adopted variations in payment. Preferred provider organizations (PPOs), for example, differentiated by using discounted fee payments instead of capitation. Other MCOs differentiated themselves according to how the medical care providers were organized. Still others offered their enrollees a choice between providers who were contractually affiliated with the organization and those who were not. MCOs also adopted various methods to control health care costs by actively monitoring utilization.

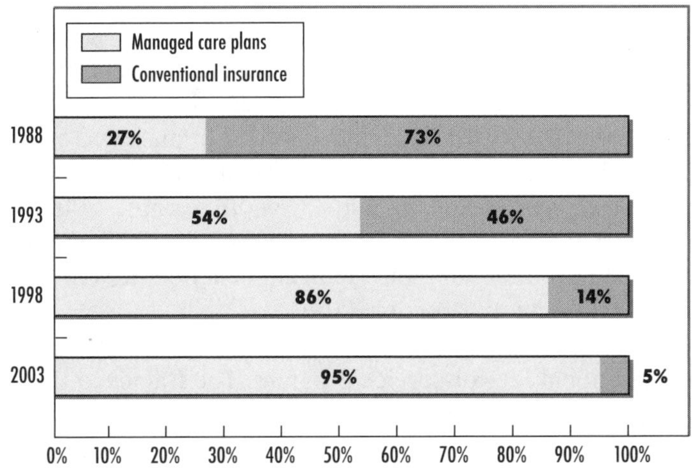

Figure 9.3 Enrollment of Workers in Employer-Sponsored Health Plans (Selected Years)

Managed Care and Private Health Insurance

Managed care has become the primary vehicle for delivering health care to the vast majority of Americans and is now a matured industry in the United States. In essence, private health insurance can now be equated to managed care, whether it is obtained through a small or large employer. High-deductible health plans (see Chapter 6) are also commonly offered in the form of managed care plans. Many employers offer their workers a choice of plans with level-dollar employer contributions, meaning workers pay more themselves—in premium contributions as well as deductibles and copayments—if they choose a more expensive conventional insurance plan.

Managed Care and Public Health Insurance

Although managed care has seen remarkable growth in the private health insurance market, the enrollment of Medicaid and Medicare beneficiaries into managed care has not met with the same degree of success. Waivers under the Social Security Act, particularly Sections 1115 and 1915(b), allowed states to enroll their Medicaid recipients in managed care plans. Later, the Balanced Budget Act of 1997 gave states the authority to implement mandatory managed care programs without federal waivers (Moscovice et al., 1998). As a result, enrollment has grown at a rapid pace. This growth has been realized particularly as MCOs were able to expand their markets into rural areas. In 2007, all states except Alaska, Mississippi, and Wyoming had Medicaid recipients enrolled in managed care plans. Of all Medicaid beneficiaries nationwide, 63.5% received health care services through managed care plans in 2007 (Sanofi-Aventis, 2008), which is somewhat lower than 65% in 2006 (Sanofi-Aventis, 2007). Approximately 15 states had 80% or more of their Medicaid beneficiaries enrolled in managed care in 2007 (Sanofi-Aventis, 2008).

For Medicare beneficiaries, enrollment in managed care is an alternative to the traditional fee-for-service program. The Balanced Budget Act of 1997 created the Medicare+Choice program (now Medicare Advantage or Part C, see Chapter 6). The program was enacted to increase Medicare enrollment into managed care. However, Medicare offers its beneficiaries the choice between Medicare Advantage and the traditional fee-for-service program, and the latter has been more popular with Medicare beneficiaries. In 2007, almost 20% of the beneficiaries were enrolled in Medicare Advantage; up from 16.6% in 2006 (Sanofi-Aventis, 2007; Sanofi-Aventis, 2008).

UTILIZATION CONTROL METHODS IN MANAGED CARE

MCOs use three main approaches to monitor and control the utilization of services: (1) Expert evaluation of what services are medically necessary in a given case. Such an evaluation ensures that only medically necessary services are actually provided. (2) Determination of how services can be provided most inexpensively while maintaining acceptable standards of quality. For example, often similar services can be obtained as an outpatient or as an inpatient. Outpatient services cost less. Similarly, generic drugs cost less than brand-name drugs. (3) Review of the process of care and changes in the patient's condition to revise the course of medical treatment if necessary. Utilization management of inpatient services takes priority because such services account for 40% or more of the total expenses in a managed care plan (Kongstvedt, 1995). The methods most commonly used for utilization monitoring and control are gatekeeping and utilization review. Generally, HMOs employ tighter utilization controls than other types of managed care plans, which are discussed later in this chapter.

Gatekeeping

Commonly used by HMOs, *gatekeeping* is an arrangement that requires a primary care physician to coordinate all health care services needed by an enrollee. The physicians usually have formal affiliations with the HMO and are referred to as in-network providers. Gatekeeping also emphasizes preventive care, routine physical examinations, and other primary care services that are delivered by the primary care gatekeeper. Secondary care services, such as diagnostic testing, consultation from specialists, and admission to a hospital, are provided only when the patient is referred by the gatekeeper. Thus, the gatekeeper controls access to higher levels of medical services.

Utilization Review

Utilization review is the process of evaluating the appropriateness of services provided. It is sometimes misunderstood to be a mechanism for denying services, but its main objective is to review each case and to determine the most appropriate level of services. There are three main types of utilization review: prospective, concurrent, and retrospective.

Prospective Utilization Review

Under this method, the medical necessity for certain treatments is determined before the care is actually delivered. An example of prospective utilization review is the decision by a primary care gatekeeper to refer or not refer a patient to a specialist. However, not all managed care plans use gatekeepers. Some plans require the enrollee or the provider to call the plan administrators for *precertification*, that is, approval before certain services are provided. Most plans use established clinical guidelines to determine the appropriateness of services. Preauthorization of hospital admissions and second opinions for surgical procedures are examples of precertification. In case of an emergency admission to an inpatient facility, plans generally require notification within 24 hours. One of the main objectives of prospective review is to prevent unnecessary or inappropriate institutionalization or other courses of treatment such as surgery.

Concurrent Utilization Review

Concurrent utilization review occurs when decisions regarding appropriateness are made during the course of health care utilization. The most common examples of this type of review involve monitoring the length of inpatient stays. When a patient is hospitalized, a certain number of inpatient days are generally preapproved. A trained nurse then monitors the patient's status and reviews the case with a physician if a longer stay is necessary. A decision is made to authorize or deny additional days.

Discharge planning is an important component of concurrent utilization review. A patient's prognosis for recovery, expected outcomes, and anticipated day of discharge are critical elements of concurrent review. *Discharge planning* deals with the patient's ongoing care and evaluates any special requirements that are necessary after discharge. For example, if a patient is admitted with a fractured hip, it is important to decide whether home health care or a skilled nursing facility would be more appropriate for convalescent care. If the patient requires care in a skilled nursing facility, then discharge planning must find out whether the appropriate level of rehabilitation services would be available and for how long insurance will pay for rehabilitation therapy in a long-term care setting.

Retrospective Utilization Review

Retrospective utilization review refers to managing utilization after services have already been delivered. The review is based on an examination of medical records to assess the appropriateness of care. The review may involve an assessment of individual cases. Large claims may be reviewed for billing accuracy. Retrospective review may also involve an analysis of data to examine patterns of excessive utilization or underutilization. *Underutilization* occurs when medically necessary care is not delivered.

TYPES OF MANAGED CARE ORGANIZATIONS

Three main factors led to the development of different types of managed care plans, the first and most important being choice of providers. HMOs were the most common type of MCOs in the 1970s, but HMO plans had inherent weaknesses, especially with regard to choice of providers. Other types of MCO plans that offered greater choice were developed mainly to compete with the more restrictive HMO plans. Second, different ways of arranging the delivery of services led to different forms of MCOs because there is no single way to arrange providers into a delivery network. Payment and risk sharing make up the third major factor.

Until about 1988, the various types of MCOs were quite distinct. Since then, the differences between traditional forms of health insurance and managed care have narrowed substantially. For example, most traditional insurance plans now incorporate some utilization management features that were once found only in MCOs (Wagner, 1995). Many commercial insurance companies have also developed their own managed care plans.

HMOs

HMOs were the first type of managed care plans to appear on the market. An HMO is distinguished from other types of plans by its focus on wellness care, capitation as the method of payment to providers, and the use of in-network providers by the enrollees. In the traditional system, health insurance pays for medical care only when a person is ill. An HMO not only provides medical care during illness but also offers a variety of services to help people maintain their health, hence the name "health maintenance" organization. HMOs place considerable emphasis on preventive and screening services through routine checkups and tests. Prevention of disease and early detection and treatment save health care costs in the long run when the course of a disease is checked before it turns into a complex case. As an incentive to the enrollees to seek wellness care, HMO plans typically do not have annual deductibles. HMOs also have lower copayments than do other types of plans.

Under capitation, HMOs pay the providers a fixed PMPM rate that covers a full range of health care services. The utilization of these services is coordinated and managed by the HMO, mainly through primary care gatekeepers.

Enrollees must obtain services from in-network hospitals, physicians, and other health care providers. Specialty services, such as mental health and substance abuse treatment, are frequently carved out. A *carve out* is a special contract outside regular capitation, which is funded separately by the HMO.

There are four common HMO models. They differ from each other according to the arrangements they make with participating physicians. The four common HMO models are the staff, group, network, and independent practice association models.

Staff Model

A staff model HMO employs its own salaried physicians. The physicians are typically paid fixed salaries, and at the end of the year, a pool of money is distributed among the physicians in the form of bonuses based on each physician's productivity and the HMO's profitability. Physicians work only for their employer HMO and provide services to that HMO's enrollees (Rakich et al., 1992, p. 281). Staff model HMOs must employ physicians in all of the common specialties to provide for the health care needs of their members. Contracts with selected subspecialties are established for infrequently needed services. The HMO operates one or more ambulatory care facilities. These contain physicians' offices, support staff, and may have ancillary support facilities, such as laboratory and radiology departments. In most instances, the HMO contracts with area hospitals for inpatient services (Wagner, 1995).

Compared with other HMO models, staff model HMOs are able to exercise a greater degree of control over the practice patterns of their physicians. Hence, it is easier to monitor utilization. Even so, the fixed salary expense can be high, which requires that these HMOs must have a large number of members to support the operating expenses. Enrollees generally have a limited choice of physicians. Because of its disadvantages, the staff model has been the least popular type of HMO. Nationwide, the number of staff model HMOs has continued to decline.

Group Model

A group model HMO contracts with a multispecialty group practice and separately with one or more hospitals to provide comprehensive services to its members. The physicians are employed by the group practice, not the HMO. The HMO generally pays an all-inclusive capitation fee to the group practice to provide physician services to its members. The group practice may be an independent practice, in which case the physicians are generally allowed to treat non-HMO patients as well. Under a different scenario, the HMO may own the group practice as a separate corporation but one that is administratively tied to the HMO. In this case, the group practice may provide services exclusively to the HMO's members. An exclusive contract with a group practice enables the HMO to exercise better control over utilization. Even when it is not an exclusive contract, the HMO brings a block of business to the group practice, which gives the HMO a fair amount of leverage regarding financial terms and utilization controls.

Network Model

Under the network model, the HMO contracts with more than one medical group practice. This model is particularly suited for operations in large metropolitan areas and across widespread geographic regions where group practices are located. Each group practice is paid a capitation fee based on the number of enrollees. The group is responsible for providing all physician services. It can make referrals to specialists but is financially responsible for reimbursing them for any referrals it makes. The network model is generally able to offer a wider choice of physicians than the staff or group models. The main disadvantage is the dilution of utilization control.

Independent Practice Association Model

Of the four HMO models, the independent practice association (IPA) model has been the most successful in terms of the largest share of enrollments. An IPA is a legal entity separate from the HMO. The IPA establishes contracts with both independent solo practitioners and group practices. Instead of establishing contracts with individual physicians or groups, the HMO contracts with the IPA for physician services. Physicians do not have a contract with the HMO, but with the IPA. Hence, the IPA functions as an intermediary representing a large number of physicians. The IPA is generally paid a capitation amount by the HMO. The IPA retains administrative control over how it pays its physicians. It may reimburse physicians through capitation or some other mechanism, such as modified fee for service. The IPA often shares risk with the physicians and assumes the responsibility for utilization management and quality assessment.

Under the IPA model, the HMO is still responsible for providing health care services to its enrollees, but the logistics of arranging physician services are shifted to the IPA. The HMO is thus relieved of the administrative burden of establishing contracts with numerous providers and controlling utilization. Financial risk is also transferred to the IPA.

The IPA model provides an expanded choice of providers to enrollees. It also allows small groups and individual physicians the opportunity to participate in managed care and to get a slice of the revenues. IPAs may be independently established by community physicians, or the HMO may create an IPA and invite community physicians to participate in it. An IPA may also be hospital based and structured so that only physicians from one or two hospitals are eligible to participate in it (Wagner, 1995). One major disadvantage of the IPA model is that if a contract is lost, the HMO loses a large number of participating physicians.

PPOs

PPO plans were created by insurance companies in response to the growth of HMOs. PPOs differentiated themselves by offering out-of-network options for enrollees. By early 1990s, PPOs became more popular and their market share began to exceed that of HMOs.

PPO enrollees agree to use preferred providers with whom the PPO has established contracts, but the enrollees are also allowed the choice of using physicians and hospitals outside the network. Higher copayments apply for using nonpreferred providers. The additional out-of-pocket expenses largely act as a deterrent to going outside the network.

Instead of capitation, PPOs make discounted fee arrangements with providers. The discounts can range between 25% and 35% off the providers' regular fees. Negotiated payment arrangements with hospitals can take any of the various forms discussed in Chapter 6, such as payments based on diagnosis-related groups, bundled charges for certain services, and discounts. Hence, no direct risk sharing with providers is involved. PPOs also apply fewer restrictions to the care-seeking behavior of enrollees. In most instances, they do not use primary care gatekeeping, which allows enrollees to see specialists without being referred by a primary care physician. Precertification (prospective utilization review) is generally employed only for hospitalization and high-cost outpatient procedures (Robinson, 2002).

Point-of-Service Plans

Point-of-service (POS) plans combine features of classic HMOs with some of the characteristics of patient choice found in PPOs. POS plans thus overcome the drawback of restricted provider choice but retain the benefits of tight utilization management. Like HMOs, they also use capitation or other risk-based reimbursement for the providers. Gatekeeping may be used to control utilization. Members may obtain specialty services without referral from in-network providers or incur higher out-of-pocket costs and obtain services from out-of-network providers. From the consumer's perspective, free choice of providers was a major selling point for POS plans, but after reaching a peak in popularity in 1998–1999, enrollment in POS plans gradually declined mainly because of the high out-of-pocket costs associated with them.

IMPACT ON COST, ACCESS, AND QUALITY

Influence on Cost Containment

Other countries assign the task of cost reduction to the government, which controls health care expenditures by budgeting systemwide expenditures and imposing limits on services and payments to providers. In the United States, the primary responsibility for cost containment falls on the private sector, but the government also has implemented various methods, mostly aimed at controlling Medicaid and Medicare costs. The private sector approach to cost containment has been the expansion of managed care, which has been widely credited for slowing down the rate of growth in health care expenditures during the 1990s. However, a backlash from consumers and providers during the 1990s also prevented managed care from achieving its full potential to control costs. Between 2001 and 2004, health insurance premiums rose at double-digit annual rates. Since then, rise in premiums has declined consistently each year. This has been achieved by shifting costs to the insured through higher cost sharing.

Impact on Access

Managed care enrollees generally have good access to primary care, preventive services, and health promotion activities (Udvarhelyi et al.,

1991). Compared to traditional fee for service, HMO enrollees also experience fewer disparities in health care access and utilization with regard to income, race, and ethnicity (Cook, 2007; DeFrancesco, 2002). Behavioral health carve outs have also been instrumental in addressing long-standing challenges in access and utilization of behavioral health care (Frank & Garfield, 2007). On a larger scale, however, it does not appear that managed care has made health insurance more affordable particularly for small employers.

Influence on Quality of Care

Despite anecdotes, individual perceptions, and isolated stories propagated by the news media, no comprehensive research to date has clearly demonstrated that the growth of managed care has been at the expense of the quality of care delivered to Americans. Actually, available evidence points to the contrary. The quality of health care provided by MCOs has improved over time (Hofmann, 2002). Early detection and treatment is more likely in a managed care plan than in a traditional fee-for-service plan (Riley et al., 1999). Financial pressures do not lead to significant changes in physician behavior because under capitation a physician takes full responsibility for the patient's overall care (Eikel, 2002).

Also, a comprehensive review of the literature by Miller and Luft (2002) concluded that HMO and non-HMO plans provided roughly equal quality of care as measured by a wide range of conditions, diseases, and interventions. At the same time, HMOs lower the use of hospital and other expensive resources. Hence, medical care delivered through managed care plans has been cost-effective. Recent evidence also suggests that race, ethnicity, and socioeconomic status of managed care enrollees have little or no effect on the quality of care they receive (Balsa et al., 2007; Brown et al., 2005). On the other hand, evaluation of the existing literature does point to lower access and lower enrollee satisfaction ratings for HMO plans compared with non-HMO plans (Miller & Luft, 2002). Also, quality of care may be lower in for-profit health plans compared to nonprofit plans (Himmelstein et al., 1999; Schneider et al., 2005). In addition, quality may not be consistent across all managed care plans. Quality of care may be lower in some managed care plans compared to commercial plans (Landon et al., 2007).

HEALTH NETWORKS

With the rapid growth of managed care, MCOs acquired enormous power. On the other hand, the bargaining power of independent health delivery organizations, such as hospitals and clinics, was being eroded. Health care organizations also came under growing pressure to reduce costs and deliver services efficiently to populations spread over large geographic areas. It became increasingly more difficult for smaller organizations, such as solo physician practices and small clinics and hospitals, to cope with external changes and stay profitable. For many health care delivery organizations, integration into networks has been a rational choice for survival. For example, even some large multispecialty physician groups often do not have adequate financial reserves. When managed care contracts are changed, huge blocks of patients may come and go. This fluctuation can result in a wild financial roller coaster ride. Joining an integrated system may help minimize such financial uncertainties (Goldfarb, 1993). Organizational integration occurred in such an environment of uncertainty that accompanied the growth of managed care.

Integrated health care organizations are commonly referred to as integrated delivery systems or health networks. They have been formed mainly by large hospitals that have acquired other health care delivery organizations. Various other legal arrangements, such as joint ventures, alliances, and contract-based affiliations, also enable organizations to combine their resources so that they can provide a full array of health care services to large communities. In other instances, hospitals have added services by building new facilities. Examples include women's health centers, specialized cardiac care clinics, outpatient surgery centers, and rehabilitation clinics. Sometimes, satellite service centers are opened or mobile delivery programs are instituted to serve smaller communities located outside an organization's primary market base. In other instances, these large full-service organizations have created their own managed care plans or have directly contracted with large employers to provide one-stop health care services to their employees. A fully integrated health network typically includes the following (DeLuca & Cagan, 1998):

- One or more acute-care hospitals
- Ambulatory-care facilities

- One or more physician group practices
- One or more long-term care facilities
- Home health and hospice services
- Ownership or contract with one or more MCOs

Organizational integration has enabled hospitals to expand into new markets. It has intensified competition among health care providers. It has enabled large health service organizations to win sizable managed care contracts or offer their own health plans. Health networks help achieve cost savings as a result of resource sharing and elimination of duplication. On the other hand, organizational networks become complex and therefore difficult to manage. Physician relations, for instance, is one area that many networks are still trying to figure out.

After a rapid growth, merger and acquisition activity has stabilized since the late 1990s. There are approximately 600 health networks operating in the United States, and nearly half of all acute-care hospitals are affiliated with an integrated network (Anonymous, 2004).

TYPES OF INTEGRATION

Integration Based on Major Participants

Physicians and hospitals have been two key participants in the formation of integrated organizations because, in almost all instances, one entity cannot function without the other. Hence, the formation of *physician–hospital organizations* (PHOs) has been a common type of integration. A PHO is a legal entity that forms an alliance between a hospital and local physicians and combines their services within one organization. It allows both entities to have greater bargaining power in contract negotiations with MCOs. Large PHOs can also contract their services directly to employers. A large number of physicians allied with a hospital can provide one-stop shopping for the enrollees. PHO formation is often initiated by the hospital, but it is unlikely to succeed without the participation of the medical staff leaders. PHOs provide the benefits of integration while preserving the independence and autonomy of physicians.

Between 1998 and 2000, the number of hospitals associated with PHOs had more than doubled, but after this initial surge, PHOs have shrunk by one-third. The percentage of hospitals with PHOs dropped from 32% in 1995 to less than 23% in 2004 (Taylor, 2006). Many failed because of poor management, undercapitalization, and federal scrutiny.

Integration Based on Type of Ownership or Affiliation

Ownership involves the purchase of a controlling interest in another company, which can be accomplished through either merger or acquisition. Ownership does not have to be an all-or-nothing deal. Joint ventures allow two or more entities to participate in joint ownership of a new entity. A third approach, which can take various forms, does not involve ownership of another company's assets. In principle, it may simply involve cooperative arrangements and joint responsibilities. There may simply be sharing of existing resources among two or more organizations or formation of an organization based on contracts.

Acquisitions and Mergers

Acquisition refers to the purchase of one organization by another. The acquired company ceases to exist as a separate entity and is absorbed under the name of the purchasing corporation. A *merger* involves a mutual agreement to unify two or more organizations into a single entity. The separate assets of two organizations are brought together, typically under a new name. Both former entities cease to exist, and a new corporation is formed.

Small hospitals may merge together to gain efficiencies by eliminating the duplication of services. Acquisitions and mergers can also help an organization expand into new geographic markets. A large hospital may acquire smaller hospitals to serve as satellites in a large metropolitan area with sprawling suburbs. A regional health care system may be formed after a large hospital has acquired other hospitals and diversified into services such as ambulatory care, long-term care, and rehabilitation.

Joint Ventures

A *joint venture* results when two or more institutions share resources to create a new organization to pursue a common purpose (Pelfrey & Theisen, 1989). Each of the participants in a joint venture continues to conduct business independently. The new company created by the participants also remains independent. Joint ventures are often used to diversify into new services when the participants can benefit by joining hands rather than competing against each other. Hospitals in a given region may engage in a joint venture to form a home health agency that benefits all partners. An acute-care hospital, a multispecialty physician group practice, a skilled nursing facility, and an insurer may join to offer a managed care plan (Carson et al., 1995, p. 209). In the latter example, each of the participants would continue to operate its own business, and all would have a common stake in the new HMO or PPO.

Alliances

In one respect, the health care industry is unique because organizations often develop cooperative arrangements with rival providers. Cooperation instead of competition, in some situations, eliminates duplication of services while ensuring that all the health needs of the community are fulfilled (Carson et al., 1995, p. 217). An *alliance* is an agreement between two organizations to share their resources without joint ownership of assets. A PHO, for example, can be formed through a merger, a joint venture, or an alliance. Each type of integration determines the extent to which the hospital controls the assets owned by the physicians or group practices.

Establishing links with one or more group practices is generally easier than establishing links with a large number of independent physicians, and alliances are relatively simpler to form than mergers. An alliance is usually a first step that gives both organizations the opportunity to evaluate the advantages of a potential merger. Alliances require little financial commitment and can be easily dissolved if the anticipated benefits do not materialize.

Virtual Organizations

When contractual arrangements between organizations form a new organization, it is referred to as a *virtual organization*, or an organization without walls. The formation of networks based on contractual arrangements is called *virtual integration*. IPAs are a prime example of virtual organizations. A PHO may also be a virtual organization. The main advantage of virtual organizations is that they require less capital to enter new geographic or service markets (Gabel, 1997). They also help bring together scattered entities under one mutually cooperative arrangement.

Integration Based on Service Consolidation

Horizontal Integration

Horizontal integration is a growth strategy in which a health care delivery organization extends its core product or service. For example, an acute-care hospital that adds coronary bypass surgery to its existing surgical services or that builds a suburban acute-care facility is integrating horizontally (Rakich et al., 1992, p. 326). Multihospital chains, nursing facility chains, or a chain of drugstores, all under the same management with member facilities offering the same core services or products, are also horizontally integrated. Horizontally linked organizations may be closely coupled through ownership or loosely coupled through alliances. The main objective of horizontal integration is to achieve geographic expansion. Diversification into new products or services is not achieved through horizontal integration.

Vertical Integration

Vertical integration links services that are at different stages in the production process of health care—for example, organization of preventive services, primary care, acute care, and postacute service delivery around a hospital. The intended purpose of vertical integration is to increase the comprehensiveness and continuity of care. Vertical integration is a diversification strategy. It may be achieved through acquisitions, mergers, joint ventures, or alliances. Health networks are formed through vertical integration. Large hospital systems are particularly attracted to group practices in the interest of vertical integration because group practices can give them a large slice of the patient market. Vertically integrated regional health systems may be the best positioned organizations to become the providers of choice for managed care or for direct contracting with self-insured employers (Brown, 1996).

CONCLUSION

Most insured Americans today receive health care through a managed care organization. MCOs have been credited with cost reductions in health care, and enrollment in managed care plans has continued to grow. Remarkably, the cost savings have been achieved while the overall quality of health care is maintained, with minor exceptions.

Health networks emerged as hospitals and physicians, in particular, faced growing pressures from managed care to deliver services at reduced costs. Integration has enabled large health care organizations to win sizable managed care contracts and, in some instances, to offer their own health insurance plans. However, the delivery of health care has become complex from the standpoint of providers and consumers. Integration of physicians into these large organizations has been particularly challenging.

REFERENCES

Anonymous. 2004. Survey identifies top IHNs, indicates stabilized growth. *Healthcare Financial Management* 58 (3):25.

Balsa, A., et al. 2007. Does managed health care reduce health care disparities between minorities and whites? *Journal of Health Economics* 26 (1):101–121.

Brown, A. F., et al. 2005. Race, ethnicity, socioeconomic position, and quality of care for adults with diabetes enrolled in managed care. *Diabetes Care* 28 (12):2864–2870.

Brown, M. 1996. Mergers, networking, and vertical integration: Managed care and investor-owned hospitals. *Health Care Management Review* 21 (1):29–37.

Carson, K. D., et al. 1995. *Management of Healthcare Organizations*. Cincinnati, OH: South-Western College Publishing.

Claxton, G., et al. 2007. *The Kaiser Family Foundation and Health Research and Educational Trust Employer Health Benefits 2007 Annual Survey*. Menlo Park, CA: Henry J. Kaiser Family Foundation and Chicago, IL: Health Research and Educational Trust.

Cook, B. L. 2007. Effect of Medicaid managed care on racial disparities in health care access. *Health Services Research* 42 (1 Pt 1):124–145.

DeFrancesco, L. B. 2002. HMO enrollees experience fewer disparities than older insured populations. *Findings Brief: Health Care Financing & Organization* 5 (2):1–2.

DeLuca, J. M., and R. E. Cagan. 1998. The integrated delivery system. In *CEO's Guide to Health Care Information Systems* (pp. 35–46). Chicago: Health Forum.

Eikel, C. V. 2002. Fewer patient visits under capitation offset by improved quality of care: Study brings evidence to debate over physician payment methods. *Findings Brief: Health Care Financing & Organization* 5 (3):1–2.

Frank, R. G., and R. L. Garfield. 2007. Managed behavioral health care carve-outs: Past performance and future prospects. *Annual Review of Public Health* 28 (1):303–320.

Gabel, J. 1997. Ten ways HMOs have changed during the 1990s. *Health Affairs* 16 (3):134–145.

Goldfarb, B. 1993. Corporate health care mergers. *Medical World News* 34 (2):26–34.

Himmelstein, D., et al. 1999. Quality of care in investor-owned vs not-for-profit HMOs. *Journal of the American Medical Association* 282 (2):159–163.

Hofmann, M. A. 2002. Quality of health care improving. *Business Insurance* 36 (38):1–2.

Iglehart, J. K. 1994. The American health care system: Managed care. In P. R. Lee and C. L. Estes (eds.). *The Nation's Health*. 4th ed., (pp. 231–237). Boston: Jones and Bartlett Publishers.

Johnson, R. L. 1994. HCMR perspective: The economic era of health care. *Health Care Management Review* 19 (4):64–72.

Kongstvedt, P. R. 1995. Managing hospital utilization. In P. R. Kongstvedt (ed.). *Essentials of Managed Health Care* (pp. 121–135). Gaithersburg, MD: Aspen Publishers.

Landon, B. E., et al. 2007. Quality of care in Medicaid managed care and commercial health plans. *Journal of the American Medical Association* 298 (14):1674–1681.

Miller, R. H., and H. S. Luft. 2002. HMO plan performance update: An analysis of the literature, 1997–2001. *Health Affairs* 21 (4):63–86.

Moscovice, I., et al. 1998. Expanding rural managed care: Enrollment patterns and prospectives. *Health Affairs* 17 (1):172–179.

Pelfrey, S., and B. A. Theisen. 1989. Joint venture in health care. *Journal of Nursing Administration* 19 (4):39–42.

Rakich, J. S., et al. 1992. *Managing Health Services Organizations*, 3rd ed. Baltimore, MD: Health Professions Press.

Riley, G. F., et al. 1999. Stage at diagnosis and treatment patterns among older women with breast cancer. *Journal of the American Medical Association* 281:720–726.

Robinson, J. C. 2002. Renewed emphasis on consumer cost sharing in health insurance benefit design. *Health Affairs Web Exclusives* W139–W154.

Sanofi-Aventis. 2007. *Managed Care Digest Series, 2007: Government Digest*. Bridgewater, NJ: Sanofi-Aventis US, LLC.

Sanofi-Aventis. 2008. *Managed Care Digest Series, 2008: Government Digest*. Bridgewater, NJ: Sanofi-Aventis US, LLC.

Schneider, E. C., et al. 2005. Quality of care in for-profit and not-for-profit health plans enrolling Medicare beneficiaries. *American Journal of Medicine* 118 (12):1392–1400.

Taylor, M. 2006. Revival of the fittest. *Modern Healthcare* 36 (26):24–26.

Udvarhelyi, I. S., et al. 1991. Comparison of the quality of ambulatory care for fee-for-service and prepaid patients. *Annals of Internal Medicine* 115 (5):394–400.

Wagner, E. R. 1995. Types of managed care organizations. In P. R. Kongstvedt (ed.). *Essentials of Managed Health Care* (pp. 24–34). Gaithersburg, MD: Aspen Publishers.

Wilson, F. A., and D. Neuhauser. 1985. *Health Services in the United States*, 2nd ed. Cambridge, MA: Ballinger Publishing.

Chapter 10

Long-Term Care Services

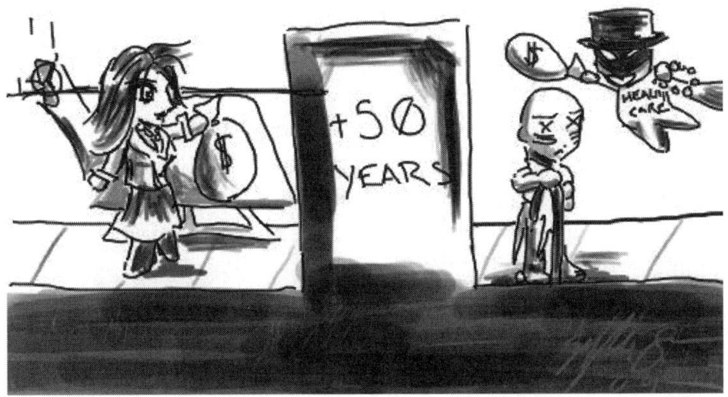

INTRODUCTION

Long-term care (LTC) is often associated with the care provided in nursing homes (skilled nursing facilities, subacute care facilities, and specialized care facilities), which is a rather narrow view because LTC services are also provided in a variety of community-based settings. Indeed, most LTC in the United States is provided informally by family and friends who receive no payment for their time and effort. There are perhaps more than 7 million Americans who provide care to over 4 million elderly persons with functional limitations. The economic value of such care may be as high as $96 billion a year (O'Keeffe & Siebenaler, 2006). It is also estimated that two of five elderly LTC users rely solely on informal care (Alecxih, 2001). Also, older people who have close access to family or surrogates (such as neighbors, friends, and church or other community organizations) often continue to live in the community much longer than those who do not have such support. Social support networks have a positive effect on physical and mental functioning status and forestall institutionalization (Wan & Weissert, 1981).

LTC includes a variety of services other than those provided in nursing homes. Examples include home health care brought to a person's own home, home-delivered meals, and minimal assistance provided in residential settings such as foster care homes and board-and-care facilities. Also, contrary to common belief, LTC is not confined to the elderly, although the elderly are the predominant users of these services, and this chapter focuses on the elderly as the primary clients of LTC.

Even though LTC services are primarily designed for the elderly, it is incorrect to presume that most elderly are in need of such care. In fact, most elderly persons are physically and mentally healthy enough to live independently. According to household surveys of the civilian noninstitutionalized population, over 73% of elderly Americans assessed their own health status as good, very good, or excellent (U.S. Department of Health and Human Services, 2007, p. 262).

Nevertheless, the aging process leads to chronic, degenerative conditions that resist cure. Hence, older people use a disproportionately large share of total health care services in the United States. Although people over age 65 represent only about 13% of the U.S. population, this group accounts for one third of all national health care spending and occupies one half of all physician time. Hence, utilization of health care services is much higher among older adults than among younger persons. This means that as people grow older, the odds increase that they will require LTC. It also means that LTC cannot be an isolated component of the health care delivery system. Non-LTC services must be closely integrated with those of LTC. To address the total health care needs of LTC patients, the delivery system must allow ease of transition among various types of health care settings and services.

Whereas medical care provided in hospitals is generally associated with acute episodes, LTC is often associated with chronic conditions. Chronic conditions are the leading cause of illness, disability, and death in the United States today. *Chronic conditions* are characterized by persistent and recurring health consequences lasting over a long period, which are generally irreversible. Arthritis, diabetes, asthma, heart disease, cancer, and dementia are some examples of chronic conditions, but a person's age or the mere presence of chronic conditions does not predict the need for LTC. However, as a person ages, chronic ailments, *comorbidity* (multiple health problems), disability, and dependency tend to follow each other. This progression increases the probability that a person will need LTC (**Figure 10.1**).

The elderly population in the United States continues to grow, and between 2000 and 2020 the number of Americans with chronic conditions is projected to increase from 125 million (45% of the population) to 157 million (Partnership for Solutions, 2002). The number of Americans who suffer from multiple chronic conditions will rise to 81 million (25% of the population) by 2020 (Anderson, 2003). It is also estimated that, with the aging of the baby-boom generation, the number of people 70 years of age and older needing LTC will increase from 10 million in 2000 to 15 million in 2020 and to 21 million in 2030 (National Academy on an Aging Society, 2000). Although the rate of institutionalization among the elderly has been falling, this trend is likely to reverse itself within the next decade. Rising levels of obesity and diabetes point to a growing need for nursing home care in the future (Lakdawalla et al., 2003). The rest of the developed world also faces aging-related problems and challenges in providing adequate LTC services very similar to those in the United States.

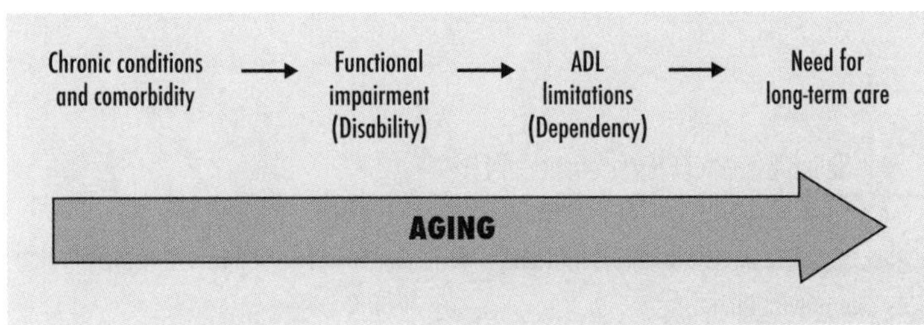

Figure 10.1 Progressive Steps Toward the Need for LTC Among the Elderly. ADL, activities of daily living.

WHAT IS LTC?

LTC can be defined as a variety of individualized, well-coordinated services that promote the maximum possible independence for people with functional limitations and that are provided over an extended period of time in accordance with a holistic approach while maximizing the quality of life. The seven essential characteristics of LTC are summarized in **Exhibit 10.1** and are explained in subsequent sections.

A Variety of Health Care Services

LTC clients need a variety of services for two main reasons. First, a variety of services are needed to fit the needs of different individuals because the need varies greatly from individual to individual. Even the elderly, who are the predominant users of LTC services, are not a homogeneous group. For example, some people just require supportive housing, whereas others require intensive treatments. Hence, LTC includes services such as housing programs, transportation, case management, recreation, nutrition, and various types of social support services.

Second, even for the same individual, the need for the various types of services generally changes over time. The change is not necessarily progressive, from lighter to more intensive levels of care. Depending on the change in condition and functioning, the individual may shift back and forth between the various levels and types of LTC services. For example, after hip surgery, a patient may require extensive rehabilitation therapy in a nursing facility for 2 or 3 weeks before returning home, where he or she receives continuing care from a home health agency. After that, the individ-

Exhibit 10.1 Seven Essential Characteristics of LTC

- It includes a variety of health care services.
- Services are individualized.
- Services must be well coordinated.
- The goal is to promote maximum possible functional independence.
- Services are needed over an extended period of time.
- Patients' physical, mental, social, and spiritual needs must be met.
- Patients' quality of life must be maximized.

ual may continue to live independently but require a daily meal from Meals on Wheels. Later, this same person may suffer a stroke and after hospitalization have to stay indefinitely in an LTC facility.

LTC often interfaces with non-LTC services, such as primary care, acute care, and rehabilitation. The LTC delivery system is not a self-contained system of comprehensive health care services, nor can it function independently of primary, acute, mental health, and rehabilitation services.

LTC must also include both therapeutic and preventive services. The primary goal of preventive services is to prevent or delay the need for institutionalization in LTC facilities. Preventive measures call for ensuring that the elderly receive good nutrition and have access to preventive medical care. For example, the elderly must have access to services such as vaccination against pneumonia, annual flu shots, glaucoma screening, diabetes screening, and cancer screening.

For those living independently, certain social support programs also serve a preventive function. Programs such as homemaker, chore, and handyman services can assist with a variety of tasks that older adults may no longer be able to perform. Examples include shopping, light cleaning, general errands, lawn maintenance, and minor home repairs.

Individualized Services

An assessment of the patient's physical, mental, and emotional condition and past medical and social history, former occupation, leisure activities, and cultural factors is used to determine appropriate services. An individualized plan of care is developed, and services are rendered according to that plan.

Coordination of Services

Just the availability of a variety of services may not sufficiently meet the varied and changing needs of LTC clients unless those services are well coordinated. As it is, many people find the health care delivery system difficult to navigate. Such difficulties compound in the case of elderly and disabled individuals. For example, acute episodes, such as pneumonia, bone fracture, or stroke, require admission to a general hospital. Many acute-care services are now delivered in a variety of outpatient settings instead of hospitals. After acute-care delivery, a patient may be transferred to a hospital-based transitional care unit for intensive rehabilitation. The patient may subsequently have to be moved to a long-term care facility for ongoing care. Depression may create a need to visit an outpatient mental health clinic. The person may also require dental or optometric care.

Maximum Possible Functional Independence

LTC becomes necessary when there is a remarkable decline in an individual's ability to perform certain common tasks of daily living independently. Among children, disabilities can result from birth defects, brain damage, or mental retardation. Younger adults may lose functional capacity as a result of an accident or a crippling disease such as multiple sclerosis. Among the elderly, complications from chronic disease or acute episodes can lead to functional impairment. Adaptive devices, such as walkers, wheelchairs, special utensils, and many other types of equipment and modification of the living environment with safety features such as grab bars, can enable many individuals to continue to live independently. However, as dependency increases, the need for LTC services also increases.

Two standard measures are available to determine a person's level of dependency. The first one is the activities of daily living (ADL) scale, which is used to assess a person's ability to perform certain common tasks of daily living referred to as *activities of daily living* (see **Exhibit 10.2**). Severe ADL limitations often indicate the need for institutional care. The second measure is the *instrumental activities of daily living* (IADL) scale. It incorporates activities that are necessary for living independently in the community, such as using the telephone, driving a car or traveling alone by bus or taxi, shopping, preparing meals, doing light housework, taking med-

Exhibit 10.2 Activities of Daily Living

The classic ADL scale includes six basic activities:

- Eating
- Bathing
- Dressing
- Using a toilet
- Maintaining bowel and bladder control
- Transferring, such as getting out of bed and moving into a chair

Sometimes grooming and walking a distance of 8 feet are also included in the scale.

icine, and handling money. IADLs are not generally used in institutional settings because institutionalized persons are not required to perform many IADLs (Ostir et al., 1999). It is estimated that approximately 40% of the elderly have some functional limitations associated with ADLs or IADLs (National Academy on an Aging Society, 2000). The progression of LTC intensity is illustrated in **Exhibit 10.3**.

The main goal of LTC is to enable the individual to maintain functional independence to the maximum level that is practicable. Restoration of function may be possible to some extent through appropriate rehabilitation therapy, but in most cases a full restoration of normal functioning is an unrealistic expectation. Caregivers must render care and assistance wherever the patient is either unable to do things for himself or herself or absolutely refuses to do so. The focus should be on maintaining whatever functional ability the patient still has and on preventing further decline of that ability. Caregivers should motivate and help patients do as much as possible for themselves.

Extended Period of Time

Compared to acute care, LTC is sustained over a longer period of time. The period of care and institutional stay when needed generally extend to weeks, months, and years instead of days. Even when institutional LTC is indicated for a short period (90 days or less), LTC services may continue in the patient's own home after the patient has been discharged from a long-term care facility. At other times, long-range confinement to a nursing home may be necessary.

Exhibit 10.3 Progression of LTC Intensity

- Independent living
- Decline in IADLs
  - Informal care for those who have adequate social support
  - Informal care supplemented by paid community-based services
- Decline in ADLs
  - For light ADLs (eating, dressing, using a toilet), informal care with supplemental services may continue
  - Institutionalization

Holistic Approach

As discussed in Chapter 2, holistic health care focuses not merely on a person's physical and mental needs, but emphasizes well-being in every aspect of what makes a person whole and complete. A patient's physical, mental, social, and spiritual needs and preferences are incorporated into medical care delivery and the living environment. The following are brief descriptions of the four aspects of holistic caregiving:

1. Physical: This refers to the technical aspects of care, such as medical examination, nursing care, medications, diet, and rehabilitation treatments. It also includes comfort factors such as appropriate temperature and cozy furnishings, cleanliness, and safety in home and institutional environments.
2. Mental: The emphasis is on the total mental and emotional well-being of each individual. It may include treatment of mental and behavioral problems, if necessary. Maintaining mental health goes beyond diagnosis and treatment of mental conditions, however. In an institutional setting, it includes appropriate layout, décor, and techniques that help overcome disorientation and confusion; mental stimulation to help overcome boredom and depression; and an environment that promotes positive feelings. For example, the living atmosphere can be enhanced through live plants, flowers, water, pleasant aromas, and soothing music. Pet animals, fish in aquariums, and birds create a vibrant living environment.
3. Social: Almost everyone enjoys warm friendships and social relationships. Visits from family, friends, or volunteers provide numerous opportunities for socializing. Many nursing homes have created indoor and outdoor spaces such as game rooms, alcoves, balconies, and patios where people can sit and enjoy each other's company.
4. Spiritual: The spiritual dimension operates at an individual level. It includes personal beliefs, values, and commitments in a religious and faith context. Spirituality and spiritual pursuits are very personal matters, but for most people, they also require continuing interaction with other members of the faith community.

Quality of Life

Quality of life refers to the total living experience that results in overall satisfaction with one's life. It is particularly relevant to LTC facilities because people typically reside there for an extended period. Quality of life factors include lifestyle pursuits, living environment, clinical palliation, and human factors.

- Lifestyle factors are associated with personal enrichment and making life meaningful through enjoyable activities. For example, many older people still enjoy pursuing their former leisure activities, such as woodworking, crocheting, knitting, gardening, and fishing.
- The living environment must be comfortable, safe, and appealing to the senses. Cleanliness, décor, furnishings, and other aesthetic features are important.
- Clinical *palliation* should be available for relief from unpleasant symptoms such as pain or nausea, for instance, when a patient is undergoing chemotherapy.
- Human factors refer to caregiver attitudes and practices that emphasize caring, compassion, and the preservation of human dignity for the patient. Institutionalized patients generally find it disconcerting to have lost their autonomy and independence. Quality of life is enhanced when residents have some latitude to govern their own lives. Residents in long-term care facilities also desire an environment that gives them adequate privacy.

COMMUNITY-BASED LTC SERVICES

Community-based LTC services have a fourfold objective: (1) to deliver LTC in the most economical and least restrictive setting whenever appropriate for the patient's health care needs, (2) to supplement informal caregiving when more advanced skills are needed to address the patient's needs, (3) to provide temporary respite to family members from caregiving stress, and (4) to delay or prevent institutionalization. These goals are accomplished through an administrative network that includes the Federal Administration on Aging, State Units on Aging, and Area Agencies on Aging. Nationally, approximately 670 Area Agencies on Aging administer funds appropriated by the federal government under the Older Americans Act of 1965.

For the financially needy, Title III of the Older Americans Act may finance such community-based services as adult day care, home maintenance, health promotion and disease prevention (e.g., medication management, nutrition, and health screening), telephone reassurance, and transportation services. States may also have some federal funds available under Title XX Social Services Block Grants. Also, community-based LTC services have grown under the Home and Community Based Services waiver program that was enacted under Section 1915(c) of the Social Security Act. Medicare and Medicaid may partially cover certain LTC services. The remainder must be covered by individual savings and private donations.

Home Health Care

Home health care refers to health care provided in the home of the patient by health care professionals. The organizational setup commonly requires a community- or hospital-based home health agency that sends health care professionals and paraprofessionals (such as home care aides) to patients' homes to deliver services approved by a physician. In 2007, there were over 9,000 Medicare-certified home health agencies in the United States. Of these, 83% were freestanding, and 17% were affiliated with an institution such as a hospital or nursing facility (National Association of Home Care and Hospice, 2008).

Home health services typically include nursing care, such as changing dressings, monitoring medications, and providing help with bathing; short-term rehabilitation, such as physical, occupational, and speech therapy; homemaker services, such as meal preparation, shopping, transportation, and some specific household chores; and certain medical supplies and equipment, such as ostomy supplies, hospital beds, oxygen tanks, walkers, and wheelchairs. Not all home health agencies provide all of these services, however.

Medicare is the largest single payer for home health services. To qualify for home care under the Medicare program, patients must be (1) homebound, (2) have a plan of treatment that is periodically reviewed by a physician, and (3) require intermittent or part-time skilled nursing and/or rehabilitation therapies.

Medicaid payments for home care are divided into three main categories: the traditional home health benefit, which is a federally mandated service provided by all states, and two optional programs, the personal care option and home- and community-based waivers. Together, services under these three programs represent a relatively small but growing portion of total Medicaid payments. The proportion of total Medicaid payments for home health care increased from 12.5% in 1998 to 16.3% in 2004 (National Association of Home Care and Hospice, 2001, 2008).

Adult Day Care

Adult day care is a daytime, community-based, group program that is designed to meet the needs of functionally and/or cognitively impaired adults and to provide partial respite to family caregivers. Adult day care is designed for people who live with their families, but because of physical or mental conditions they cannot remain alone during the day when the family members are working.

There are three main types of adult day centers: (1) social, which provide meals, recreation, and some health-related services; (2) medical/health, which provide social activities as well as more intensive clinical and therapeutic services; and (3) specialized, which provide specialized services such as dementia care or care for those with developmental disabilities (dysfunctions that begin in early childhood and are often accompanied by diminished mental capacity).

There are over 3,400 adult care centers in the United States. Seventy percent of these centers are affiliated with larger organizations such as skilled nursing facilities, medical centers, or multipurpose senior organizations. The average capacity is 40, and over half of the clients have some cognitive impairment (National Adult Day Services Association, 2008).

Adult Foster Care

Adult foster care is defined as a service characterized by small, family-run homes providing room, board, oversight, and personal care to nonrelated adults who are unable to care for themselves (AARP studies adult foster care, 1996). Foster care generally provides services in a community-based dwelling in an environment that promotes the feeling of being part of a family unit (Stahl, 1997). Participants in the program are elderly or disabled individuals who require assistance with one or two ADLs. Many of the residents have a psychiatric diagnosis.

Typically, the caregiving family resides in part of the home. To maintain the family environment, most states license fewer than 10 beds per family unit. Each state has established its own standards for the licensing of foster care homes. As states have continued to shift Medicaid funds from institutional to community-based services, adult foster care use has grown.

Senior Centers

Senior centers are local community centers for older adults. They are places where seniors can congregate and socialize. Many centers serve a noon meal daily. Others sponsor wellness programs, health education, counseling services, recreational activities, information and referral, and some limited health care services. Typical health care services offered at senior centers include health screening, especially for glaucoma and hypertension.

There are approximately 15,000 senior centers across the country, serving close to 10 million older adults annually. Many are supported by government and local non-profit organizations, while others receive funds from organizations such as the YMCA, United Way, and Catholic Charities. The Older Americans Act provides some funding support to over 6,000 senior centers through service contracts for program activities (National Council on Aging, 2005).

Home-Delivered and Congregate Meals

The Elderly Nutrition Program operates under the U.S. Administration on Aging to serve congregate meals in senior centers and home-delivered meals to those who want to stay at home. The goal of this program is to improve the dietary intake of older Americans. The program generally provides one hot noon meal for 5 days a week to people aged 60 and older (and their spouses) who are unable to prepare a nutritionally balanced noon meal for themselves.

Home-delivered meals for homebound persons are commonly referred to as Meals on Wheels. Meals are prepared by local institutions and delivered by volunteers. The volunteers also offer an important opportunity to check on the welfare of homebound elderly and are encouraged to report any health or other problems that they may note during their visits.

Homemaker and Handyman Services

Some older adults are relatively healthy but cannot carry out a few simple tasks necessary for independent living. These tasks may be as urgent as repairing a burst plumbing pipe or as mundane as cleaning the house. Some tasks, such as grocery shopping, must be performed often, whereas others, such as replacing storm windows, require attention just once or twice a year. Homemaker, household chore, and handyman services can assist older adults with a variety of such tasks, including shopping, light cleaning, general errands, and minor home repairs. Homemaker programs may be staffed largely or entirely by volunteers.

Personal Emergency Response

A personal emergency response system (PERS), also called a medical emergency response system, requires an electronic device that enables people to summon help in an emergency. The system is specifically designed for disabled or elderly people who live alone and may not otherwise need ongoing medical or supportive care. Other patients, after returning home from hospitals and nursing homes, are plagued by anxiety about relapses or accidents because they are often unprepared to self-manage after returning home. Usually they either wear or carry a transmitter unit that enables them to send a medical alert to a local 24-hour monitoring and response center. The system is available for a reasonable fee.

Case Management

Case management refers to a method of linking, managing, and coordinating services to meet the varied and changing health care needs of elderly clients (Zawadski & Eng, 1988). Case management services are designed to assess the special needs of older adults, to prepare a care plan to address those needs, to identify services that are most appropriate, to determine eligibility for services, to make referrals and coordinate delivery of care, to arrange for financing, and to ensure that clients are receiving services. Case managers often assist the adult children of disabled elderly who may be living far from each other.

INSTITUTIONAL LTC

Generally, institutional LTC is more appropriate for patients whose needs cannot be adequately met in a less clinical, community-based setting. However, a variety of institutional options are available to meet the varying needs of the elderly who no longer can live alone safely. Available options today include retirement centers, residential or personal care facilities, assisted living facilities, and nursing homes. These facilities provide varying levels of assistance.

An evaluation of the extent of functional impairment often determines which services are best suited, but personal preferences, and often the availability of financing, can also play a significant role. Most people prefer to receive care in their own home, and when institutionalization becomes necessary, they prefer a home-like, nonclinical setting. However, medical needs must often override personal preferences, especially when severe physical or mental problems develop. Figure 10.2 illustrates, on a continuum, six types of elder care institutions that can be classified under three general categories: retirement homes, personal care homes, and nursing homes. Continuing-care retirement communities (CCRCs) offer all three options within one campus-like setting. Based on the concept of aging-in-place, CCRCs can address people's changing needs.

Retirement Facilities

Retirement facilities do not deliver nursing care services but emphasize privacy, security, independence, and active lifestyles. Some very basic personal care such as assistance with bathing may be available in some retirement facilities, but in most instances, when additional nursing or rehabilitation services are needed, arrangements are made with a local home health agency.

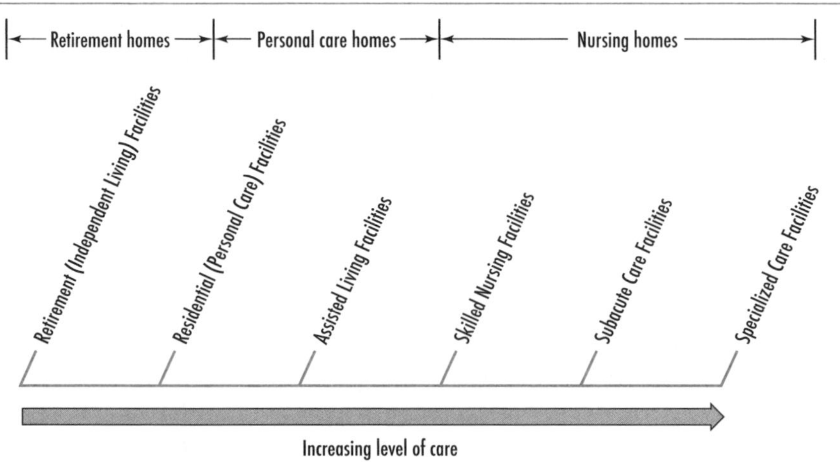

Figure 10.2 LTC Institutions for the Elderly

The special features and amenities in retirement facilities are designed to create a physically supportive environment that promotes independence. For example, the living quarters are equipped with emergency call systems. Many provide monthly blood pressure and vision screenings. Most of these facilities organize programs for socializing, physical fitness, recreation, and local outings for shopping and entertainment. Some basic hotel services, such as one meal a day and periodic housekeeping, are generally provided. Apartment units or detached cottages equipped with kitchenettes and private baths are the most common types of retirement facilities. Common laundry rooms are often shared with other residents. Many upscale retirement centers abound, in which one can expect to pay a fairly substantial entrance fee plus a monthly rental or maintenance fee. On the other hand, many communities have government-subsidized housing units for the low-income elderly and disabled individuals.

Personal Care Facilities

Personal care can be defined as nonmedical custodial care. *Custodial care* is confined to basic assistance provided in a protected environment and does not include active medical or rehabilitative treatments that would improve health or function.

Facilities providing personal care may be called by different names such as domiciliary care facilities, board-and-care homes, foster care homes, residential care facilities, or personal care facilities. These facilities provide physically supportive dwelling units, monitoring and/or assistance with medications, oversight, and light assistance with certain ADLs such as bathing and grooming. To maintain a residential rather than an institutional environment, many such facilities limit the admission of residents who use wheelchairs. Most of these facilities are relatively small and can be viewed as community-based alternatives rather than institutions. Staff members are mostly nursing paraprofessionals, such as personal care aides, who do not require a license or professional certification to deliver care. Similar workers employed in nursing homes must be certified by the state.

Assisted Living Facilities

An assisted living facility is generally described as a residential setting that provides personal care services, 24-hour supervision, scheduled and unscheduled assistance, social activities, and some nursing care services (Citro & Hermanson, 1999). The most common areas of assistance with ADLs are bathing, dressing, and toileting. The majority of residents also require help with medications. Some facilities have a skeleton staff of licensed nurses, generally licensed practical nurses (LPNs) (referred to as licensed vocational nurses [LVNs] in some states), to do admission assessments and deliver basic nursing care. Hence, these facilities border between personal care homes and nursing homes. Advanced nursing care and rehabilitation therapy can be arranged through a home health agency. Approximately one third of the residents are discharged because their functional status has declined to the extent that they need a higher level of services, which are provided in skilled nursing facilities (National Center for Assisted Living, 2006).

Skilled Nursing Facilities

A skilled nursing facility provides a full range of clinical LTC services, from skilled nursing care to rehabilitation to assistance with all ADLs. *Skilled nursing care* is medically oriented care provided by a licensed nurse. The plan of treatment is authorized by a physician. The majority of direct care with ADLs is delivered by paraprofessionals, such as certified nursing assistants and therapy assistants, but under the supervision of licensed nurses and therapists.

A variety of disabilities, including problems with ambulation, incontinence, and behavior, often coexist among a relatively large number of patients in need of skilled care. Compared to other types of facilities, these nursing homes have a significant number of patients who are cognitively impaired because of confusion, delirium, loss of memory, or dementia. The social functioning of many of the patients is also in severe decline.

Licensed professionals in skilled care facilities include registered nurses (RNs), licensed practical/vocational nurses (LPNs/LVNs), and registered therapists (physical therapists, occupational therapists, respiratory therapists, and speech/language pathologists). Rehabilitation is often an important component of skilled care, and so are therapeutic diets and nutritional supplements. The patient's assessment requires multidisciplinary input from various health care professionals, and the treatment plan is highly individualized.

Subacute Care Facilities

Subacute care is a blend of intensive medical, nursing, and other services that are technically complex. Examples include wound care, intravenous therapy, blood transfusion, ventilator support, and AIDS care. Subacute care is a substitute for services that were previously provided in acute-care hospitals and has grown because it is a cheaper alternative to a hospital stay. The severity of a patient's condition often requires active physician contact, professional nursing care, rehabilitative services, and the involvement of a multidisciplinary team in total care management (National Subacute Care Association, 1996).

Subacute care generally follows hospitalization and is required for a relatively short period of time, such as between 20 and 90 days. Services are generally delivered via three main avenues.

1. Long-term care hospitals (LTCHs). According to federal regulations, LTCHs must be certified as acute-care hospitals and must have an average length of stay greater than 25 days.
2. Many skilled nursing facilities have opened subacute care units by raising the staff skill mix by hiring additional RNs and having therapists on staff.
3. Some subacute-type services are rendered by community-based home health agencies. Thanks to new technology, certain subacute services can be provided in a patient's own home.

Specialized Care Facilities

By their very nature, both subacute care and specialized care place high emphasis on medical and nursing services. Some skilled nursing facilities have opened specialized care units for patients requiring ventilator care, wound care, services for Alzheimer's disease, intensive rehabilitation, or closed head trauma care. Other freestanding facilities have chosen a niche, specializing only in Alzheimer's care, rehabilitation, or AIDS care.

LICENSING AND CERTIFICATION OF NURSING HOMES

Nursing homes are heavily regulated through licensure and certification requirements. In the United States, it is illegal to operate a nursing facility without a license. Medicare and Medicaid funding involves certification of facilities by the federal government.

Licensing

Every state requires nursing homes to be licensed by the state. By approving or denying a license for a proposed new facility or additional beds at an existing facility, a state can control the total number of nursing home beds. Annual renewal of a license is required for existing nursing homes. To keep their licenses in good standing, it is essential that facilities comply with the state's standards for nursing homes. The standards vary from state to state, except for national fire safety regulations. The Life Safety Code, published by the National Fire Protection Association, encompasses national building and fire safety rules that have been made a part of licensure standards. In addition, each state has crafted basic standards for nursing care and other services. Compliance with standards is verified through periodic inspections, generally once a year. A state's department (board or division) of health or department of human services generally has nursing home licensing and oversight responsibilities.

Certification

If a nursing home wants to serve Medicaid and/or Medicare clients, it must be certified by the Centers for Medicare and Medicaid Services (CMS), an agency of the U.S. Department of Health and Human Services. To be certified, a nursing home must first be licensed by the state. Thus, licensure and certification serve different purposes. A license allows a facility to operate and do business. Certification allows a nursing home to admit patients who are on public assistance. It is possible for a facility to only have a license, but in that case, it cannot receive payments from Medicaid or Medicare.

There are three distinct federal certification categories, and facilities in all three categories are generically referred to as nursing homes.

1. SNF (skilled nursing facility) certification allows a facility to admit patients whose care is financed by Medicare and pays only for post-acute skilled care after a patient has stayed in a hospital for a minimum of 3 days. The maximum coverage in an SNF-certified facility is 100 days, but in actual practice, people receive an average of only 23 days of care per admission (Centers for Medicare and Medicaid Services,

2002). This is due to complex Medicare rules that the facility must use for determining length of stay. Also, Medicare pays the full cost of skilled nursing care only for the first 20 days. The beneficiary must pay a substantial copayment ($133.50 per day in 2009) for days 21 through 100.

2. NF (nursing facility) certification allows a facility to admit patients whose care is financed by Medicaid. Unlike Medicare, Medicaid is a comprehensive health care program that allows patients to stay in an NF-certified nursing home indefinitely as long as the patient's physician authorizes the need for nursing care and the patient qualifies for Medicaid assistance. The beneficiary is required to turn over most of his or her monthly income to the facility; Medicaid pays the remaining costs. Many patients are initially admitted to a facility with a private pay source of funding. When private funds are exhausted, these patients generally become eligible for Medicaid assistance.
3. ICF/MR (intermediate care facility for the mentally retarded) certification allows a nursing facility to serve patients who are mentally retarded/developmentally disabled. Developmental disability is a physical incapacity that generally accompanies mental retardation and often arises at birth or in early childhood. These institutions provide specialized programming and care modules for patients suffering from mental retardation and associated disabilities. The reimbursement is derived mostly from Medicaid.

Certification is granted on the basis of compliance with federal standards. The same standards apply to both SNF and NF certifications, but different standards apply to ICF/MR certification. A facility may be dually certified as both an SNF and an NF. Facilities having *dual certification* can admit Medicare and/or Medicaid patients to any part of the facility.

In 2005, 62.3% of nursing home expenditures were attributed to government sources (U.S. Department of Health and Human Services, 2007, p. 380). With an increasing share of nursing home revenues coming from public sources, the number of nursing homes that have elected to be certified has grown over time. In 2004, only about 1.2% of the nation's nursing homes had opted not to obtain federal certification (U.S. Census Bureau, 2008, Table 183). The small number of facilities that have elected not to be certified can admit only those patients who have a private source of funding for nursing home care. On the other hand, *private-pay patients*—those not covered by either Medicare or Medicaid for long-term nursing home care—are not restricted to noncertified facilities. In most certified nursing homes, private-pay patients are placed alongside those who depend on Medicare and Medicaid.

OTHER LTC SERVICES

Respite Care

Family caregivers often experience physical and emotional problems. Caregiving responsibilities can ignite family conflicts and encroach on caregivers' employment and leisure activities. Under these circumstances, caregivers experience stress and burnout. *Respite care* is the most frequently suggested intervention to address family caregivers' feelings of stress and burden. Virtually any kind of service—adult day care, home health care, and temporary institutionalization—can be viewed as respite care as long as the focus is on giving informal caregivers some time off while meeting disabled persons' needs for assistance (Doty et al., 1996).

Restorative Care

Restorative care is based on the philosophy of caregiving in which patients are viewed as participants capable of reaching their maximum potential in physical and mental functioning. Restorative services include, but go beyond, the typical rehabilitation therapies (physical, occupational, and speech therapy). Restoration of functioning is incorporated into the daily care routine. Examples include range of motion exercises, bowel and bladder training, and assisted walking, all provided by paraprofessionals. Restorative care is often provided by home health agencies, rehabilitation hospitals, outpatient rehabilitation clinics, adult day care centers, and assisted living and skilled nursing care facilities.

Hospice Care

Approaches to terminal illness and death with the objective of maintaining the patient's dignity and comfort have received increased attention in the delivery of health care. Roughly 75% of all deaths occur at age 65 or older. Among the elderly, 35% of all deaths are related to heart disease, and 22% are related to cancer. Other diseases that are often fatal to the elderly are cerebrovascular disease (stroke), chronic obstructive pulmonary disease, diabetes, pneumonia, and influenza (Sahyoun et al., 2001). Hence, dealing with death and dying is very much a part of LTC.

End-of-life care is commonly associated with *hospice*, a cluster of comprehensive services for the terminally ill who have a life expectancy of 6 months or less. Hospice is a method of care, not a location, although there are some freestanding hospice facilities. Hospice can be a part of home health care when the services are provided in the patient's home. In other instances, hospice services (described in Chapter 7) are taken to patients in nursing homes, retirement centers, or hospitals.

STATE OF THE NURSING HOME INDUSTRY

Between 1995 and 2006, the number of nursing home beds declined by 2% and the number of residents receiving care in these facilities declined by 3% (Table 10.1). It is mainly because of the growth of community-based LTC alternatives that earlier predictions of a boom in nursing homes did not materialize. For example, home health care and assisted living facilities have experienced remarkable growth and popularity. On the other hand, more recent evidence indicates that occupancy rates in nursing homes may be gradually creeping up (Kramer, 2003). This trend is expected to continue as the community-based LTC industry matures. A growing population with chronic conditions, comorbidities, and subsequent disability, but with increased lifespan, will eventually need nursing home care.

The nursing home industry in the United States is dominated by private for-profit nursing home chains. Chain nursing homes are members of a group of nursing homes operated under a corporate ownership. Approximately 54% of all nursing home beds in the United States are chain affiliated because chains have acquired an increasing number of independent facilities. About 62% of all nursing home beds are operated by proprietary (for-profit) nursing homes, and 29% are operated by private nonprofit entities (U.S. Census Bureau, 2008, Table 183). Only about 9% are government owned, and most of these are owned and operated by local counties. The average size of a nursing home (108 beds) has changed little over time. (See Table 10.1.)

Nursing home expenditures are shown in Table 10.2. Medicaid is the largest single source of payment for nursing home services. Medicare pays

Table 10.1 Nursing Home Trends (Selected Years)

	1995	2000	2006
Number of nursing homes	16,389	16,886	15,899
Number of beds	1,751,302	1,795,388	1,716,102
Average beds per nursing home	107	106	108
Number of residents	1,479,550	1,480,076	1,433,523
Occupancy rate*	84.5%	82.4%	83.5%

*Percentage of beds occupied (number of residents per 100 beds). These data do not include long-term care facilities that are not classified as nursing homes (Figure 10.2). Data from U.S. Department of Health and Human Services. *Health, United States, 2007* (pp. 370–371).

Table 10.2 Nursing Home Expenditures, 2004

Total Medicare payments to SNF-certified facilities	$17.1 billion
Total Medicaid payments to nursing homes	
NF-certified facilities	$42.0 billion
ICF/MR facilities	$11.1 billion
Medicaid payments per recipient of nursing home care	
NF-certified facilities	$24,475
ICF/MR facilities	$97,497
Average monthly charges	
Dually certified beds	$ 5,654
SNF-certified beds	$ 7,541
NF-certified beds	$ 6,206
Noncertified beds	$ 4,117

Data from U.S. Department of Health and Human Services. *Health, United States* 2007 (pp. 396, 408, 414, 415). Hyattsville, MD: U.S. Department of Health and Human Services.

for eligible beneficiaries under Part A, but the coverage is for a short duration. Only 8% of institutional LTC services are paid through private insurance. LTC insurance policies are generally expensive and cover only a portion of the total expenses, especially when long-range care in a nursing home is needed. Coverage for nursing home expenditures from private insurance has increased slightly in recent years, but less than 10% of people age 50 and over have purchased private insurance policies for LTC coverage (Seff, 2003).

CONCLUSION

LTC must be viewed not as an isolated component of the health care delivery system but as a continuum of both community-based and institution-based services that must be rationally linked to the rest of the health care delivery system. LTC includes medical care, social services, and housing alternatives. Hence, it involves a range of services that can vary according to individual needs. Chronic conditions and comorbidities can lead to physical and/or mental disability. Such disabilities may impair the performance of ADLs and/or IADLs. LTC services often complement what people with impaired functioning can do for themselves. Informal caregivers provide the bulk of these services. Respite care can provide family members temporary relief from the burden of caregiving. When the required intensity of care exceeds the capabilities of informal caregivers, available alternatives include professional community-based services to supplement informal care or admission to a long-term care facility. Services offered at these facilities vary from basic personal assistance to more complex skilled nursing care and subacute care. Specialized facilities caring for patients with Alzheimer's, AIDS, or head trauma have also grown in numbers. Some LTC patients may require long-range custodial care without the prognosis of a cure. Others may require short-term postacute convalescence and therapy. Still others may need end-of-life care through a hospice program. With the aging of the baby boom population, LTC services are expected to grow at a rapid rate beginning around 2015.

REFERENCES

AARP studies adult foster care for the elderly. 1996. *Public Health Reports* 111 (4):295.

Alecxih, L. 2001. The impact of sociodemographic change on the future of long-term care. *Generations* 25 (1):7–11.

Anderson, G. F. 2003. Physician, public, and policymaker perspectives on chronic conditions. *Archives of Internal Medicine* 163 (4):437–442.

Centers for Medicare and Medicaid Services. 2002. *Program Information.* Retrieved from http://www.cms.hhs.gov/charts/series/sec3-D.ppt.

Citro, J., and S. Hermanson. 1999. *Fact Sheet: Assisted Living in the United States*. Washington, DC: AARP.

Doty, P., et al. 1996. Informal caregiving. In C. J. Evashwick (ed.). *The Continuum of Long-Term Care: An Integrated Systems Approach* (pp. 125–141). Albany, NY: Delmar Publishers.

Kramer, R. G. 2003. Financial benchmarks: Signs of struggle and hope. *Nursing Homes Long Term Care Management* 52 (9):68–69.

Lakdawalla, D., et al. 2003. Forecasting the nursing home population. *Medical Care* 41 (1):8–20.

National Academy on an Aging Society. 2000. *Caregiving: Helping the Elderly with Activity Limitations*. Washington, DC: National Academy on an Aging Society.

National Adult Day Services Association. 2008. *Adult Day Services: Overview and Facts*. Retrieved August 2008 from http://www.nadsa.org/adsfacts/default.asp.

National Association of Home Care and Hospice. 2001. *Basic Statistics About Home Care*. Retrieved from http://www.nahc.org.

National Association of Home Care and Hospice. 2008. *Basic Statistics About Home Care*. Retrieved August 2008 from http://www.nahc.org/facts/08HC_Stats.pdf.

National Center for Assisted Living. 2006. *Assisted Living Resident Profile*. Retrieved August 2008 from http://www.ncal.org/about/resident.cfm.

National Council on Aging. 2005. *Fact Sheets: Senior Centers*. Retrieved October 2008 from http://www.ncoa.org/content.cfm?sectionID=103&detail=1177&increaseText=true.

National Subacute Care Association. 1996. Definition of subacute care as developed and approved by the NSCA board of directors, June 27, 1996. Retrieved from http://www.nsca.net/info/definition.htm.

O'Keeffe, J. and K. Siebenaler. 2006. *Adult Day Services: A Key Community Service for Older Adults*. Washington, DC: U.S. Department of Health and Human Services.

Ostir, G. V., et al. 1999. Disability in older adults 1: Prevalence, causes, and consequences. *Behavioral Medicine* 24 (4):147–156.

Partnership for Solutions. 2002. *Chronic Conditions: Making the Case for Ongoing Care*. Baltimore, MD: Johns Hopkins University.

Sahyoun, N. R., et al. 2001, March. Trends in causes of death among the elderly. *Aging Trends*. Hyattsville, MD: National Center for Health Statistics.

Seff, M. K. 2003, January–March. Clearing up health care myths. *Golden Lifestyles* 7.

Stahl, C. 1997, September 29. Adult foster care: An alternative to SNFs? *ADVANCE for Occupational Therapists*.

U.S. Census Bureau. 2008. *Statistical Abstract of the United States, 2008*. Washington, DC: Government Printing Office.

U.S. Department of Health and Human Services. 2007. *Health, United States, 2007*. Hyattsville, MD: U.S. Department of Health and Human Services.

Wan, T., and W. G. Weissert. 1981. Social support networks, patient status, and institutionalization. *Research on Aging* 3:240–256.

Zawadski, R. T., and C. Eng. 1988, December. Case management in capitated long-term care. *Health Care Financing Review Annual Supplement* 75–81.

Chapter 11

Underserved Populations

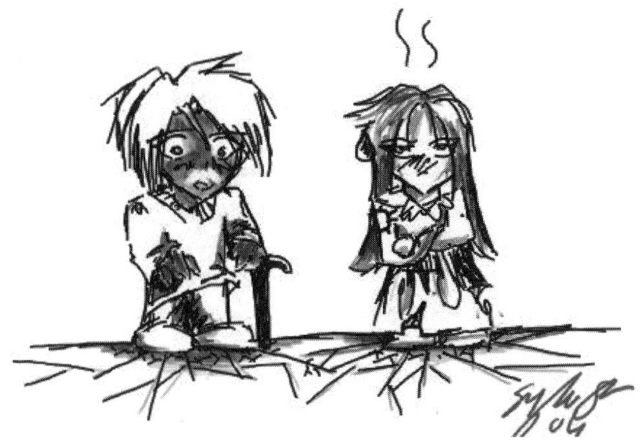

INTRODUCTION

Certain population groups in the United States face greater challenges than the general population in accessing timely and needed health care services. They are at greater risk of poor physical, psychological, and/or social health (Aday, 1994). Various terms are used to describe these populations, such as "underserved populations," "medically underserved," "medically disadvantaged," "underprivileged," and "American underclasses." The causes of their vulnerability are largely attributable to unequal social, economic, health, and geographic conditions. These population groups consist of racial and ethnic minorities, uninsured children, women, those living in rural areas, the homeless, the mentally ill, the chronically ill and disabled, and those with HIV/AIDS. These population groups are more vulnerable than the general population and experience greater barriers in access to care, financing of care, and racial or cultural acceptance. This chapter defines these population groups, describes their health needs, and summarizes the major challenges faced by them.

FRAMEWORK TO STUDY VULNERABLE POPULATIONS

The vulnerability model (see Figure 11.1) is an integrated approach to studying vulnerability. *Vulnerability* denotes susceptibility to negative events. From a health perspective, vulnerability refers to the likelihood of experiencing poor health or illness. Poor health can be manifested physically, psychologically, and/or socially. Because poor health along one dimension is likely to be compounded by poor health along others, the health needs are greater for those with problems along multiple dimensions than those with problems along a single dimension. Vulnerability does not represent a personal deficiency of special populations but rather the interaction effects of multiple factors, over many of which individuals have little or no control (Aday, 1999). It also justifies the role of society as a whole to address the concerns of vulnerable populations.

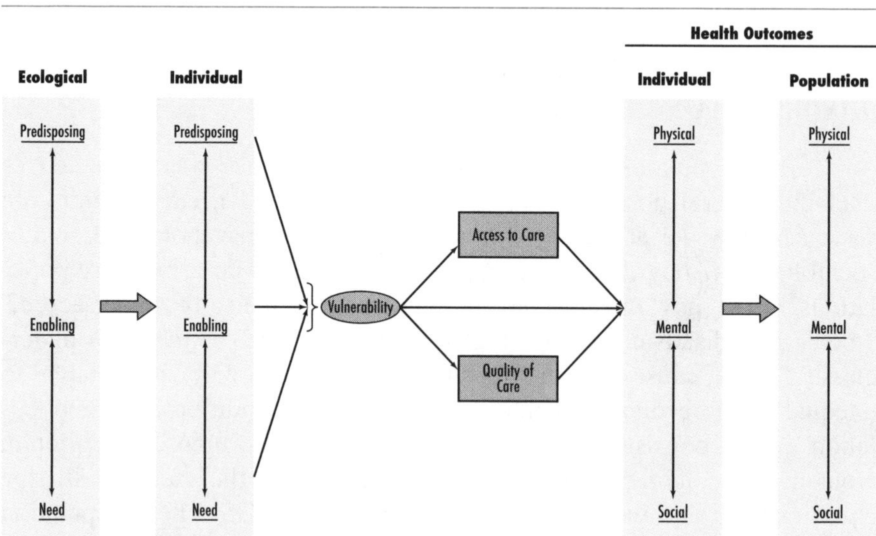

Figure 11.1 A General Framework to Study Vulnerable Populations

Vulnerability is determined by a convergence of (1) predisposing, (2) enabling, and (3) need characteristics at both individual and ecological (contextual) levels (**Exhibit 11.1**). Not only do these predisposing, enabling, and need characteristics converge and determine the access of individuals to health care, they also ultimately influence individuals' risk of contracting illness or, for those already sick, recovering from illness. Individuals with multiple risks (i.e., a combination of two or more vulnerability traits) typically experience worse access to care, care of lesser quality, and inferior health status than do those with fewer vulnerability traits.

Understanding vulnerability as a combination or convergence of disparate factors is preferred over studying individual factors separately because vulnerability, when defined as a convergence of risks, best captures reality. This approach not only reflects the co-occurrence of risk factors but underscores the belief that it is difficult to address disparities in one risk factor without addressing others.

The vulnerability model presented above has a number of distinctive characteristics. First, it is a comprehensive model, including both individual and ecological attributes of risk. Second, this is a general model focusing on the attributes of vulnerability for the total population rather than focusing on vulnerable traits of subpopulations. Although we recognize individual differences in exposure to risks, we also think there are common, crosscutting traits affecting all vulnerable populations. Third, a major distinction of our model is the emphasis on the convergence of vulnerability. The effects of experiencing multiple vulnerable traits may lead to cumulative vulnerability that is additive or even multiplicative. Examining vulnerability as a multidimensional construct can also demonstrate gradient relationships between

Exhibit 11.1 Predisposing, Enabling, and Need Characteristics of Vulnerability

- Predisposing Characteristics
  - Racial/ethnic characteristics
  - Gender and age (women and children)
  - Geographic location (rural health)
- Enabling characteristics
  - Insurance status (uninsured)
  - Homelessness
- Need characteristics
  - Mental health
  - Chronic illness/disability
  - HIV/AIDS

vulnerability status and outcomes of interest and thus improve our understanding of the patterns and factors related to the outcomes of interest.

Attributes that predispose to vulnerability include demographic characteristics, belief systems, and social structure variables. These attributes influence vulnerability status because they are associated with social position, status, access to resources, health behaviors, and variations in health status. Individuals have relatively little control over predisposing attributes, which are difficult to change. Predisposing attributes are often sources of discrimination. Patients may be discriminated against by health care providers and the health care delivery system because of their race, gender, financial status, or sexual preference. The following section discusses some of these predisposing characteristics, including race and ethnicity, gender, age, and geographic distribution.

Racial/Ethnic Minorities

In October 1997, the United States Office of Management and Budget (OMB) announced revised standards for federal data on race and ethnicity to better reflect the growing diversity in the country (U.S. Census Bureau, 2000). As such, the minimum categories for race in the U.S. population are black, Asian, American Indian or Alaska Native, Native Hawaiian or other Pacific Islander, and white. Instead of allowing a multiracial category, as was originally suggested in public and congressional hearings, the OMB adopted the Interagency Committee's recommendation to allow respondents to select one or more races when they self-identify.

Now, with the approval of the OMB, the Census 2000 questionnaires also included a sixth racial category: some other race. Effective January 1, 2003, the seven official racial categories are white alone, black alone, American Indian and Alaska Native alone, Asian alone, Native Hawaiian or other Pacific Islander alone, some other race alone, and two or more races. Two categories for ethnicity were also created: Hispanic or Latino and not Hispanic or Latino. Hispanic or Latino Americans include Mexicans, Puerto Ricans, Central or South Americans, Cubans, and persons from other Spanish cultures or origins.

Asian refers to persons originating from the Far East, Southeast Asia, or the Indian subcontinent, including, for example, Cambodia, China, India, Japan, Korea, Malaysia, Pakistan, the Philippine Islands, Thailand, and Vietnam. Native Hawaiians or other Pacific Islanders include persons originating from Hawaii, Guam, Samoa, or other Pacific Islands. American Indian or Alaska Natives include persons originating from North and South America (including Central America) who maintain tribal affiliation or community attachment. Close to 30% of the U.S. population is made up of minorities: black (12.2%), Hispanics or Latinos (14.8%), Asians (4.4%), Native Hawaiian and other Pacific Islanders (0.14%), and American Indian and Alaska Natives (0.8%). In addition, 2.0% identified themselves as being of two or more races.

Significant differences exist across the various racial/ethnic groups on health. Minority race and ethnicity usually serves as a proxy for other factors such as socioeconomic status, language ability, or cultural behaviors that are correlated with health status and health care experiences. The available evidence consistently suggests that racial/ethnic minorities have poorer access to health care, receive poorer quality care, and experience greater deficits in health status (see **Exhibit 11.2**).

Exhibit 11.2 Predisposing Racial and Ethnic Characteristics and Services

Black Americans

- More likely than whites to be economically disadvantaged
- Shorter life expectancies than whites
- Higher age-adjusted death rates for leading causes of death
- Higher neonatal, infant, and postneonatal mortality rates
- More likely than whites to report fair or poor health status
- Males more likely than white males to smoke cigarettes (U.S. Department of Health and Human Services, 2002)

Hispanic Americans

- Nearly one third have less than 9th-grade education.
- Over one quarter of families live below the poverty line (U.S. Census Bureau, 2007).
- They are more likely to be uninsured and underinsured than non-Hispanic whites.
- AIDS is the leading cause of death.
- Homicide rate remains the second leading cause of death for young males (National Center for Health Statistics, 2002).
- Among individuals 18 years or older, a higher proportion of Hispanics are overweight and/or obese.
- Alcoholism is 30.3% in Hispanics versus 7.9% in all races (National Center for Health Statistics, 1995).
- Twenty-eight percent of Hispanic individuals age 18–25 years smoke versus 24% of non-Hispanic blacks (National Center for Health Statistics, 2002).

(continued)

Exhibit 11.2 *(Continued)*

Asian Americans

- There is a bipolar distribution of education, income, and health status.
- Asian/Pacific Islander category is extremely heterogeneous, encompassing 21 subgroups with different health profiles.
- In 1999, median family income was $35,353, a higher percentage (11.9%) live in poverty than non-Hispanic whites (10.3%) (U.S. Census Bureau, 2002).
- Cambodian refugees have extremely high rates of posttraumatic stress disorder, dissociation, depression, and anxiety.
- As a whole, Asian/Pacific Islanders have the lowest smoking rates in the United States, but certain groups have smoking rates of
  - 92% of Laotians
  - 71% of Cambodians
  - 65% of Vietnamese (Yoon & Chien, 1996)
- Korean-Americans have a fivefold incidence of stomach cancer and eightfold incidence of liver cancer compared with whites.

American Indians and Alaska Natives

- They are at the bottom of the socioeconomic strata.
- Poverty is associated with high injury-related mortality rate among these children.
- The rate of death due to alcohol is seven times greater and suicide rate is 3.5 times greater than national averages (Pleasant, 2003).

One of the most consistent findings across decades of research is that minorities continue to have poor access to health services compared with their white counterparts, even after taking into account insurance, socioeconomic, and health status. Various studies document that minority Americans experience higher rates of illness and mortality than do white Americans. Disparities in health exist between white and nonwhite Americans in terms of perceived health status as well as traditional indicators of health such as the infant mortality rate, the general population mortality rate, and birth weight.

The most commonly used measure of access to care is whether a person has a regular or usual source of care. In most research studies, a usual source of care is defined as a single provider or place where patients obtain, or can obtain, the majority of their health care. Having a usual source of care is associated with greater coordination of care.

The majority of federal initiatives have served primarily to generate national attention on racial disparities in health care (see **Exhibit 11.3**). The creation of the Office of Minority Health was particularly important because it plays a coordinating role for other federal agencies and the minority health initiatives they support. The programs offering services at both the federal and state level provide extensive services that address some of the key pathways leading to racial disparities in Hispanic and Indian health and health care.

Although these service programs are designed to address specific needs of the minorities in their target populations, they nonetheless reflect a somewhat fragmented approach to addressing disparities in minority health and health care. The creation of the Federal Office of Minority Health may overcome this problem by coordinating future

Exhibit 11.3 Federal Programs to Eliminate Racial and Ethnic Disparities

U.S. Department of Health and Human Services Initiative to Eliminate Racial and Ethnic Disparities in Health (1998)

- To reduce disparities in six key topic areas: infant mortality, cancer screening and management, cardiovascular disease, diabetes, HIV/AIDS, immunizations

U.S. Office of Minority Health (1985)

- Mission is to "improve the health of racial and ethnic minority populations through the development of effective health policies and programs that help eliminate disparities in health" (Racial and Ethnic Approaches to Community Health, 2010)
- Program launched by the Centers for Disease Control in 1999
- To support the goals of Healthy People 2010 to eliminate racial disparities in health and health care

Minority Health Initiative (1992)

- Launched by the Office for Research on Minority Health at the National Institutes of Health (NIH) to improve the national research agenda on minority health issues and strengthen the national commitment and responsiveness to the health and training needs of minority Americans

Indian Health Service

- Is an agency within the U.S. Department of Health and Human Services with the mission to be the principal advocate and provider of health services to American Indians and Alaska Natives

Migrant Health Center Program

- Was established by the Migrant Health Act (1962) to provide medical and support services to migrant farm workers and their families efforts to improve health, access to health care, and quality of health services. Yet it will remain important to balance national efforts to improve racial/ethnic equity in health and health services delivery with the ability to address the specific cultural barriers and unique needs of each racial and minority group.

Women and Children

Women in the United States now enjoy a life expectancy almost 8 years longer than that of men, but they suffer greater morbidity and poorer health outcomes. They also have a higher prevalence of certain health problems than men over the course of their lifetimes (Sechzer et al., 1996). Compared with men of comparable age, women develop more acute and chronic illnesses, resulting in a greater number of short- and long-term disabilities (NIH, 1992). Heart disease and stroke account for a higher percentage of deaths among women than men at all stages of life. In contrast to 31% of men, 49% of women who have heart attacks die within a year. Women also represent the fastest growing population diagnosed with AIDS.

The differences between men and women are equally pronounced for mental illness. For example, anxiety disorders and major depression affect twice as many women as men (Rodin & Ikovics, 1990). Approximately 90% of all cases occur in young women, and eating disorders account for the highest mortality rates among all mental disorders (Weissman & Klerman, 1977).

The Office on Research on Women's Health, administered under the NIH (under the U.S. Department of Health and Human Services), has a mission to stimulate, coordinate, and implement a comprehensive women's health agenda on research, service delivery, and education across the agencies of the U.S. Department of Health and Human Services, as well as other government agencies.

Children's health has certain unique aspects in the delivery of health care. Among these are children's developmental vulnerability, dependency, and differential patterns of morbidity and mortality. *Developmental vulnerability* refers to the rapid and cumulative physical and emotional changes that characterize childhood and the potential effects that illness, injury, or untoward family and social circumstances can have on a child's life-course trajectory. *Dependency* means the special circumstances children face in that others often have to recognize and respond to their health needs. Children depend on their parents, school officials, caregivers, and sometimes neighbors to discover their need for health care, seek health care services on their behalf, authorize treatment, and comply with recommended treatment regimens. These relationships can affect the utilization of health services by children.

Children are increasingly affected by a broad and complex array of conditions collectively referred to as "new morbidities." *New morbidities* include drug and alcohol abuse, family and neighborhood violence, emotional disorders, and learning problems from which older generations did not suffer. Such conditions require a continuum of comprehensive services that includes multidisciplinary assessment, treatment, and rehabilitation, as well as community-based prevention strategies.

Geographic Distribution: Rural Health

Poverty is a consistent dimension of life in rural areas. Poor economic conditions are often reflected in diminished access to health care and the poor health status of rural citizens (Cohen et al., 1994). Access to health care is affected by poverty, long distances, rural topography, weather conditions, and limited availability of personal transportation.

Geographic maldistribution that creates a shortage of health care professionals in rural settings is another dimension of poor health care delivery. An estimated 51 million Americans live in places classified as nonmetropolitan, about one fifth of the population, and over 20 million of nonmetropolitan residents live in designated areas of primary health care provider shortages. Low population density makes it difficult for communities to attract physicians and for physicians to establish financially viable practices. As a result, rural populations face greater barriers in access to care.

Various measures have been undertaken to improve access to care in rural America, including the promotion of the National Health Service Corps (defined in a later section), the designation of Health Manpower Shortage Areas and Medically Underserved Areas, the development of the Community and Migrant Health Centers, and the enactment of the Rural Health Clinics Act.

ENABLING CHARACTERISTICS

Enabling characteristics include socioeconomic status, individual assets, and mediating factors. Socioeconomic status is associated with social position, access to resources, and variations in health status (e.g., income, education, employment status, and occupation). Individual assets (human capital) contribute to one's ability to be economically self-sufficient (e.g., inheritance, wealth, skills). Mediating factors are associated with the use of health care services (e.g., health insurance, access to health care, quality of health care). The following section discusses enabling characteristics such as insurance status and homelessness.

Uninsured

According to recent estimates, a little more than 17% of civilian noninstitutionalized Americans may be without health care coverage (National Center for Health Statistics[JBA1], 2007, Table 139). For the most part, the uninsured tend to be poor and less educated, and they work in part-time jobs and/or are employed by small firms. The uninsured also tend to be younger (25–40 years old) because most of the elderly (age 65 and over) is covered by Medicare. Ethnic minorities are also more likely to lack health insurance.

The plight of the uninsured affects those who have insurance. Costs to hospitals and health centers for providing uncompensated care to the uninsured were estimated at between $5 and $28 billion in 1995. Much of this cost is shared by Medicaid, federal grants to nonprofit hospitals, and charitable organizations. If uncompensated care remains at the current levels, these costs are likely to be at least partly passed on to the U.S. public at large through an increased need for (and decreased ability to pay for) more expensive emergency health care.

Homelessness

Nationally, approximately 3.5 million people experience homelessness each year (1% of the U.S. population). Thirty percent of the homeless population consists of families with children. About 40% of all homeless men have served in the armed forces. Single women constitute about 17% of the U.S. homeless adult population. Approximately 16% of the single adult population suffer from some form of severe and persistent mental disorder, yet only 5% to 7% require institutionalization, whereas the rest can live in the community with appropriate help (National Coalition for the Homeless, 2006a & b).

The homeless face several barriers to adequate and appropriate health care. They have financial barriers and problems in satisfying eligibility requirements for health insurance. Accessible transportation to medical facilities is often unavailable to this population. The homeless usually have a lack of proper sanitation, lack of a stable place to store medications safely, and have an inability to obtain the proper food for a medically indicated diet necessary for conditions such as diabetes mellitus or hypertension. The homeless, adults and children, have a high prevalence of untreated acute and chronic medical, mental health, and substance abuse problems. Homeless persons are also at a greater risk of assault and victimization, as well as exposure to harsh environmental elements.

Federal Initiatives to Eliminate Socioeconomic Disparities

Several federal programs have been established to help eliminate socioeconomic differences that jeopardize health.

- The Community Health Center Program was established in 1969 to improve access to health care services for low-income families.
- The National Health Service Corps works with communities and health care clinics in federally designated health professional-shortage areas to provide medical care to individuals living in these underserved areas.
- The Public Housing Primary Care Program is administered by the Bureau of Primary Health Care to support health centers and other community providers in delivering care to residents of public housing, individuals living near public housing, and anyone benefiting from public rent subsidies.
- The Healthy Schools, Healthy Communities Program, established in 1994, became the first federal program to encourage the development of new comprehensive full-time school-based primary care programs that serve vulnerable children.
- The Health Care for the Homeless Program, administered by the Bureau of Primary Health Care, supports grantees from community health centers, local health departments, community coalitions, and other nonprofit organizations to provide services to homeless individuals.

NEED CHARACTERISTICS

The need attributes of individuals include their self-perceived or professionally evaluated health status and their quality-of-life indicators. Self-perceived or professionally evaluated health status refers to self-perceived physical and mental health status and diagnoses of disease and illness from health professionals. Quality-of-life indicators include such factors as activity of daily living (ADL) performance, instrumental activity of daily living (IADL) performance, social limitations, cognitive limitations, and limitations in work, housework, or school.

Certain subpopulation groups are known to be at higher health risk. These include risks to physical health (high-risk mothers and infants, chronically ill and disabled individuals, and persons with HIV/AIDS), mental health (the mentally ill and disabled, alcohol or substance abusers, those who are suicide- or homicide-prone), and social well-being (abusive families, the homeless, and immigrants and refugees).

Mental Health

Mental illness ranks second, after ischemic heart disease, as a burden on health and productivity. It is estimated that one in five Americans has a mental disorder in any one year (Satcher, 1999). Mental disorders are common psychiatric illnesses affecting adults and present a serious public health problem in the United States. National studies have concluded that the most common mental disorders include phobias, substance abuse (including alcohol and drug dependence), and affective disorders (including depression). Schizophrenia is considerably less common, affecting perhaps 0.5% to 1% of the population. These illnesses affect an estimated 11 million persons each year at a cost of approximately $69 billion (Pear, 1999). Mental illness is a risk factor for death from suicide, cardiovascular disease, and cancer.

Most mental health services are provided in the general medicine sector—a concept first described by Regier et al. (1988) as the de facto mental health service system—rather than through formal mental health specialist services. The de facto system combines specialty mental health services with general counseling services, such as those provided in primary care settings, nursing homes, and community health centers by ministers, counselors, self-help groups, families, and friends. The nation's mental health system is composed of two subsystems, one primarily for individuals with insurance coverage or private funds and the other for those without private means of coverage.

Chronic Illness/Disability

Every person is vulnerable to chronic illness and/or disability during his or her lifetime. Overall, chronic diseases are responsible for 7 of 10 deaths (totaling 1.7 million Americans) and are largely attributable to preventable chronic illnesses. Tobacco use, a lack of physical activity, poor nutrition, and a lack of regular screening for cancers of the breast, cervix, colon, and rectum contribute to the major chronic disease killers: cardiovascular disease, cancer, diabetes, and chronic obstructive pulmonary disease (Centers for Disease Control, 1998, p. vii; U.S. Department of Health and Human Services, 1990). An illness is considered chronic if a disease or injury with long-term (noticed for 3 months or more) conditions or symptoms is present. Other illnesses—namely, congenital anomalies, asthma, diabetes, and heart disease—have been specifically classified as chronic by the National Center for Health Statistics, regardless of duration (National Center for Health Statistics, 1999b, p. 5). Chronic illness and disability also pose unique challenges to a health care system that is primarily oriented toward treating acute illness.

HIV/AIDS

Acquired immunodeficiency syndrome (AIDS) is caused by the human immunodeficiency virus (HIV). HIV is an unusual type of virus, called a retrovirus, that causes immune system suppression leading to AIDS. Certain widely recognized risk factors promote the transmission of HIV, including male-to-male sexual contact, male-to-female sexual contact, drug use by injection, exposure to contaminated blood products, and perinatal transmission from mother to infant (during pregnancy, delivery, or breastfeeding).

Many public health experts believe that cases of AIDS are still underreported. The reasons for such underreporting include poor reporting standards in U.S. health departments (Selike et al., 1993), patients' denial of the risk behaviors that are likely to transmit HIV, and absence or decreased access to health care (Robertson et al., 1974), which prevents the diagnosis of HIV. With the advent of combination antiretroviral therapy, AIDS surveillance data no longer reflect trends in HIV transmission because this therapy has been effective in delaying the progression of HIV to AIDS (Centers for Disease Control, 1999).

The cost of $12,000 or more per year makes the treatment unavailable to many patients in the United States and keeps it out of reach in developing countries where more than 90% of the new HIV infections occur. Also, the complicated drug regimen requires coordination of many pills and doses, which makes it easier to skip medications or doses so that some patients temporarily stop treatment. Other HIV problems in the United States include issues of urban home health care; HIV infection in rural communities, children, and women; lack of HIV prevention programs; discrimination; and the need for more HIV/AIDS-related research and health care provider training.

CONCLUSION

This chapter examines the major characteristics of certain U.S. population groups that face challenges and barriers in accessing health care services. These population groups are organized along predisposing, enabling, and need characteristics and include racial/ethnic minorities, children and women, those living in rural areas, the homeless, the mentally ill, and those with HIV/AIDS. The gaps that currently exist between these population groups and the rest of the population indicate the need for significant efforts to address the unique health concerns of U.S. subpopulation groups.

REFERENCES

Aday, L. A. 1994. Health status of vulnerable populations. *Annual Review of Public Health* 15:487–509.

Aday, L. A. 1999. Vulnerable populations: A community-oriented perspective. In J. G. Sebastian and A. Bushy (eds.). *Special Populations in the Community* (pp. 313–330). Gaithersburg, MD: Aspen.

Centers for Disease Control and Prevention. 1998. Update: HIV counseling and testing using rapid tests—United States, 1995. *MMWR Morbidity and Mortality Weekly Report* 47 (11):211–215.

Centers for Disease Control and Prevention. 1999. Guidelines for national human immunodeficiency virus case surveillance, including monitoring for human immunodeficiency virus infection and acquired immunodeficiency syndrome. *MMWR Morbidity and Mortality Weekly Report* 48(RR-13):2–7.

Cohen, S. E., et al. 1994. The geography of AIDS: Patterns of urban and rural migration. *Southern Medical Journal* 85 (6):599.

Kraus, L. E., S. Stoddard, and D. Gilmartin. 1996. *Chartbook on Disability in the United States, 1996. An InfoUse Report*. Washington, DC: US National Institute on Disability and Rehabilitation Research.

National Center for Health Statistics. 1999a. *Health, United States, 1999*. Hyattsville, MD: U.S. Department of Health and Human Services.

National Center for Health Statistics. 1999b. *Healthy People 2000 Review, 1998–99* (pp. 163–167). Hyattsville, MD: Public Health Series.

National Center for Health Statistics. 2002. *Health, United States, 2002*. Hyattsville, MD: U.S. Department of Health and Human Services.

National Coalition for the Homeless. 2006a. NCH fact sheet #2: How many people experience homelessness? http://www.nationalhomeless.org/publications/facts/How_Many.pdf

National Coalition for the Homeless. 2006b. NCH fact sheet #3: Who is homeless? http://www.nationalhomeless.org/publications/facts/Whois.pdf

National Institutes of Health. Office of Research on Women's Health. 1992. *Report of the National Institutes of Health: Opportunities for research on women's health*. (NIH Publ. No. 92–3457). Washington, DC: Government Printing Office.

Pear, R. 1999, December 13. Mental disorders common, U.S. says, many not treated. *New York Times*.

Pleasant, R. 2003. Minority health. In The Department of Health and Human Services: 50 Years of Service. DHHS, pp.92–95.

Regier, D. A., et al. 1988. One month prevalence of mental disorders in the United States: Based on five epidemiologic catchment area sites. *Archives of General Psychiatry* 45 (11):977–986.

Robert Wood Johnson Foundation. 1996, November. *Chronic Care in America: A 21st Century Challenge*. Retrieved from http://www.rwjf.org/library.

Robertson, L. S., et al. 1974. *Changing the Medical Care System: A Controlled Experiment in Comprehensive Care*. New York: Praeger Publishers.

Rodin, J., and J. Ikovics. 1990. Women's health: Review and research agenda as we approach the 21st century. *American Psychologist* 45:1018–1034.

Satcher, D. 1999. *Mental Health: A Report of the Surgeon General.* Retrieved January 4, 2000, from http://www.surgeongeneral.gov/library/mental health/home.html.

Sechzer, J. A., et al. 1996. *Women and Mental Health.* New York: New York Academy of Sciences.

Selike, R. M., et al. 1993. HIV infection as leading cause of death among young adults in U.S. cities and states. *Journal of the American Medical Association* 269:2991–2994.

U.S. Census Bureau, 2002. Statistical Abstract of the United States, 2002. The National Data Book. Washington, DC: Government Printing Office.

U.S. Census Bureau, 2007. Statistical Abstract of the United States, 2007. The National Data Book. Washington, DC: Government Printing Office.

U.S. Department of Health and Human Services. 1990. *Health Status of the Disadvantaged.* Department of Health and Human Services Publication No. (HRSA) HRS-P-DV 90–1. Washington, DC: Government Printing Office.

U.S. Census Bureau, 2000. Racial and ethnic classifications used in Census 2000 and beyond. Washington, DC: Government Printing Office.

U.S. Department of Health and Human Services. 2002. *Health, United States, 2002.* Hyattsville, MD: U.S. Department of Health and Human Services.

Weissman, M. M., and G. L. Klerman. 1977. Sex differences and the epidemiology of depression. *Archives of General Psychiatry* 34 (1):98–111.

Yoon, E., and F. Chien. 1996. Asian American and Pacific Islander health: A paradigm for minority health. *Journal of the American Medical Association* 275 (9):736–737.

Chapter 12

Cost, Access, and Quality

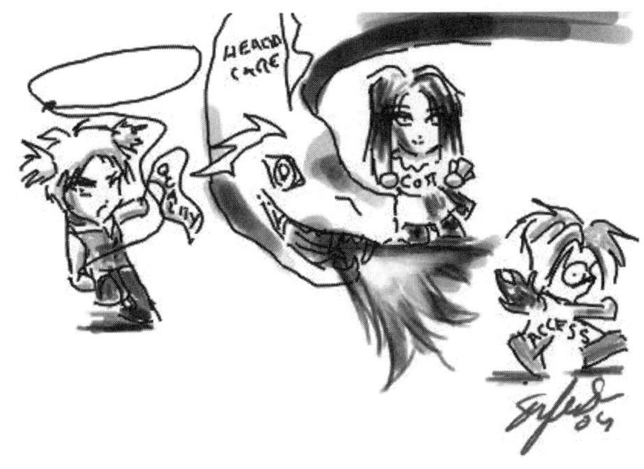

INTRODUCTION

Cost, access, and quality are three major cornerstones of health care delivery (Al-Assaf, 1993a). For many years, employers and third-party payers in the United States have been preoccupied with controlling the growth of health care expenditures. One reason that past attempts to bring universal access to the United States have failed is the concern that such a move would be extremely costly in terms of national health care expenditures. Such a fear is founded on the premise that cost and access go hand in hand. Although cost and access have remained the primary concerns within the U.S. health care delivery system, the quality of health care is increasingly taking center stage. At the same time, rising systemwide costs will remain the focus of attention for many years to come.

An interactive relationship exists between the cost of health care, people's ability to obtain health care when needed, and the quality of services delivered. From a macroperspective, the costs are commonly viewed in terms of national expenditures for health care. A widely used measure for national health expenditures is the proportion of the gross domestic product (GDP) a country spends on the delivery of health care services. In simple terms, it refers to the proportion of its national income a country spends on health care. From a microperspective, health care costs refer to both costs incurred by employers to purchase health insurance and out-of-pocket costs incurred by individuals when they receive health care services. The improvement of access to health care and equal access to quality health care are contingent on expenditures at both the macro and micro levels. High-quality care should also be the most cost-effective care. Hence, cost is an important factor in the evaluation of quality. On the other hand, quality is achieved when accessible services are provided in an efficient, cost-effective, and acceptable manner (Al-Assaf, 1993a).

This chapter discusses some of the major reasons for the dramatic rise in health care expenditures. Costs are compared with those of other countries, and the impact of various cost-containment measures is examined. The government has played a significant role in cost containment and quality improvement, but the extension of universal access to all Americans has remained an elusive dream.

COST OF HEALTH CARE

"Cost" can carry different meanings in the delivery of health care. The meaning depends on the perspective one takes. Three different meanings are presented here.

1. When consumers and financiers speak of the cost of health care, they most often mean the "price" of health care, such as the physician's bill or the premiums employers pay for purchasing employee health insurance.
2. From a national perspective, health care costs refer to how much a nation spends on health care services, commonly referred to as "health care expenditures" or "health care spending." These terms primarily reflect the consumption of economic resources in the delivery of health care. The economic resources include health insurance, the skills of health care professionals, organizations and institutions of health care delivery, pharmaceuticals, medical equipment and supplies, public health functions, and new medical discoveries. Because expenditures equal price times quantity, $E = (P)(Q)$, growth in health care spending can be

accounted for by growth in prices charged by the providers of health services as well as increases in the utilization of services.

3. A third perspective is that of the providers, where the notion of cost refers to staff salaries, capital costs for building and equipment, rental of space, purchase of supplies, and other costs of production.

Regardless of perspective, it is useful to understand which factors drive costs in the health care delivery system and thus identify which can be controlled to ensure that health care is delivered at an optimal value.

HIGH IN COST

Health care spending spiraled upward at double-digit rates during the 1970s after a massive growth in access created by the Medicare and Medicaid programs in 1965. By 1970, government expenditures for health care services and supplies had grown by 140%, from $7.9 to $18.9 billion (National Center for Health Statistics [NCHS], 1996). During the 1980s, the rate of increase began slowing down. In the 1990s, medical inflation was finally brought under control to a single-digit rate of growth, mostly because medical care costs and use were controlled through managed care. For example, the rate of growth in health spending slowed to its lowest levels in four decades (5.7% average annual growth) between 1993 and 2000, as managed care proliferated; however, the rate of growth has once again started to accelerate, albeit at a relatively slow pace. Annual growth in 2001, at 8.7%, was the fastest since 1991. The main culprits for this recent rise in expenditures are hospital services, prescription drugs, and physician services (Levit et al., 2003).

Trends in national health expenditures are commonly evaluated by comparing medical inflation to general inflation in the economy (measured by annual changes in the consumer price index or CPI) and by comparing changes in national health spending to changes in the GDP. Typically, the rates of change in medical inflation have remained consistently above the rates of change in the CPI, and health care spending growth rates have consistently surpassed growth rates in the general economy. When spending on health care grows at a faster rate than the GDP, this means that a growing share of total economic resources is devoted to the delivery of health care.

Table 12.1 compares U.S. health spending with that of 30 other developed countries. In 2005, the United States spent $6,401 per capita on health, about $1,500 per capita more than the second highest country,

Table 12.1 Health Spending in Organization for Economic Cooperation and Development Countries

	Total Health Spending per Capita 2005			GDP per Capita 2005			Health Spending as % of GDP	
	U.S. $ PP	% of U.S. Level	AAG 1995–2005 (5)	U.S. $ PPP	% of U.S. Level	AAG 1995–2005 (%)	% of GDP	% of U.S. Level
United States	6,401	100.0	3.6	41,789	100.0	3.2	15.3	100.0
Luxembourg	5,352	83.6	7.6	70,245	168.1	4.3	7.6	49.7
Norway	4,364	68.2	3.4	47,207	113.0	3.0	9.2	60.4
Switzerland	4,177	65.3	2.8	35,650	85.3	1.4	11.7	76.5
Austria	3,519	55.0	2.4	34,393	82.3	2.2	10.2	66.8
Iceland	3,443	53.8	5.0	36,183	86.6	4.1	9.5	62.1
Belgium	3,389	52.9	3.2	32,998	79.0	2.1	10.3	67.0
France	3,374	52.7	2.3	30,266	72.4	2.2	11.1	72.8
Canada	3,326	52.0	3.2	34,058	81.5	3.3	9.5	63.8
Germany	3,287	51.4	1.8	30,777	73.6	1.4	10.7	69.7
Australia	3,128	48.9	4.7	34,240	81.9	3.7	9.1	59.6
Denmark	3,108	48.6	2.8	34,137	81.7	2.2	9.1	59.4
Netherlands	3,094	48.3	3.0	35,120	84.0	2.6	8.8	57.5
Greece	2,981	46.6	4.7	29,578	70.8	3.7	10.1	65.8
Ireland	2,926	45.7	7.2	38,850	93.0	7.6	7.5	49.2

Sweden	2,918	45.6	3.8	32,111	76.8	2.9	9.1	59.3
United Kingdom	2724	42.6	4.2	32,860	78.6	2.8	8.3	54.1
Italy	2,532	39.6	3.2	28,094	67.2	1.4	9.0	58.8
Japan	2,358	36.8	2.6	30,842	73.8	1.3	7.6	49.9
New Zealand	2,343	36.6	4.3	25,950	62.1	3.2	9.0	58.9
Finland	2,331	36.4	3.5	30,959	74.1	3.7	7.5	49.2
Spain	2,255	35.2	3.0	27,400	65.6	3.6	8.2	53.7
Portugal	2,033	31.8	3.8	19,889	47.6	2.5	10.2	66.7
Czech Republic	1,479	23.1	2.5	20,606	49.3	2.9	7.2	46.9
Hungary	1,337	20.9	4.9	17,483	41.8	3.9	7.6	49.9
Korea	1,318	20.6	7.6	22,098	52.9	5.0	6.0	38.9
Slovak Republic	1,137	17.8	3.7	15,983	38.2	4.3	7.1	46.4
Poland	867	13.5	5.2	13,894	33.2	4.4	6.2	40.7
Mexico	675	10.5	3.6	10,627	25.4	2.8	6.4	41.5
Turkey	586	9.2	6.3	7,711	18.5	4.5	7.6	49.6
Organization for Economic Cooperation and Development Median	2,922	45.6	3.6	30,901	73.9	3.1	9.0	58.9

Sources: *OECD Factbook 2007* (pp. 26–33); *Health at a Glance 2007* (p. 87). Paris: Organization for Economic Cooperation and Development.

Luxembourg. National health care expenditures have been projected to reach $2.8 trillion in 2011 and are expected to constitute 17% of the GDP by 2011 (Heffler et al., 2002). These forecasts portend that the health care sector will remain one of the fastest growing components of the U.S. economy. In addition to an increased demand for services that will expand job opportunities, we can also expect to see policy debates and new initiatives to keep costs from spiraling out of control in the future.

REASONS FOR HIGH COST

The rising health care expenditures have been attributed to the complex interaction of numerous factors. General inflation in the economy is a more visible cause of health care spending because it affects the cost of producing health care services through higher wages, cost of supplies, and so forth; however, apart from the effects of general inflation, there are nine major areas that influence medical cost inflation (see **Exhibit 12.1**).

Third-Party Payment

Health care is among the few services for which a third party, not the consumer, pays the lion's share for most of the services used. Whether the government or a private insurance company foots the bill, individual patients pay a price far lower than the actual cost of the service (Altman & Wallack, 1996). As a result, moral hazard and provider-induced demand (discussed in earlier chapters) lead to excessive utilization of health care services. The patient and provider have little incentive to be cost conscious when someone else is paying the bill.

Exhibit 12.1 Reasons for the High Cost of Health Care

- Third-party payment
- Imperfect market
- Growth of technology
- Increase in the elderly population
- Medical model of health care delivery
- Multipayer system and administrative costs
- Defensive medicine
- Waste and abuse
- Practice variations

Imperfect Market

Prices charged by providers for health care services are likely to be much closer to the cost of producing the services in a highly regulated market or in a highly competitive market (Altman & Wallack, 1996); the U.S. health care market is neither. Because the U.S. health care delivery system does not consist of a national health care program, it is not as highly regulated as are single-payer systems in other countries. Health care delivery in the United States also does not represent a highly competitive market because of various market imperfections discussed in Chapter 1. In an imperfect market, the use of health care is driven by need rather than economic demand; the quantity of health care services produced and delivered is likely to be much higher than in a competitive market, and the prices charged for health care services will be permanently higher than the true economic costs of production (Altman & Wallack, 1996).

Growth of Technology

In the adoption and diffusion of intensive procedures, the United States follows an early-start, fast-growth pattern (TECH Research Network, 2001). Growth and intensive use of technology have a direct impact on the escalation of health care costs (see Chapter 5). New technology is expensive to develop, and costs incurred in research and development are included in the total health care expenditures. Once technology is developed, it creates demand for its use. The development of new technology raises the expectations of consumers about what medical science can do to diagnose and treat disease and prolong life. Attempts to limit the diffusion of certain expensive technologies in the United States have been largely unsuccessful.

Increase in the Elderly Population

During the past 100 years, life expectancy in the United States has risen substantially. Life expectancy at birth increased by almost 30 years from 47.3 years in 1900 to almost 77 years in 2000 (NCHS, 2002a). With increased life expectancy and the aging of the baby-boomer generation, the United States is experiencing a notable increase in its elderly population. The number of elderly is projected to continue to rise through the middle of the 21st century. The elderly consume more health care than other age groups, with costs 3.5 times as high. In 1998, the average medical expenses for a person 65 years or over came to $6,265 per person compared with $1,810 per person for those under the age of 65 (NCHS, 2002a, p. 295).

Medical Model of Health Care Delivery

As discussed in Chapter 2, the Medical Model emphasizes medical intervention after a person has become sick. Prevention and lifestyle/behavior changes to promote health are de-emphasized. Although health promotion and disease prevention are not the answer to every health problem, these principles have not been accorded their rightful place in the U.S. health care delivery system. Consequently, more costly health care resources are to be employed to treat health problems that could have been prevented.

Multipayer System and Administrative Costs

Administrative costs are costs associated with the management of the financing, insurance, delivery, and payment functions. These costs include management of the enrollment process, setting up contracts with providers, claims processing, utilization monitoring, denials and appeals, and marketing and promotional expenses. Because of the complexity of a multipayer system, costs are often duplicated and may be as high as 24% to 25% of total health care expenditures in the United States. A single-payer health care system might cut health care administrative costs by one half (Hellander et al., 1994).

Defensive Medicine

The U.S. health care delivery system is riddled with legal risks for providers that promote defensive medicine (see Chapter 1). The practice of *defensive medicine* leads to tests and services that are not medically justified but are performed by physicians to protect themselves against potential malpractice lawsuits. Unrestrained malpractice awards by the courts and increased malpractice insurance premiums for physicians significantly add to the cost of health care.

Waste and Abuse

In general terms, *fraud* involves a knowing disregard of the truth and typically occurs when billing claims or cost reports are intentionally falsified. Health care fraud has been identified as a major problem in the

Medicare and Medicaid programs. Fraud may also occur when more services are provided than are medically necessary or when services not provided are billed. The latter practice may include billing for a higher priced service when a lower priced service is actually delivered.

Practice Variations

The work of John Wennberg and others brought to the forefront a disturbing aspect of physician behavior accounting for wide variations in treatment patterns for similar patients. These practice variations are referred to as *small area variations* because the observed differences in practice patterns have been associated only with geographic areas of the country. This variation, which can be as great as twofold, cannot be explained by age, gender, race, pricing variations, demand inducements, or health status (Baucus & Fowler, 2003). Small area variations signal gross inefficiencies in the U.S. health care delivery system because they increase costs without appreciably better outcomes.

COST CONTAINMENT

Even though rising health care expenditures may seem innocuous to some, they need to be controlled for several reasons. First, rising health care costs mean that Americans have to forgo other goods and services when more is spent on health care. Second, economic resources should be directed to their highest valued uses, even though consumers decide how much should be spent on purchasing a product or service based on their perception of the value they expect to receive (Feldstein, 1994, p. 13).

The United States has made many attempts to control health care spending, using a combination of government regulation and market-based competition; however, most of these undertakings have met only limited success, mainly because implementing a systemwide cost-control initiative has not been feasible in such a fragmented system. In contrast, national health care programs in other countries have an *all-payer system* in which centralized controls allow cost-containment efforts to sweep through the entire health care delivery system. Cost-containment measures in the United States can only be applied in a piecemeal fashion and affect only certain targeted sectors of the health care delivery system at a time.

Another reason that cost-control efforts in the United States have not proven very successful is because of cost shifting between programs and/or sectors. *Cost shifting* refers to the ability of providers to make up for lost revenues in one area by increasing use or charging higher prices in other areas that are free of controls. Providers are able to shift costs when cost-control measures are not applied systemwide. Regulatory approaches to cost containment typically control the capacity of the supply side, through what is referred to as health planning, and the demand side, in the form of price and utilization control.

Health Planning

Health planning refers to an undertaking by the government to align and distribute health care resources in a manner that, in the eyes of the government, would achieve desired health outcomes for all people. Health planning employs supply-side rationing (see Chapter 2) to control health care expenditures. The central planning function does not fit so well in a system that is largely private because of the absence of a central administrative agency to monitor the system (see Chapter 1). Instead, market forces are allowed to govern the system. The types of health care services, their geographic distribution, access to these services, and the prices charged by providers develop independently of any preformulated plans.

Price Controls

In 1971, President Nixon imposed the Economic Stabilization Program (ESP), which placed limits on the amount hospitals could raise their prices from year to year (Williams & Torrens, 1993). The ESP controls did generate a moderating influence on price increases for most medical services; however, the program placed no limits on the quantity of services or costs of production (Altman & Eichenholz, 1976); therefore, after controls were lifted, inflation returned to its precontrol levels (Altman & Eichenholz, 1976).

Perhaps the most important undertaking to control prices for inpatient hospital care was the conversion of hospital Medicare reimbursement from a retrospective to a prospective system based on diagnosis-related groups (DRGs) as authorized under the Social Security Amendments of 1983 (see Chapter 6). It reduced the growth in inpatient hospital spending but had little impact on total per capita Medicare cost inflation; costs mainly shifted from the inpatient to the outpatient sector.

Another rate-setting mechanism was the Omnibus Budget Reconciliation Act (OBRA) of 1989, which helped establish a national Medicare fee schedule described in Chapter 6 (see Resource-Based Relative Value Scale). With the fee schedule, physicians are paid according to relative value units established for more than 7,000 covered services, and a volume performance standard was implemented to contain the annual rate of growth in Medicare physician payments. The program seems to have achieved some success. Between 1992 and 1997, the average annual growth in total Part B expenditures was 9.2%, compared with 6.1% for physician services.

Peer Review

The term "peer review" refers to the general process of medical review of utilization and quality carried out directly by, or under the supervision of, physicians (Wilson & Neuhauser, 1985, p. 270). Under the Medicare program, a new system of peer review organizations (PROs) was established in 1984 to determine whether care is reasonable, necessary, of adequate quality, and provided in the most appropriate setting. PROs are statewide private organizations composed of practicing physicians and other health care professionals who are paid by the federal government to review the care provided to Medicare beneficiaries. They can deny payment if care does meet with their standards (Health Care Financing Administration, 1996). PROs are also referred to as quality improvement organizations.

Competitive Approaches

Competition refers to rivalry among sellers for customers (Dranove, 1993). In health care delivery, it means that providers of health care services try to attract patients who have the ability to choose from several different providers. Although competition more commonly refers to price competition, it may also be based on technical quality, amenities, access, or other factors (Dranove, 1993). In the United States, competitive reforms were given preference because of the growing interest in market-oriented approaches across many sectors of the economy during the Reagan presidency in the 1980s. Market-oriented reforms were accompanied by mounting cost-containment efforts in the private sector and the growth of managed care. Competitive strategies can be divided into four broad types:

demand-side incentives, supply-side regulation, payer-driven price competition, and utilization controls.

Demand-side incentives refer to cost-sharing mechanisms that place a larger cost burden on consumers, thus encouraging consumers to be more cost conscious in selecting the insurance plan that best serves their needs and more judicious in their utilization. *Supply-side regulation* typically refers to antitrust laws in the United States, which prohibit business practices that stifle competition among providers, such as price fixing, price discrimination, exclusive contracting arrangements, and mergers deemed anticompetitive by the Department of Justice. This forces health care organizations to be cost-efficient to survive. Payer-driven price competition occurs when employers shop for the best value in terms of the cost of premiums and the benefits package (competition among insurers) and when MCOs shop for the best value from providers of health services (competition among providers). The utilization controls used in managed care (discussed in Chapter 9) have cut through some of the unnecessary or inappropriate services provided to consumers by intervening in the decisions made by care providers to ensure that only appropriate and necessary services are provided and that services are provided efficiently.

Electronic Health Records

Electronic health records (EHR) are patients' medical records in digital format accessed over a computer on a network. There is heavy support for implementation from policy makers to convert from paper-based health records to electronic because of cost-containment benefits. Paper records rely heavily on the photo copying, faxing, and transporting of records in order to share information between providers, involving much time and money as well as the possibility of missing paper work because of the storage of information at different locations. These costs and problems can be eliminated by interoperable EHRs that could be shared easily from one provider to another as well as contain a patient's complete history in the health care system, eliminating the problem of missing records or paperwork within the file. Electronic records will result in a more coordinated health care system with the potential to improve clinicians' use of unnecessary tests and treatments. A reduction in the use of health care services will also reduce both baseline costs and cost trends. The conversion is a difficult task to undertake, however, because of critical barriers involved.

Health Care Delivery

The delivery of health care in the United States is inefficient in regards to chronic conditions such as diabetes and cardiovascular disease. The system often fails to deliver preventive programs to patients who are headed toward such conditions as well as interventions to maintain health and avoid hospitalizations. About 70% of health carc costs are generated by 10% of patients, who mostly have one or more chronic diseases; thus, the potential for cost containment through the improvement of the delivery of care for chronic conditions is large. The difficulty in implementing more preventive programs is the fragmented system of independent practitioners that makes it tough to maintain programs as well as the money lost by reducing preventable hospitalizations since proactive care management is not covered in the current health care system.

UNEQUAL IN ACCESS

In broad terms, *access* to care can be defined as the ability to obtain needed, affordable, convenient, acceptable, and effective personal health services in a timely manner. Access is one of the key determinants of health status, along with environment, lifestyle, and heredity factors (see Chapter 2). It also helps to benchmark the effectiveness of the medical care delivery system and is increasingly linked to quality of care and the efficient use of needed services.

Although "access" is a familiar term and is often used by popular and academic media, it is often used to indicate numerous and differing concepts. It may refer to whether an individual has a usual source of care, the actual use of health services, or it may reflect the acceptability of particular services. **Figure 12.1** illustrates the system, provider, and individual characteristics that influence utilization or access to care.

Data on Access

Population-based surveys supported by federal statistical agencies are the major data sources for conducting analyses on access to care. Large

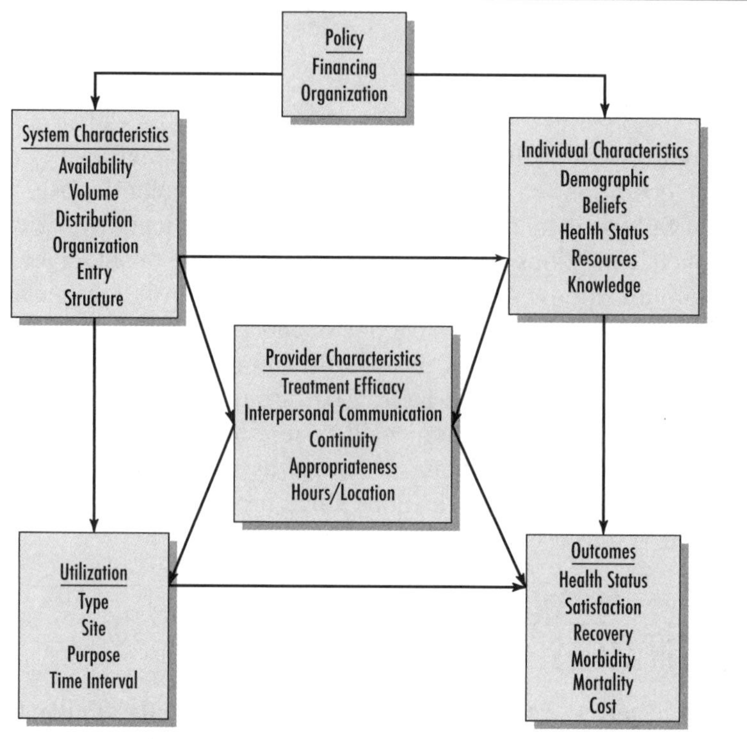

Figure 12.1 Determinants of Access

national surveys such as the National Health Interview Survey (NIHS) and the Medical Expenditure Panel Survey (MEPS) are the leading data sources used to monitor access trends as well as other issues of interest. The latter is a series of surveys that contain data on health care use and expenditures (e.g., inpatient, outpatient, and office-based care; dental care; and prescription medications), health insurance coverage, access to care, sources of payment, health status and disability, medical conditions, health care quality, and measures of socioeconomic and demographic characteristics.

Other well-known national surveys can be found in **Table 12.2** and include national surveys and surveys on special topics.

Table 12.2 National Surveys

Survey Title	Survey Author	Survey Function
Current Population Survey and Survey of Income and Program Participation	U.S. Census Bureau	Information on population characteristics
Area Resource File	Bureau of Health Professions	Pools information on characteristics of population and health care delivery system
National Health and Nutrition Examination Survey	NCHS	Information on demographics, prevalence of selected diseases, nutrition, and behavioral risk factors
National Hospital Discharge Survey	NCHS	Data on short-stay hospital discharges and utilization
Ambulatory Medical Care Survey	NCHS	Data on ambulatory medical encounters
National Hospital Ambulatory Medical Care Survey	NCHS	Data on ambulatory hospital encounters
National Nursing Home Survey	NCHS	Data on nursing homes and utilization, nursing home residents, and nursing home staff
Behavioral Risk Factor Survey National Immunization Survey National Survey of Ambulatory Surgery National Home and Hospice Care Survey	CDC	Data on health practices and behavioral risks of illness
National Health Provider Inventory	CDC	Data on inpatient facilities
Longitudinal Survey on Aging	CDC	Data on older individuals
National Nursing Home Survey Follow-Up	CDC	Data on nursing homes
National Employer Health Insurance Survey	CDC	Data on insurance
Vital Statistics of the United States	CDC	Vital statistics information

CDC, Centers for Disease Control and Prevention.

The federal government also collects data on special topics such as community health centers (Bureau of Common Reporting Requirement and Uniform Data System); HIV/AIDS (HIV Cost and Services Utilization Study 1994–1998); managed care (Consumer Assessment of Health Plans Study 1996); and mental health (Mental Health Care Services Study). The Medicare Current Beneficiary Survey, the Medicare Statistical System, the Medicaid Data System, and the Medicaid Demonstration Projects (1983–1984, 1992–1996) have collected data relevant to Medicare and Medicaid.

States, associations, and research institutions also regularly collect data on topics of interest to them. Examples include state health services utilization data (all-payer hospital discharge data systems), state-managed care data (managed care encounter data), state Medicaid enrollee satisfaction data (Medicaid enrollee satisfaction surveys), physician data from the American Medical Association's Physician Masterfile, and hospital data from the American Hospital Association's Annual Survey of Hospitals 1946 to present. Examples of research institution-based initiatives include collecting data on the health care delivery system (Center for Evaluative Clinical Sciences: Dartmouth Atlas of Health Care in the U.S.), women's health (Commonwealth Fund: Women's Health Survey 1993), minority health (Commonwealth Fund: Health Care Services and Minority Groups: A Comparative Survey of Whites, African Americans, Hispanics, and Asian Americans 1994), health insurance (Mathematica Policy Research/Robert Wood Johnson Foundation: Family Survey on Health Insurance 1993–1994), and access to care (Robert Wood Johnson Foundation National Access Surveys, Mathematica Policy Research: Access to Care Pilot Survey of Medicaid Beneficiaries 1994).

With the growth of managed care, encounter databases have become increasingly critical in recording and evaluating access. In addition to the federal government, private nonprofit research centers also collect information on managed care. Examples include the National Health Maintenance Organization Census (1977 to the present, sponsored by Interstudy) and the Health Plan Employer Data and Information Set (sponsored by the National Committee for Quality Assurance).

Access Disparities

In the United States, both low socioeconomic status and minority group membership are associated with lower overall health care usage and access. Data from the 1998 National Health Interview Survey reveal that nonwhite persons under the age of 65 years were 5% to 22% less likely than their white counterparts to be insured. Among nonelderly middle-to-high income individuals, only 9% reported being uninsured compared with their near-poor (31%) and poor (34%) counterparts. These differences/discrepancies are particularly significant, given the predominant role of insurance in the U.S. health care delivery system.

Among NHIS measures of primary care access, racial/ethnic minorities are less likely than their white counterparts to have a specific source of ongoing care. A similar trend is observed among lower income individuals and their higher income counterparts. Among those who had a usual source of care, blacks and Hispanics were more likely than whites to have hospital-based (as opposed to office-based) care. Hispanics in particular are less likely to have a usual primary care provider than their non-Hispanic white counterparts (36% vs. 21%). Similar trends are observed among Medicare beneficiaries, for whom many preventive services (e.g., flu shots, cancer screenings) require no cost sharing. Nonwhite beneficiaries have fewer cancer screenings, flu shots, and ambulatory and physician visits than their nonwhite counterparts (Gornick, 2000).

Geographic disparities in access are also present, and individuals from rural areas face greater access barriers than those residing in urban areas. Rural Americans have higher mortalities and morbidities and shorter life expectancies than their urban counterparts (Cordes, 1989; DeFriese & Ricketts, 1989; Rowland & Lyons, 1989; Sherman, 1991). Rural Americans are more likely to be poor, suffer from chronic impairment, to be uninsured if under 65 years, and more likely to be elderly than their urban counterparts (Norton & McManus, 1989). The health care system available to address these problems, however, faces severe limitations, including maldistribution of physicians, lack of sufficient primary care services, and lack of access to care for geographic, financial, or discrimination/cultural reasons (Freeman et al., 1982; Sardell, 1988).

Reasons for Unequal Access

In the United States, significant barriers to access still exist at both the individual and system levels. Individually, it is those with minority origins, low income, less education, special needs defined by disability and chronic illness, and no health insurance coverage who continue to face greater barriers to access than the rest of the population. Access is best predicted by race, income, and occupation. These three factors are interrelated: those belonging to minority groups tend to be poorer, less educated, and more likely to work in job environments that pose greater health risks.

Access Initiatives

Access to care has been incrementally addressed by the U.S. government through a variety of public programs. Although a preventive- and chronic-care model of health care delivery in the United States is an evolving departure from the traditional acute-care system, the concepts of prevention and comprehensive primary care are clearly established in legislative history. The Sheppard-Towner Act of 1921 exemplifies early federal attempts to provide direct primary care health services to economically disadvantaged mothers and children. Screening and other preventive care programs followed suit in subsequent Social Security Amendments. Government interest in assuring access to other lower-income populations grew during World War II, when comprehensive care was extended to the wives and children of low-grade armed forces personnel. The issue of health care access among disadvantaged populations paved the way for the Great Society programs of the 1960s. Rising health care costs, along with disproportionately high individual cost-sharing among the elderly, prompted Congress to create the Medicare program (which later expanded coverage to people with disabilities and end-stage renal disease) and Medicaid for the poor.

In the latter portion of the 20th century, services such as cancer screening and immunizations were added to the Medicare program, and $24 million was allocated to states in 1997 to create State Children's Health Insurance Programs (SCHIPs) for low-income children in families that did not otherwise qualify for Medicaid. In addition to health insurance programs, the U.S. government has also provided funding to strengthen community health centers and other safety net providers.

Critique and Prospect

It is society's duty to ensure equitable access to an adequate level of health care for all. According to one view, economic scarcity is a relative measure. Scarcity in the U.S. medical delivery system is largely the result of distributive practices that limit access for those who are poor and those who live in rural areas. In the overall system, a surplus exists—for example, of hospital beds and physicians practicing in urban areas. The problem is that these surpluses are not generally shifted to respond to need (Brown, 1992).

Earlier chapters discussed the lack of access for the uninsured. Access, however, is also limited because of underinsurance and, for a few people, because of lifetime caps on health insurance. For years, these lifetime caps have been arbitrarily set at around 1 or 2 million dollars. A number of Americans who are otherwise insured are affected by lifetime caps because of a costly catastrophic injury or illness. For example, the average lifetime cost of care for a person with a spinal cord injury who is ventilator dependent can be more than $5 million. After the cap is reached, insurance companies stop coverage, although the need for medical care continues.

Access to health care has considerable influence on population health. The prospects of universal access in the United States are contingent on drastic reductions in health care expenditures. Without significant improvements in access, the U.S. health care delivery system will continue to be rated behind most others in the developed world. From a systems standpoint, this situation is a predicament. The problem requires national policy initiatives, but it does not diminish the need to pursue quality improvements at the micro level in which practitioners, ancillary workers, and health care managers have more control.

AVERAGE IN QUALITY

Quality can be appreciated from both microperspectives and macroperspectives. See **Exhibit 12.2** for examples of micro and macro quality indicators. The microview focuses on services at the point of delivery and their subsequent effects. It is associated with the performance of individual caregivers and health care organizations. The macroview looks at quality from the standpoint of populations. It reflects the performance of the entire health care delivery system.

The Institute of Medicine has defined quality as "the degree to which health services for individuals and populations increase the likelihood of

Exhibit 12.2 Quality Indicators

Micro:	Macro:
• Small area variations	• Cost
• Medical errors	• Access
• Patient satisfaction	• Population health
• Quality of life	
• Health outcomes	

desired health outcomes and are consistent with current professional knowledge" (McGlynn, 1997). The definition has several implications.

1. Quality performance occurs on a continuum, theoretically ranging from unacceptable to excellent.
2. The focus is on services provided by the health care delivery system (as opposed to individual behaviors).
3. Quality may be evaluated from the perspective of individuals and populations or communities.
4. The emphasis is on desired health outcomes; research evidence must be used to identify the services that improve health outcomes.
5. In the absence of scientific evidence regarding appropriateness of care, professional consensus can be used to develop criteria for the definition and measurement of quality (McGlynn, 1997).

Although complete in many respects, the definition of quality proposed by the Institute of Medicine leaves out the roles of cost and access in the evaluation of quality. Even though the United States spends more of its national income on health care than other nations, Americans are not the healthiest people in the world. Perhaps a key reason why the United States, despite its tremendous advances in medical technology, trails behind other industrialized nations in broad population measures of health is widespread lack of access to basic health care. Clearly, more health care expenditures or more intense medical services do not produce better health. In other words, more is not better, and more does not represent better quality.

In his well-known model to help define and measure quality in health care organizations, Donabedian (1980) proposed three domains in which health care quality should be examined: structure, process, and outcomes. Donabedian noted that all three domains are important in measuring the quality of care. He also emphasized that these three approaches are complementary and should be used collectively to monitor quality of care (Al-Assaf, 1993b).

Structure, process, and outcomes are closely linked (**Figure 12.2**). The three domains are also hierarchical. Structure is the foundation of the quality of health care. Good processes require a good structure. In other words, deficiencies in structure generally have a negative effect on the processes (defined in "Process" section following) of health care delivery. Structure and processes together influence quality outcomes. Structure primarily influences process and has only a secondary direct influence on outcome. The model views quality strictly from the delivery system's perspective. It does not account for social and individual lifestyle and behavioral factors that also have a significant influence on health status.

Structure

Structure has been defined as "the relatively stable characteristics of the providers of care, of the tools and resources they have at their disposal, and of the physical and organizational settings in which they work" (Donabedian, 1980, p. 81). Structural measures indicate the extent to which health care organizations are capable of providing adequate levels of care (Williams & Torrens, 1993). Hence, structure provides an indirect measure of quality under the assumption that a good structure enables health delivery professionals to employ good processes that would lead to good outcomes.

A significant initiative towards improving structure are electronic health records (EHRs), which are digital formats of a patient's medical record that when implemented into the health care system should reduce cost and provide greater coordination across the system. The Agency for Healthcare Research and Quality (AHRQ) is currently funding projects across the nation to implement and evaluate electronic medical and health records to determine their impact on quality, safety, efficacy, and cost on health care. Analysis on the national level has shown a savings to physicians of almost $10 billion when the resulting safety and efficiency improvements from the use of EHRs are considered yet a study for small practices show a net loss of $20,000 per physician per year.

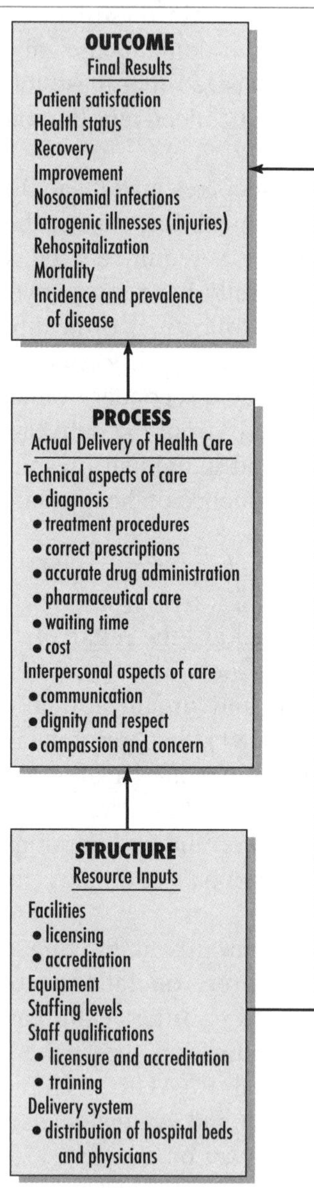

Figure 12.2 The Three Domains of Health Care Quality

Process

"Process" refers to the specific way in which care is provided. Examples of process are correct diagnostic tests, correct prescriptions, accurate drug administration, pharmaceutical care (see Chapter 4), waiting time to see a physician, and interpersonal aspects of care delivery. Just as with structure, it is important to relate process to patient care outcomes. In other words, structures and processes should be employed with the objective of achieving better outcomes. Some significant initiatives toward process improvement have occurred in recent years. Some of the main developments in this area are clinical practice guidelines, cost-efficiency, critical pathways, and risk management, which are discussed in the "Developments in Process Improvement" section that follows.

Outcomes

Outcomes refer to the effects or final results obtained from utilizing the structure and processes of health care delivery. Outcomes are viewed by many as the bottom line measure of the effectiveness of the health care delivery system (McGlynn & Brook, 1996). Positive outcomes suggest recovery from disease and improvement in health. They also suggest an overall improvement in health status through health promotion and disease prevention efforts and adequate access to health care services. Outcome measures include postoperative infection rates, nosocomial infections, iatrogenic illnesses, rates of rehospitalization, and patient satisfaction.

DEVELOPMENTS IN PROCESS IMPROVEMENT

Clinical Practice Guidelines

In response to findings of small area variations, various professional groups, MCOs, and the government have embarked on the development of standardized practice guidelines. Clinical practice guidelines (also called medical practice guidelines) are explicit descriptions representing preferred clinical processes. A clinical practice guideline constitutes a plan for managing a clinical problem based on evidence, whenever possible, and on consensus in the absence of evidence (Larsen, 1996). Hence, clinical practice guidelines are designed to provide scientifically based protocols to guide physicians' clinical decisions. These guidelines are intended to promote lower costs and better outcomes.

Cost-Efficiency

Also referred to as cost-effectiveness, cost-efficiency (discussed in Chapter 5 in conjunction with technology assessment) is an important concept in quality assessment. A service is cost-efficient when the benefit received is greater than the cost incurred in providing the service. In economic terms, additional services beyond the optimum point produce diminishing marginal returns. This point also represents optimal quality, which serves as a point of demarcation between underutilization and overutilization. *Underutilization* (underuse) occurs when the benefits of an intervention outweigh the risks or costs and yet the intervention is not used (Chassin, 1991). On the other hand, *overutilization* (overuse) occurs when the costs or risks of treatment outweigh the benefits and yet additional care is delivered. When health care is overused, precious resources are wasted.

Critical Pathways

Critical pathways are outcome-based and patient-centered case management tools that are interdisciplinary and that facilitate coordination of care among multiple clinical departments and caregivers. A critical pathway is a time line that identifies planned medical interventions along with expected patient outcomes for a specific diagnosis or class of cases, often defined by a diagnosis-related group. In addition to technical outcomes, pathways may measure factors such as patient satisfaction, self-reported health status, mental health, and activities of daily living. Use of critical pathways reduces costs and improves quality by reducing errors, improving coordination among interdisciplinary players, streamlining case management functions, providing systematic data for assessing care, and reducing variation in practice patterns (Giffin & Giffin, 1994).

Risk Management

Risk management consists of proactive efforts to prevent adverse events related to clinical care and facilities operations, and is especially focused on avoiding medical malpractice (Orlikoff, 1988). Initiatives undertaken by a health care organization to review clinical processes and establish protocols for the specific purpose of reducing malpractice litigation can actually enhance quality. Because malpractice concerns also result in defensive medicine, risk-management approaches should employ the principles of cost-efficiency along with standardized practice guidelines and critical pathways; however, fear of litigation actually leads to a reluctance of hospitals and physicians to disclose preventable harm and actual medical errors. In this respect, fear of litigation may actually conceal problems that may compromise patient safety (Lamb et al., 2003).

CONCLUSION

Increasing costs, lack of access, and concerns about quality pose the greatest challenges to health care delivery in the United States. To some extent, the three issues are interrelated. Increasing costs limit the system's ability to expand access and without universal coverage for all Americans, it is doubtful that the United States will ever match other developed countries in population health status.

Health care costs in the United States are the highest in the world. A move toward prospective payments and the growth of managed care can be largely credited with the brakes put on rising health care spending during the 1990s; however, the best current forecasts are for accelerated spending growth in the future, which means that a larger share of the economic resources will be devoted to the delivery of health care.

Access to medical care is one of the determinants of health status, along with environmental, lifestyle, and heredity factors. Access is also regarded as a significant benchmark in assessing the effectiveness of the medical care delivery system. Access is explained in terms of enabling and predisposing factors, as well as factors related to health policy and health care delivery.

One reason that the pursuit of quality in health care has trailed behind the emphasis on cost and access is the difficulty in defining and measuring quality. On the other hand, growth of managed care and the emphasis on cost containment have produced a heightened interest in quality because of the intuitive concern that control of costs may have a negative impact on quality; however, there is still a long way to go in specifying what constitutes good quality in medical care, how to ensure it for patients, and how to reward providers and health plans whose outcomes indicate successes in quality improvement. One challenge in achieving such a goal is that patients, providers, and payers each define quality differently, which translates into different expectations of the health care delivery system and thus differing evaluations of its quality (McGlynn, 1997).

REFERENCES

Al-Assaf, A. F. 1993a. Introduction and historical background. In A. F. Al-Assaf and J. A. Schmele (eds.). *The Textbook of Total Quality Management* (pp. 3–12). Delray Beach, FL: St. Lucie Press.

Al-Assaf, A. F. 1993b. Outcome management and TQ. In A. F. Al-Assaf and J. A. Schmele (eds.). *The Textbook of Total Quality Management* (pp. 221–237). Delray Beach, FL: St. Lucie Press.

Altman, S. H., and J. Eichenholz. 1976. Inflation in the health industry: Causes and cures. In M. Zubkoff (ed.). *Health: A Victim or Cause of Inflation?* (pp. 1–32). New York: Milbank Memorial Fund.

Altman, S. H., and S. S. Wallack. 1996. Health care spending: Can the United States control it? In S. H. Altman and U. E. Reinhardt (eds.). *Strategic Choices for a Changing Health Care System*. Chicago: Health Administration Press.

Baucus, M., and E. J. Fowler. 2003. Geographic variation in Medicare spending and the real focus of Medicare reform. *Health Affairs* Web Exclusive. Retrieved from http://content.healthaffairs.org/cgi/content/abstract/hlthaff.w2.115v1.

Brown, K. 1992. Death and access: Ethics in cross-cultural health care. In E. Friedman (ed.). *Choices and Conflict: Explorations in Health Care Ethics*. Chicago: American Hospital Publishing.

Chassin, M. R. 1991. Quality of care—Time to act. *Journal of the American Medical Association* 266:3472–3473.

Cordes, S. M. 1989. The changing rural environment and the relationship between health services and rural development. *Health Services Research* 23 (6): 757–784.

DeFriese, G. H., and T. C. Ricketts. 1989. Primary health care in rural areas: An agenda for research. *Health Services Research* 23 (6):931–974.

Donabedian, A. 1980. *Explorations in Quality Assessment and Monitoring: The Definition of Quality and Approaches to Its Assessment*. Vol. 1. Ann Arbor, MI: Health Administration Press.

Dranove, D. 1993. The case for competitive reform in health care. In R. J. Arnould, R. F. Rich, and W. D. White (eds.). *Competitive Approaches to Health Care Reform* (pp. 67–82). Washington, DC: Urban Institute Press.

Feldstein, P. 1994. *Health Policy Issues: An Economic Perspective on Health Reform*. Ann Arbor, MI: AUPHA Press/Health Administration Press.

Freeman, H. E., et al. 1982. Community health centers: An initiative of enduring utility. *Milbank Memorial Fund Quarterly/Health and Society* 60 (2): 245–267.

Giffin, M., and R. B. Giffin. 1994. Market memo: Critical pathways produce tangible results. *Health Care Strategic Management* 12 (7):1–6.

Gornick, M. E. 2000. *Vulnerable Populations and Medicare Services: Why Do Disparities Exist*. New York: Century Foundation Press.

Health Care Financing Administration. 1996. Overview of the Medicare program. *Health Care Financing Review: Medicare and Medicaid Statistical Supplement* 5.

Heffler, S., et al. 2002. Health spending projections for 2001–2011: The latest outlook. *Health Affairs* 21 (2):207–218.

Hellander, I., et al. 1994. Health care paper chase, 1993: The cost to the nation, the states, and the District of Columbia. *International Journal of Health Services* 24 (1):1–9.

Lamb, R. M., et al. 2003. Hospital disclosure practices: Results of a national survey. *Health Affairs* 22 (2):73–83.

Larsen, R. R. 1996. Narrowing the gray zone: How clinical practice guidelines can improve the decision-making process. *Postgraduate Medicine* 100 (2):17–24.

Levit, K., et al. 2003. Trends in U.S. health care spending, 2001. *Health Affairs* 22 (1):154–164.

McGlynn, E. A. 1997. Six challenges in measuring the quality of health care. *Health Affairs* 16 (3):7–21.

McGlynn, E. A., and R. H. Brook. 1996. Ensuring quality of care. In R. M. Andersen, T. H. Rice, and G. F. Kominski (eds.). *Changing the U.S. Health Care System: Key Issues in Health Services, Policy, and Management*. San Francisco: Jossey-Bass Publishers.

National Center for Health Statistics. 1996. *Health, United States, 1995*. Hyattsville, MD: U.S. Department of Health and Human Services.

National Center for Health Statistics. 2002a. *Health, United States, 2002*. Hyattsville, MD: U.S. Department of Health and Human Services.

National Center for Health Statistics. 2002b. *National Vital Statistics Reports* 49 (12). Atlanta, GA: Centers for Disease Control and Prevention.

Norton, C. H., and M. A. McManus. 1989. Background tables on demographic characteristics. *Health Services Research* 23 (6):807–848.

Orlikoff, J. E. 1988. *Malpractice Prevention and Liability Control for Hospitals*, 2nd ed. Chicago: American Hospital Publishing.

Rowland, D., and B. Lyons. 1989. Triple jeopardy: Rural, poor, and uninsured. *Health Services Research* 23 (6):975–1004.

Sardell, A. 1988. *The U.S. Experiment in Social Medicine, the Community Health Center Program, 1965–1986*. Pittsburgh, PA: University of Pittsburgh Press.

Sherman, A. 1991. *Falling By the Wayside: Children in Rural America*. Washington, DC: Children's Defense Fund.

TECH Research Network. 2001. Technology change around the world: Evidence from heart attack care. *Health Affairs* 20 (3):25–42.

Williams, S. J., and P. R. Torrens. 1993. Influencing, regulating, and monitoring the health care system. In S. J. Williams and P. R. Torrens (eds.). *Introduction to Health Services*, 4th ed. (pp. 421–429). Albany, NY: Delmar Publishers.

Wilson, F. A., and D. Neuhauser. 1985. *Health Services in the United States*, 2nd ed. Cambridge, MA: Ballinger Publishing Co.

Chapter 13

Health Policy

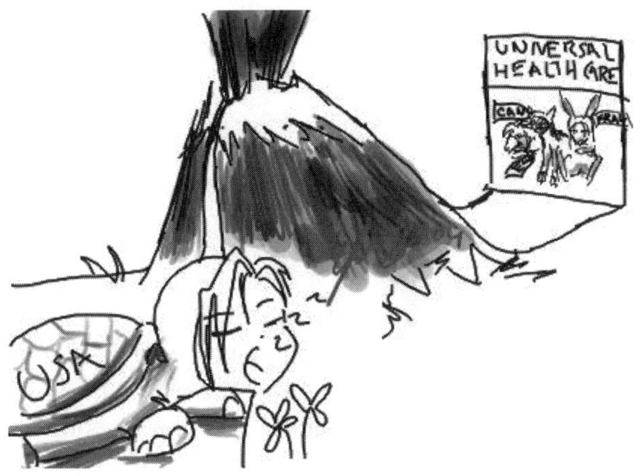

INTRODUCTION

Even though the United States does not have a centrally controlled system of health care delivery, it does have a history of federal, state, and local government involvement in health care and health policy. Americans possess an incredible desire to be healthy. They contend that their individual health contributes to the overall health of the nation and, consequently, to the economy. It is not surprising, therefore, that the government is keenly interested in health policy. This chapter first defines what health policy is and explores the principal features of health policy in the United States. Next, it describes the development of legislative policy and gives examples of critical health policy issues. Finally, an outlook for the future of health policy in the United States is provided.

WHAT IS HEALTH POLICY?

Public policies are authoritative decisions made in the legislative (congressional), executive (presidential), or judicial (court including the Supreme Court) branches of government that are intended to direct or influence the actions, behaviors, or decisions of others (Longest, 1994). When public policies pertain to or influence the pursuit of health, they become health policies. Thus, health policy can be defined as "the aggregate of principles, stated or unstated, that . . . characterize the distribution of resources, services, and political influences that impact on the health of the population" (Miller, 1987, p. 15).

Different Forms of Health Policies

Health policies often come as a byproduct of public social policies enacted by the government. A relevant example is the expansion of health care insurance coverage. Policies that excluded fringe benefits from income or Social Security taxes and a Supreme Court ruling that employee benefits, including health insurance, could be legitimately included in the collective bargaining process led to important changes in the health care system (see Chapter 3). As a result, employer-provided health insurance benefits grew rapidly in middle decades of the 20th century (Health Insurance Association of America, 1992). In 1965, adoption of the Medicare and Medicaid legislation expanded the health sector by providing publicly subsidized health insurance to the elderly and indigent.

The American health care system has developed under extraordinarily favorable public policies. For example, the federally funded National Institutes of Health (NIH) had a budget of about $10 million when the agency was established in the early 1930s. Today, following exponential growth, the NIH annual budget is about $10 billion. Also, encouraged by policies that permit businesses to recoup their investments in research and development from the government, private industry spends a significant amount on biomedical research and development (NIH, 1991).

Health policies pertain to health care at all levels, including policies affecting the production, provision, and financing of health care services. Health policies affect groups or classes of individuals, such as physicians, the poor, the elderly, or children. They can also affect types of organizations, such as medical schools, health maintenance organizations (HMOs), nursing homes, producers of medical technology, or employers. In the United States, each branch and level of government can influence health policy. For example, both the executive and legislative branches at the federal, state, and local levels can establish health policies, and the judicial branch can uphold, strike down, or modify existing laws affecting health and health care at any level.

Statutes or laws, such as the statutory language contained in the 1983 Amendments to the Social Security Act that authorized the prospective payment system (PPS) for reimbursing hospitals for Medicare beneficiaries, are also considered policies. Another example is the certificate-of-need (CON) programs through which many states seek to regulate capital expansion in their health care systems (see Chapters 5 and 12).

Regulatory Tools

Health policies can be used as regulatory tools (Longest, 1994). They call on the government to prescribe and control the behavior of a particular target group by monitoring the group and imposing sanctions if it fails to comply. Federally funded peer review organizations, for instance, develop and enforce standards concerning appropriate care under the Medicare program (see Chapter 12). State insurance departments across the country regulate health insurance companies in an effort to protect the customers from excessive premiums, mendacious practices, and defaults on coverage in case of financial failure of an insurance company.

Some health policies are self-regulatory. For example, physicians set standards of medical practice, and schools of public health decide which courses should be part of their graduate programs in public health (Weissert & Weissert, 1996).

Allocative Tools

Health policies can also be used as allocative tools (Longest, 1994). They involve the direct provision of income, services, or goods to certain groups of individuals or institutions. Allocative tools in the health care arena are of two main types: distributive and redistributive. Distributive policies spread benefits throughout society. Typical distributive policies include funding of medical research through the NIH, the construction of facilities (e.g., hospitals under the Hill-Burton program during the 1950s and 1960s), and the initiation of new institutions (e.g., HMOs).

Redistributive policies, on the other hand, take money or power from one group and give it to another. This system often creates visible beneficiaries and payers. For this reason, health policy is often most visible and politically charged when it performs redistributive functions. Redistributive policies include the Medicaid program, which takes tax revenue from the public and spends it on the poor in the form of free health insurance.

PRINCIPAL FEATURES OF U.S. HEALTH POLICY

Several features characterize U.S. health policy, including government being a subsidiary to the private sector; fragmented, incremental, and piecemeal reform; pluralistic (interest group) politics; a decentralized role for the states; and the impact of presidential leadership. These features often act or interact to influence the development and evolution of health policies.

Government as Subsidiary to the Private Sector

In the United States, health care is not seen as a right of citizenship or a primary responsibility of government. Instead, the private sector plays a dominant role. Similar to many other public policy issues, Americans generally prefer market solutions over government intervention in health care financing and delivery, and for this reason, they have a strong preference for keeping the government's role in the delivery of health care to a minimum. One result is that Americans have developed social insurance programs far more reluctantly than most industrialized democracies. In addition, public opinion regarding such programs in the United States often presumes such programs to be overly generous.

Generally speaking, the role of government in U.S. health care has grown incrementally, mainly in response to perceived problems and negative consequences. Some of the most cited problems associated with government involvement include escalating costs, bureaucratic inflexibility and red tape, excessive regulation, irrational paperwork, arbitrary and sometimes conflicting public directives, inconsistent enforcement of rules and regulations, fraud and abuse, inadequate reimbursement schedules, arbitrary denial of claims, insensitivity to local needs, consumer and provider dissatisfaction, and charges that such efforts tend to promote welfare dependence rather than a desire to seek employment (Longest, 1994).

The most credible argument for policy intervention begins with the identification of situations in which markets fail or do not function efficiently. Health care in the United States is a big industry, but certain specific characteristics and conditions of the health care market distinguish it from other types of businesses. The market for health care services in the United States violates the conditions of a competitive market in several ways.

The complexity of health care services almost eliminates the ability of the consumer to make informed decisions without guidance from the sellers (providers). The entry of sellers into the health care market is heavily regulated. Widespread insurance coverage also affects the decisions of both buyers and sellers in these markets. These and other factors mean that the markets for health care services do not operate competitively, thus inviting policy intervention.

Government spending for health care has been largely confined to filling the gaps in the private sector. This intervention includes environmental protection, preventive services, communicable disease control, care of special groups, institutional care of the mentally and chronically ill, provision of medical care to the indigent, and support for research and training. With health coverage considered a privilege or even a luxury for those who are offered insurance through their employers, the government is left in a gap-filling role for the most vulnerable of the uninsured population.

Fragmented, Incremental, and Piecemeal Reform

The subsidiary role of the government and the attendant mixture of private and public approaches to the provision of health care also results in a complex and fragmented pattern of health care financing in which (1) the employed are predominantly covered by voluntary insurance provided through contributions made by themselves and their employers; (2) the aged are insured through a combination of coverage financed out of Social Security tax revenues (Medicare Part A), voluntary insurance for physician and supplementary coverage (Medicare Part B), and voluntary purchase of Medigap plans; (3) the poor are covered through Medicaid via federal, state, and local revenues; and (4) special population groups, such as veterans, Native Americans, and members of the armed forces, have coverage provided directly by the federal government.

Health policies in the United States have been incremental and piecemeal. An example is the gradual reforms in the Medicaid program since its establishment in 1965. In 1984, the first steps were taken to mandate coverage of pregnant women and children in two-parent families who met income eligibility requirements and also to mandate coverage for all children 5 years old or younger who met financial eligibility requirements. In 1986, states were given the option of covering pregnant women and children up to 5 years of age in families with incomes below 100% of federal poverty income guidelines. In 1988, that option was increased to cover families at 185% of federal poverty income. In 1988, as part of the Medicaid Catastrophic Act that remains in effect today, Congress mandated coverage for pregnant women and infants in families with incomes below 100% of federal poverty guidelines. (In 1989, it was expanded to 133% of the poverty income, and coverage of children was expanded to include the age of 6 years.) In 1988, Congress required that Medicaid coverage be continued for 6 months for families leaving the Aid to Families with Dependent Children (AFDC) program and allowed states the option of adding six months to that extension. The recently enacted State Children's Health Insurance Program (SCHIP) allows states to use Medicaid expansion to extend insurance coverage to uninsured children who otherwise are not qualified for existing Medicaid programs.

These examples illustrate how a program is reformed and/or expanded through successive legislative enactments over several years. In a typical American fashion, the Medicaid program has been reformed through incremental change but without ensuring access to medical care for all of the nation's uninsured. Among the uninsured are millions of Americans who are not categorically eligible for services. These uninsured consist mostly of adults under age 65 with no dependent children. Congress has demonstrated the desire and political will to address the needs of a small number of the uninsured perceived to be the most vulnerable (e.g., pregnant women and children) but has not developed a consensus on more dramatic steps to move beyond incremental adjustments to existing programs.

The process of legislative health policy development offers another vivid case of institutional fragmentation. Thirty-one different congressional committees and subcommittees try to claim some fragment of jurisdiction over health legislation. The reform proposals that emerge from these committees face a daunting political challenge because of the process of separate consideration and passage in each chamber, negotiations in a joint conference committee to reconcile the bills passed by the two houses, then back to each chamber for approval. In the Senate, 41 of the 100 members can thwart the entire process at any point.

After a specific bill has passed in Congress, however, its journey is far from complete. Multiple levels of federal and state bureaucracy must interpret the legislation. Rules and regulations must be written for its implementation. During this process, political actors, interest groups, or project beneficiaries may influence the ultimate design of the program. At times, the final result can differ significantly from the initial intent of its congressional sponsors. This complex and seemingly anarchic process of policy formulation and implementation makes fundamental, comprehensive policy reform extremely difficult. Ideology and the organization of government reinforce the tendency toward a standstill. It usually takes a great political event—a landmark election, a mass popular upheaval, a war, or a domestic crisis—to shake off the normal tilt temporarily toward inaction and the status quo.

Pluralistic and Interest Group Politics

Perhaps the most common explanation for health policy outcomes in the United States is one based on the role of interest groups and the incremental policies that result from compromises designed to satisfy their demands. Traditionally, the membership of the policy community has included (1) the legislative committees with jurisdiction in a policy domain, (2) the executive branch agencies responsible for implementing policies in the public domain, and (3) the interest groups in the private domain. The first two categories are the suppliers of the policies demanded by the third category.

Innovative, nonincremental policies are resisted by the established groups because such measures undermine the bargaining practices designed to reduce threats to established interests. The stability of the system is ensured because most groups are satisfied with the benefits that they receive; however, the result for any single group is less than optimal.

Interest Groups

The most effective demanders of policies are the well-organized interest groups. Interest groups' pluralism affects health policy just as it does any other policy debate in American politics. Powerful interest groups involved in health care politics are adamant about resisting any major change (Alford, 1975). Each group fights hard to protect its best interests.

By combining and concentrating the resources of their members, organized interest groups can dramatically change the ratio between the costs and benefits of participation in the political markets for policy change. Such interest groups represent a variety of individuals and entities, such as physicians in the American Medical Association, senior citizens allied with the AARP (American Association of Retired Persons), institutional providers such as hospitals belonging to the American Hospital Association, nursing homes belonging to the American Health Care Association or the American Association of Homes and Services for the Aging, and the member companies in the Pharmaceutical Research and Manufacturers of America. In recent years, physicians have often found it difficult to establish a unified voice to lobby for their interests because of the many specialty groups that exist among them.

The policy agenda of interest groups is typically reflective of their own interests. For example, the AARP advocates programs to expand financing for long-term care for the elderly. Organized labor was among the staunchest supporters of national health insurance during the 1950s and again in the 1990s. Educational institutions and accrediting bodies have their primary concerns embedded in policies that would enable them to receive higher funding to educate health professionals.

Employers

The health policy concerns of American employers are mostly shaped by the degree to which employers are involved in the provision of health insurance benefits for their employees, their dependents, and their retirees. Many small business owners adamantly oppose health policies that would mandate them to provide coverage for employees because they believe they cannot afford to do so. Health policies that affect the health of workers or the health of the labor-management relations experienced by employers also attract their attention. For example, employers have to comply with federal and state regulations regarding the health and well-being of their employees and to prevent job-related illnesses and injuries. Employers are often subject to inspection by regulatory agencies to ensure that they are adhering to health and safety policies applicable to the workplace.

Consumer Groups

The interests of consumers are not uniform, nor are the policy preferences of their interest groups. Also, consumers often do not have sufficient financial means to organize and advocate for their own best interests.

The health policy concerns of consumers and the groups that represent them reflect the rich diversity of the American people. Blacks and, more recently, the rapidly growing numbers of Hispanic Americans face special health problems. Both groups are underserved for many health care services and are underrepresented in all of the health professions in the United States. Their health policy interests include getting their unique health problems (e.g., higher infant mortality, higher exposure to violence among adolescents, higher levels of substance abuse among adults, and earlier deaths from cardiovascular disease and various other causes) adequately addressed.

Manufacturers of Technology

The health policy concerns of pharmaceutical and medical technology organizations include discerning changes in health policy areas and exercising influence on the formulation of policies. Health policy concerns regarding medical technology (including pharmaceuticals) are driven by three main factors: (1) medical technology plays an important role in rising health costs, (2) medical technology often provides health benefits to people, although not always, and (3) the use of medical technology provides economic benefits aside from its potential to provide health benefits. These factors are likely to remain important determinants of the nation's policies toward medical technology. Another factor driving the nation's current medical technology policy is the policy makers' desire to develop cost-saving technology and to expand access to it. The government is spending an increasing amount of money on technology assessment. The goal is to identify the relative values among alternative technologies, presumably so that the government can support the best values in technology.

Alliances

To overcome pluralistic interests and maximize policy outcome, diverse interest groups form alliances among themselves and with members of the legislative body to protect and enhance the interests of those receiving benefits from government programs. Each member of the alliance receives benefits from current programs. The legislators are able to demonstrate to their constituencies the economic benefits from government spending in their districts, agencies are able to expand their programs, and interest groups are the direct recipients of benefits bestowed by the government programs.

Decentralized Role of the States

In the United States, individual states play a significant role in the development and implementation of health policies. The importance of the role of individual states can be seen in programs involving the following:

- Financial support for the care and treatment of the poor and chronically disabled, which includes the primary responsibility for the administration of the federal/state Medicaid program and the recently enacted SCHIP
- Quality assurance and oversight of health care practitioners and facilities (e.g., state licensure and regulation)
- Regulation of health care costs and insurance carriers
- Health personnel training (states provide the major share of the cost for the training of health care professionals)
- Authorization of local government health services

States are vested with broad legal authority to regulate almost every facet of the health care system. They license and regulate health care facilities and health professionals; restrict the content, marketing, and price of health insurance (including professional liability or malpractice insurance); set and enforce environmental quality standards; and enact a variety of controls on health care costs. All states bear a large responsibility for financing health services for the poor, primarily through the Medicaid program, for which financing is shared with the federal government. In addition, most states also help subsidize some of the costs of delivering health services to those without any coverage at all, public or private. Personal health services funded or provided by states, often in cooperation with local government, range from public health nursing and communicable disease control to family planning and prenatal care to nutrition counseling and home health services.

Most of the incremental policy actions of recent years originated in state governments. One action, taken by 24 states, was to create a special program called an "insurance risk pool." These programs are intended to help persons acquire private insurance who are otherwise unable to do so because of the medical risks that they pose to insurance companies. Most of these programs are financed by a combination of individual premiums and taxes on insurance carriers.

Other state-initiated programs have addressed additional vulnerable populations. New Jersey developed a program to ensure access to care for all pregnant women. Florida began a program, called Healthy Kids Corporation, that linked health insurance to schools. Massachusetts, Hawaii, and Oregon have experimented with more comprehensive programs designed to provide universal access to care within their jurisdictions.

Arguments have been made against too much state control over health policy decisions. The greater control the states have, the more difficult it becomes to develop a coordinated national strategy. For example, it is difficult to plan a national disease control program if all states do not participate in the program or if they do not collect and report data in the same way. Moreover, some argue that disparities among states may lead to inequalities in access to health services. This might, in turn, lead to migration from states with poor health benefits to those with more generous programs. Finally, states may interpret federal incentives in ways that jeopardize the policy's original intent. For example, many states took advantage of federal matching grants for Medicaid programs by including a number of formerly state-funded services under an "expanded" Medicaid program. This allowed states to gain increased federal funding while providing exactly the same level of services as before. This phenomenon, called Medicaid maximization, although pursued by only a few states, had an impact outside of those states and may have contributed nationally to rising health care costs in the early 1990s (Coughlin et al., 1999).

Impact of Presidential Leadership

Americans often look to strong presidential leadership in the search for possible sources of major change in health policies, and presidents have important opportunities to influence congressional outcomes through their efforts to develop compromises that allow bills with at least some of their preferred agendas to be passed.

President Lyndon Johnson's role in the passage of Medicare and Medicaid is often cited as a prime example. Johnson achieved the passage of Medicare and Medicaid in 1965 in the context of an unusually favorable level of political opportunity and by effectively using his leadership skills.

Some important health policies have been passed since President Harry Truman's time in office. The major piece of health legislation that passed under Truman was the Hill-Burton Hospital Construction Act. Two major pieces of health legislation were passed during Nixon's presidency: (1) the actions leading to federal support of HMOs in 1973 and (2) the enactment of the National Health Planning and Resources Development Act of 1974. Under President Reagan, new Medicare cost-control approaches for hospitals and physicians were created, and additional Medicare coverage for the elderly was established. Even though President Clinton's comprehensive reform efforts failed, his incremental initiatives succeeded. Examples include the Health Insurance Portability and Accountability Act of 1996 and the SCHIP.

Many political lessons are to be learned from the failure of Clinton's health care reform initiative (Litman & Robins, 1997). Presidential leadership in achieving landmark changes in health policies can be successful only when a convergence of political opportunity, political skill, and commitment occurs. Opportunities were uniquely abundant for Johnson in 1965, and he effectively handled his legislative role. Presidents Truman, Kennedy, and Carter might have promoted their proposals with greater skill, but they were fundamentally thwarted by the lack of a true window of opportunity. Clinton enjoyed a uniquely high level of public interest in health care reform but failed in part because of other weaknesses in his level of opportunity, especially his failure to act within the first 100 days after his election. The complexity of the ever-changing details of his proposal was another major flaw and ultimately proved too much for the general public to comprehend and too easy for adversaries to distort.

Results of the 2008 presidential election, with Obama victorious, offers another opportunity for Democrats to learn from the lessons of the past and take up health care reform once again. Although the extent and timetable for the reform remain uncertain given the current economic recession that the country is experiencing, campaign speeches by Mr. Obama did suggest a new direction in U.S. health care reform in the coming years. While campaigning for the presidency, Mr. Obama presented a framework for health care reform to achieve three goals: modernize the health care system to improve quality and reduce costs, expand coverage to all Americans, and improve prevention and public health.

DEVELOPMENT OF LEGISLATIVE HEALTH POLICY

The making of health policy in the United States is a complex process involving both private and public sectors (including multiple levels of government).

Policy Cycle

The formation and implementation of health policy occur in a policy cycle comprising five components: (1) issue raising, (2) policy design, (3) building of public support, (4) legislative decision making and building of policy support, and (5) legislative decision making and policy implementation. These activities are likely to be shared with Congress and interest groups in varying degrees.

Issue-raising activities are clearly essential in the policy formation cycle. The enactment of a new policy is generally preceded by a variety of actions that first create a widespread sense that a problem exists and needs to be addressed. The president may form policy concepts from a variety of sources, including campaign information; recommendations from advisers, cabinet members, and agency chiefs; personal interests; expert opinions; and public opinion polls.

The second component of policy-making activity involves the design of specific policy proposals. Presidents have substantial resources at their disposal for developing new policy proposals. They may call on segments of the executive branch of government, such as the Health Care Financing Administration and policy staffs within the U.S. Department of Health and Human Services.

In building public support, presidents can choose from a variety of strategies, including major addresses to the nation, and efforts to mobilize their administrations to make public appeals, and organized attempts to increase support among interest groups.

To facilitate legislative decision making and the building of policy support, presidents, key staff, and department officials interact closely with Congress. Presidents generally meet with legislative leaders several mornings each month in an effort to shape the coming legislative agenda and to identify possible problems as bills move through various committees.

Legislative Process

When a bill is introduced in the House of Representatives, it is assigned to an appropriate committee by the Speaker. The committee chair forwards the bill to the appropriate subcommittee. The subcommittee forwards proposed legislation to agencies that will be affected by the legislation, holds hearings ("markup") and receives testimony, and may add amendments. The subcommittee and committee may recommend the bill, not recommend it, or recommend that it be tabled. Diverse interest groups, individuals, experts in the field, and business, labor, and professional associations often exert influence over the bill through campaign contributions and intense lobbying. The full House then hears the bill and may add amendments. The bill can be approved with or without amendments. The approved bill is sent to the Senate.

In the Senate, the bill is sent to an appropriate committee and next forwarded to an appropriate subcommittee. The subcommittee may send the bill to agencies that will be affected. It also holds hearings and testimonies from all interested parties (e.g., private citizens, business, labor, agencies, experts). The subcommittee votes on and forwards the proposed legislation with appropriate recommendations. Amendments may or may not be added. The full Senate hears the bill and may add amendments. If the bill and House amendments are accepted, then the bill goes to the President. If the Senate adds amendments that have not been voted on by the House, then the bill must go back to the floor of the House for a vote.

If the amendments are minor and noncontroversial, the House may vote to pass the bill. If the amendments are significant and controversial, the House may call for a conference committee to review the amendments. The conference committee consists of members from equivalent committees of the House and Senate. If the recommendations of the conference committee are not accepted, then another conference committee is called.

After the bill has passed both the House and Senate in identical form, it is then forwarded to the President for signature. If the President signs the legislation, it becomes law. If the President does not sign it, at the end of 21 days it becomes law unless the president vetoes it. If less than 21 days are left in the congressional session, then inaction on the part of the President results in a veto. This is called a "pocket veto." The veto can be overturned by a two thirds majority of the Congress; otherwise, the bill is dead.

After legislation has been signed into law, it is forwarded to the appropriate agency for implementation. The agency publishes proposed regulations in the Federal Register and then holds hearings regarding how the law is to be implemented. A bureaucracy only loosely controlled by either the president or Congress writes (publishes, gathers comments about, and rewrites) regulations. Then the program goes on to the 50 states for enabling legislation, if appropriate. There, organized interests hire local lawyers and lobbyists, and a whole new political cycle begins. Finally, all parties may adjourn to the courts, where long rounds of litigation shape the final outcome.

CRITICAL POLICY ISSUES

Government health policies have been enacted to resolve or prevent perceived deficiencies in health care delivery. Over the last 4 decades, most health policy initiatives and legislative efforts have focused on access to care (e.g., expanding insurance coverage, outreach programs in rural areas), cost of care (e.g., PPS, resource-based relative-value scale), and quality of care (e.g., creating the Agency for Health Care Policy and Research, later renamed as the Agency for Health Research and Quality, and calling for clinical practice guidelines).

Access to Care

Policies on access are aimed primarily at providers and financing mechanisms, with the purpose of expanding care to the most needy and underserved populations, including the elderly, minorities, rural residents, those with low incomes, and persons with AIDS (see Chapter 11).

Providers

Several groups of providers are involved in delivering health care. Policy issues include ensuring that there are a sufficient number of providers and that their geographic distribution is desirable. The debate over the supply of physicians is an important public policy issue because policy decisions influence the number of persons entering the medical profession, and that number, in turn, has implications on other policies. The number of new entrants into the profession is influenced by programs of government assistance for individual students and by government grants given directly to educational institutions. An increasing supply of physicians may result in increased health care expenditures because of provider-induced demand. An increasing supply of physicians may also help alleviate shortages in certain regions of the country. Policy approaches to expanding access have included the National Health Service Corps, legislation supporting rural health clinics to expand geographic access, student assistance programs to expand the pool of health care workers, legislation to expand a system of emergency medical services, and establishment of community health centers in inner cities and rural areas to extend medical care services to those underserved areas.

Public Financing

Although a national health care program is seen by many people as the best means of ensuring access, the United States focuses instead on the needs of particular groups. Medicare and its companion program Medicaid (care for the poor was added to Medicare in part to compromise with a physician-drafted proposal) established the precedent that government should facilitate access to health care among those unable to secure it for themselves. Over the years, policies have been enacted to provide access to health care for specific groups otherwise unable to pay for and receive care. These groups include the elderly (Medicare), poor children (Medicaid), poor adults (Medicaid and local or state general assistance), the disabled (Medicaid and Medicare), veterans (Veterans Health Administration), Native Americans (Indian Health Service), and patients with end-stage renal disease (Social Security benefits for kidney dialysis and transplants). Access continues to be a problem in many communities, partly because health policies enacted since 1983 have focused on narrowly defined elements of the delivery system. The fact that many Americans remain uninsured is reason to expect ongoing debate toward a public policy response concerning this issue; however, in policy debates, the need to expand access often overshadows how the expanded access will be financed.

Access and the Elderly

Two main concerns dominate the debate about Medicare policy. First, spending must be restrained to keep the program viable. Second, the program must be made truly comprehensive by adding services not currently covered or covered inadequately (e.g., comprehensive nursing home coverage).

Access and Minorities

Minorities are more likely than whites to face access problems. Hispanics, blacks, Asian Americans, and Native Americans, to name the most prevalent minorities, all experience difficulties accessing the health care delivery system. In some instances, the combination of low income and minority status creates difficulties; in others, the interaction of special cultural habits and minority status causes problems in accessing health care. Resolving the problems confronting these groups would require policies designed to encourage professional education programs sensitive to the special needs of minorities and programs to expand the delivery of services to areas populated by minorities. Many of these areas have been designated as having shortages of health care workers.

Access in Rural Areas

Delivery of health care services in rural communities has always posed the problems of how to make advanced medical care available to residents of sparsely settled areas. Financing high-tech equipment for a few people is not cost-efficient, and finding physicians who want to reside in rural areas is difficult. Thus, specialists and expensive diagnostic equipment are not readily available in rural medical practices. Reimbursement systems based on average costs make it difficult for rural hospitals with few patients to survive financially.

Funding the National Health Service Corps is one step toward redressing the problem of personnel shortages in rural areas; however, the Corps affects only the percentage of graduating physicians practicing in shortage areas, and only for a limited time period for each student. Additional programs that increase the total supply of physicians and create incentives for permanent practice in rural areas are needed.

Access and Low Income

Low-income mothers and their children have problems accessing the health care system, both because they lack insurance and because they generally live in medically underserved areas. Pregnant women in low-income families are far less likely to receive prenatal care than are women in higher income categories. Limited access among children creates problems of untreated chronic health conditions that lead to both increased medical expenditures and loss of productivity in society. The SCHIP, signed into law in 1997, has given states some flexibility in how they spend the $24 billion in federal funds that has been invested in children's health coverage in 5 years (States face a welcome dilemma, 1997).

Access and Persons with AIDS

Persons with AIDS, those who have progressed from infection with HIV to actually having the disease and therefore needing more expensive treatment, also have problems obtaining health care. People with AIDS experience difficulty obtaining insurance coverage, and their illness leads to catastrophic health care expenditures. Financial access can be a barrier, particularly for persons without adequate health insurance benefits. The AIDS epidemic presents a special challenge to policy makers committed to universal access to health care services. The services required are expensive, and the population in need is relatively small. Furthermore, the care is directed toward patients who are terminally ill.

Universal Health Coverage

Universal health coverage is health care extended to all eligible citizens and noncitizens in a country often funded publicly through taxes. Among all of the industrialized countries in the world, the United States is the only one lacking a universal health care system, which is slowly becoming an issue with the growing number of uninsured. In 2003, the number of uninsured adults reached 45 million, about 15% of the population, whereas another 16 million adults were underinsured, meaning that their insurance plans did not provide sufficient protection in the event of a catastrophic health care expense (Schoen et al., 2005). In response to the lack of national action for universal health coverage, movement has begun at the state and municipal level. For example, Massachusetts enacted health care reforms in April 2006 that involved an individual health insurance mandate for all state residents 18 years and older confirmed and enforced by state tax returns and the creation of a central agency, the Commonwealth Health Insurance Connector, to administer insurance reforms

Smoking and Tobacco Use

In the United States, lung cancer is the leading cancer cause of death, killing 160,000 people annually. The American Cancer Society has estimated that 87% of these deaths are a result of smoking and exposure to secondhand smoke. This is in addition to the 100,000 deaths from lung diseases and over 140,000 from heart disease and stroke also from smoking and exposure to secondhand smoke. In 2007, the IOM released *Ending the*

Tobacco Problem: A Blueprint for the Nation with the purpose of reducing smoking rates in the country. This goal is to be achieved through a two-pronged strategy involving strengthening and fully implementing traditional tobacco control measures and changing the regulatory landscape to permit policy innovations. The report concluded that if states maintained a comprehensive integrated tobacco control strategy at the CDC-recommended level of $15 to $20 per capita, tobacco use could be reduced effectively. Research has shown that more capital and time invested in tobacco control programs result in greater and quicker impact. For example, in California, the state with the longest running tobacco control program, smoking rates have fallen from 22.7% in 1988 to 13.3% in 2006 and, since 1998, has had a decline rate four times faster than the rest of the nation. These comprehensive tobacco control programs run by the states have several goals to reduce disease, disability, and death caused by smoking, such as preventing use among youth and young adults, promoting quitting, eliminating exposure to secondhand smoke, and identifying and eliminating tobacco-related disparities among population groups.

In addition to control programs, the government also teams up with national partners to run nationwide campaigns. The American Legacy Foundation administers the truth campaign that supports state-based youth prevention efforts. The American for Nonsmokers' Rights provides states and municipalities with assistance and guidance in the process of passing and implementing smoke-free indoor air policies. The American Cancer Society, American Heart Association, and American Lung Association provide advocacy leadership on tobacco control policy issues, while also providing support at the community level through offices across the nation.

Fighting HIV/AIDS

The CDC estimated that 850,000 to 950,000 persons are positive for HIV in the United States, a quarter of whom are unaware of their own infection. Annually, 40,000 are infected with a disproportionate amount among the black and Hispanic populations. The Department of Health and Human Services supports research, prevention initiatives, and efforts to expand access to quality health care and services for those in need of them. Research initiatives include vaccine development, prevention research, clinical trials of potential therapies, and effective drugs for treatment. Prevention strategies involve funding programs for high risk populations, promoting safety in the blood supply, monitoring the spread of AIDS/HIV, and running a national AIDS hotline. In the 2003 fiscal year budget, $16 billion went to the fight against AIDS/HIV at home and abroad, with a significant part of the budget targeted at reducing the disproportionate impact of the infection among racial and ethnic minorities.

Cost Containment

To a large extent, the strengths of the U.S. health care delivery system also contribute to its weaknesses. The United States has the latest developments in medical technology and well-trained specialists, but these advances amount to the most expensive means possible to provide care to patients, making the U.S. health care system the most costly in the world. No other aspect of health care policy has received more attention during the past 20 years than efforts to contain increases in health care costs. Two major policy initiatives enacted by the federal government have targeted first hospitals (PPS) and then physicians' services (resource-based relative value scale) for price control.

The National Health Planning and Resources Development Act of 1974 became law in 1975. This act marked the transition from improvement of access to cost containment as the principal theme in federal health policy. Health planning, through CON review, was used as a policy tool to contain hospital costs. One major change in the health policy environment was a new system of paying hospitals for Medicare clients, the PPS, enacted in 1983 (Mueller, 1988). In lieu of the tight regulation of charges established by individual hospitals, the PPS serves as a general fee schedule and establishes a prospective payment for general categories of treatment (based on diagnosis-related groups) that applies to all short-stay hospitals. PPS has proved to be the most successful tool for controlling hospital expenditures (Wennberg et al., 1984). Government programs, especially Medicare and Medicaid, federal employee benefit programs, and those of the Veterans Health Administration and armed services as well are under constant pressure from Congress to keep costs down.

Expenditures are a function of the price of services times the quantity of services delivered (see Chapter 12). Most policies enacted, to date, have focused on the price of services. Policy makers are reluctant to consider restricting the quantity of services, fearful of interpretations that they are sacrificing quality of care for cost containment. Such concerns are warranted because the media fuel the frenzy over denial of services by managed care organizations.

Increased debate over the right to die and the value of life-extending services provides an opportunity to discuss limiting reimbursable services. So far, the federal government has been reluctant to adopt an explicit rationing strategy to contain expenditures, but state governments can be expected to experiment with various means of cost containment.

The private sector also influences the policy focus on cost containment. Major corporations are now aggressively pursuing ways to restrain the escalation of medical costs. These large purchasers are buying medical services in volume, at wholesale prices, and even dictating the terms of service provision. Institutional buyers want to know what they are getting for their money. The answers require detailed data, close scrutiny, and, ultimately, outside judgment of whether the services are worth their value.

Quality of Care

Along with access and cost, quality of care is the third main concern of health care policy. The federal government began its actions to relieve the malpractice crisis and devoted greater attention to policing the quality of medical care with the Health Care Quality Act of 1986. This legislation mandated the creation of a national database within the U.S. Department of Health and Human Services to provide data on legal actions against health care providers. This information allows people recruiting physicians in one state to know of actions against those physicians in other states.

In 1989, the federal government embarked on a major effort to sponsor research to establish guidelines for medical practice. In the OBRA of 1989, Congress created a new agency, the National Center for Health Services Research (now called the Agency for Healthcare Research and Quality), and mandated it to conduct and support research with respect to the outcomes, effectiveness, and appropriateness of health care services and procedures (U.S. House of Representatives, 1989). The AHRQ has established funding for patient outcomes research teams (PORTs) that focus on particular medical conditions. The PORTs are part of a broader effort, the medical treatment effectiveness program, which "consists of four elements: medical treatment effectiveness research, development of databases for such research, development of clinical guidelines, and the dissemination of research findings and clinical guidelines" (Salive et al., 1990).

Presidential Candidates' Positions on Healthcare Reform 2008

Increasingly, health care reform has been one of the major concerns for politicians. Because of the growing numbers of uninsured individuals and skyrocketing health care costs, the 2008 presidential campaigns of candidates Barack Obama and John McCain focused heavily on this issue.

Democratic candidate, Barack Obama, shaped his health care policy toward decreasing the number of uninsured through a national health insurance program and a government agency named the National Health Insurance Exchange that would act as a watchdog group and assist in the reform of the private insurance market. Obama proposed forming a government sold insurance plan similar to the plan offered to members of Congress that would feature: guaranteed eligibility; affordable premiums, copays, and deductibles; easy enrollment; portability and choice; and comprehensive benefits, including preventive, maternity, and mental health care. The proposed agency, National Health Insurance Exchange, would then ensure equality among the private insurance groups by enforcing companies to become more affordable and accessible while providing services as generous as the public plan. In addition, reforms would be implemented to help lower costs and improve health care quality, which would include health and wellness promotions, such as worksite wellness programs, school efforts to address childhood obesity, education for health care professionals, and individual and community initiatives to help Americans make healthy choices.

On the other hand, Republican candidate, John McCain planned to reform the health care system through free market tactics of open market competition rather than more government programs. He planned to provide a direct refundable tax credit of $2,500 for individuals and $5,000 for families to compensate for the cost of insurance. He proposed making insurance more portable so that the coverage follows an individual from job changes to early retirement and even when an individual desires extended time off. He also wanted to assist in establishing a Guaranteed Access Plan (GAP) with the states to ensure traditionally uninsurable patients—individuals without prior group coverage or suffer from pre-existing conditions that prevent them from acquiring affordable coverage—have access to health coverage.

Research and Policy Development

The research community can influence the making of health policy through documentation, analysis, and prescription (Longest, 1994). The first role of research in policy making is documentation, that is, the gathering, cataloging, and correlating of facts that depict the state of the world that policy makers face. This process may help define a given public policy problem or raise its political profile.

A second way in which research informs, and thus influences, policy making is through analysis of what does and does not work. Program evaluation and outcomes research fall under this domain. Often taking the form of demonstration projects intended to provide a factual basis for determining the feasibility, efficacy, or practicality of a possible policy intervention, analysis can help define solutions to health policy problems.

The third way in which research influences policy making is through prescription. Research that demonstrates that a particular course of action being contemplated by policy makers may (or may not) lead to undesirable or unexpected consequences can make a significant contribution to policy making.

CONCLUSION

Health policies are developed to serve the public's interests; however, public interests are diverse. Members of the public often hold conflicting views. Although the public consistently supports the goal of national health insurance, it also rejects the idea of the federal government running the health care delivery system. Similarly, although the public wants the government to control health care costs, it also believes that the federal government already controls too much of Americans' daily lives. The challenge for policy makers is to find a balance between governmental provisions and control, and the private health care market to improve coverage and affordability of care. Successful health policies are more likely to be couched in terms of cost containment (a market-justice, economic, business, and middle-class concern) than in improved or expanded access and reducing or eliminating health disparities (a social-justice, liberal, labor, low-income issue); however, cost-related policies are likely to have very little impact on improving the quality of care or reducing health disparities.

REFERENCES

Alford, R. R. 1975. *Health Care Politics: Ideology and Interest Group Barriers to Reform*. Chicago: University of Chicago Press.

Coughlin, T., et al. 1999. A conflict of strategies: Medicaid managed care and Medicaid maximization. *Health Services Research* 34 (1):281–293.

Health Insurance Association of America. 1992. *Source Book of Health Insurance Data*. Washington, DC: Health Insurance Association of America.

Institute of Medicine (IOM). 2007. *Ending the Tobacco Problem: A Blueprint for the Nation*. Washington DC: Author.

Litman, T., and L. Robins. 1997. The relationship of government and politics to health and health care—A sociopolitical overview. In T. Litman and L. Robins (eds.). *Health Politics and Policy*, 3rd ed. (pp. 3–45). New York: John Wiley and Sons.

Longest, B. B. 1994. *Health Policymaking in the United States*. Ann Arbor, MI: Health Administration Press.

Miller, C. A. 1987. Child health. In S. Levine and A. Lillienfeld (eds.). *Epidemiology and Health Policy*. New York: Tavistock Publications.

Mueller, K. J. 1988. Federal programs do expire: The case of health planning. *Public Administration Review* 48:719–735.

National Institutes of Health. 1991. *NIH Data Book*. Washington, DC: U.S. Department of Health and Human Services.

Salive, M. E., et al. 1990. Patient outcomes research teams and the Agency for Health Care Policy and Research. *Health Services Research* 25:697–708.

Schoen et al., 2005. Taking the pulse of health care systems: experiences of patients with health problems in six countries. *Health Aff.* Web Exclusives(suppl):W5-509-25.

States face a welcome dilemma: How to best spend $24 billion to cover nation's uninsured children. 1997. *State Health Watch* 4 (8):1, 4.

U.S. House of Representatives. 1989, 21 November. *Omnibus Budget Reconciliation Act of 1989: Conference report to accompany H.R. 3299*. Washington, DC: Government Printing Office.

Weissert, C., and W. Weissert. 1996. *Governing Health: The Politics of Health Policy*. Baltimore, MD: Johns Hopkins University Press.

Wennberg, J. E., et al. 1984. Will payment based on diagnosis-related groups control hospital costs? *New England Journal of Medicine* 311 (5):295–300.

Chapter 14

The Future of Health Services Delivery

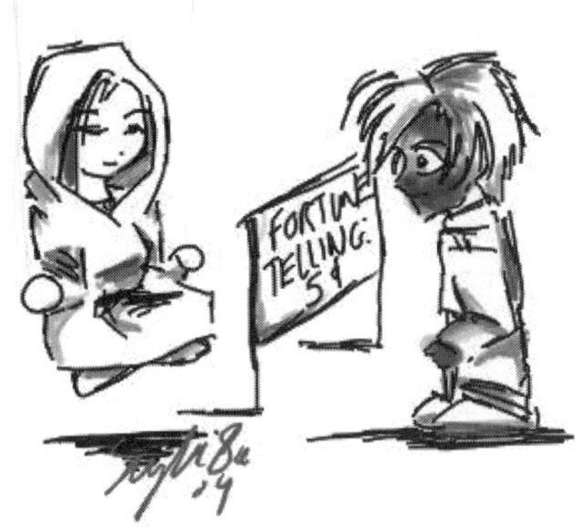

INTRODUCTION

Historical precedents and current developments can project future directions in U.S. health care delivery. In discussing the future, one key question is often raised: How close are we to having a national health care system in the United States? Various plans and proposals have been put forth since the early 1900s to move the nation toward a national health care plan, but they have failed. One main reason why Americans have thus far not favored such a move is that it runs contrary to the beliefs and values prevalent in the United States. Americans have traditionally maintained a strong belief in capitalism and individual achievement. They have preferred relatively little government involvement in private affairs. Americans have also become disenchanted by such national programs as the public education system, which has failed to deliver on its promise of scholastic excellence for America's youth. As an example, a 1993 report by the U.S.

Department of Education estimated that functional illiteracy—a person's incompetence in using such basic skills as reading, writing, and simple computations in everyday life situations—plagued as many as one in four American adults (Carvin, 2000). The situation in the government-controlled educational system has not become any better. Given the grim record of performance of tax-supported programs in the United States and abroad, most Americans have not been comfortable turning over critical issues of life and health to the government. On the other hand, the lack of insurance for about 45 million Americans remains a social concern.

CONFLICTING REALITIES OF COST AND COVERAGE

The United States is plagued by two major issues: increasingly unaffordable cost of health care and a lack of insurance coverage for a relatively large segment of the population. A report released in January 2004 by the Institute of Medicine advocated that the United States adopt universal health insurance in the form of continuous health care coverage for all Americans by 2010 (American Public Health Association, 2004). While America has been contemplating how to expand and pay for health care coverage, other nations that already have universal coverage are grappling with the impending dilemma of how they can keep their systems solvent without having to curtail services.

The United States has been at the cutting edge of technological innovation. By absorbing the full cost of research and development for technology that other nations later adopt and use, the United States indirectly subsidizes the cost of health care in other countries. Unlike most other advanced nations, the United States also assimilates into its society a disproportionate share of immigrants, both legal and illegal. U.S. hospitals, particularly in the South where a high number of illegal immigrants from Mexico and Central American countries find refuge, end up bearing the cost of providing free care to many of the uninsured immigrants. A large portion of these costs is passed on to the rest of American society. Those who criticize the high cost of delivering health care in the United States often downplay these unique factors that other nations do not have to contend with on the same scale.

Universal health care in America remains a worthy goal, but it cannot be achieved without a massive escalation in total health care expenditures.

Americans are not opposed to expanding coverage to the uninsured, but most middle-class Americans have been reluctant to pay additional taxes to expand health insurance under the auspices of the federal government.

Besides cost, an unknown factor is the availability of health care services if a large segment of the population that is currently uninsured is given health insurance. Contrary to popular belief, health insurance is not necessarily equivalent to access. A person has access to health care only if that person, insured or uninsured, can obtain health care services when needed. The United States currently has a shortage of primary care physicians, nurses, and other health professionals. Expanding health insurance can actually diminish access for most Americans.

Managed care made significant headway during the decade of the 1990s and achieved notable success in slowing down the growth of national health care expenditures. Remarkably, this was achieved without noticeable declines in the quality of health care, as some had feared. The rising costs of health care were contained by closely monitoring utilization and managing reimbursement to providers, but toward the latter half of the 1990s, both practices drew a backlash from consumers and providers. The American media also played a role in shaping public opinion against managed care by presenting, in many instances, one-sided and subjective "news" stories.

For the enrollees, dissatisfaction with managed care was associated mostly with the erosion of choice resulting from the limited number of providers associated with the plans and some restrictions in direct access to specialized services. Dissatisfaction on the part of physicians, hospitals, and other providers was related to the control that managed care organizations (MCOs) exerted over utilization and limits on reimbursement. However, in the process, all parties had to make certain adjustments.

In response to the backlash, HMOs in particular moved away from tight management of health care services but without totally abandoning utilization controls. Preferred provider organizations (PPOs) offered greater choice of access to providers. Both enrollees and providers welcomed these adjustments. Consolidation by providers and the emergence of integrated delivery systems gave providers greater bargaining power to negotiate reimbursement rates, which put significant pressure on MCOs. On the other side, MCOs retained their bargaining power as enrollments in managed care plans continued to increase. In the end, the enrollees had to give up unconditional freedom over choice, the providers had to accept some controls over how they would practice medicine and settle for lower rates of reimbursement than what they were getting under fee for service, and MCOs had to relax tight management of health care utilization. Although the managed care industry has developed plan choices, to some degree relaxed controls and flexibility have become common features of all plans. Managed care has evolved quite differently from what it was initially intended to be: an organizational mechanism that would tightly control the financing and delivery of health care.

Of the twin problems of cost and coverage, cost escalation is the primary issue. American health care is unaffordable without insurance coverage. The high costs also interfere with the nation's ability to expand health insurance.

Massachusetts crafted a universal coverage program for its residents. The program went into effect in July 2007 and has already run into problems. On the positive side, the program has enrolled roughly half of the previously uninsured population in the state. But, double-digit cost increases plague the new system. One reason for the cost increases is the program's failure to attract enough of the wealthier, healthier uninsured. The program is underfunded for 2008 by perhaps $100 million and needs $1.5 billion over the next 3 years from the federal government to meet the needs of subsidized enrollees. For those low-income people who earned too much for Medicaid but finally got covered under the new plan, unpleasant surprises awaited. Premiums were expected to rise 10% in July 2008. The state hopes to raise additional revenues by implementing a major increase in the tobacco tax and by extracting more money from everyone involved in the health care system (Sloane, 2008). The cost to employers of the additional coverage take up has been substantial and many employers have expressed concern that unless the state seriously addresses the underlying factors driving costs, the current trajectory of the reform is financially unsustainable. Particularly, small employers' motivations and ability to continue health benefits may be waning (Draper et al., 2008). On the other hand, the program's impact on access to health care still remains to be seen.

FUTURE OF MANAGED CARE, HEALTH CARE COSTS, AND SYSTEM REFORM

Managed care has become a mature industry in the United States. Over 95% of privately insured individuals, a little over 60% of Medicaid beneficiaries, and almost 20% of Medicare beneficiaries are now enrolled in managed care plans. Hence, managed care will continue to dominate the financing and delivery of health care, but it will also continue to evolve. Managed care's ability to squeeze excesses from the health care system has been stalled. As employers, employees, and the government face mounting cost pressures, the managed care industry as well as providers of health care will have to step up to the plate. The managed care industry will have to create well-differentiated offerings: cheaper plans that also tightly manage utilization and more liberal plans that also cost much more. Health care providers will also have to share the increased costs by accepting lower reimbursement and, in turn, lowering the costs of production.

National health expenditures are projected to rise at an average annual rate of 6.9% (**Figure 14.1**). They will continue to outpace growth in the Gross Domestic Product. In simple terms, it means that health care expenditures will continue to rise beyond people's ability to pay for them because wage increases will not keep up with medical cost inflation. A well-recognized factor associated with any discussion of future costs is the aging of the population. It is estimated that health care will consume almost

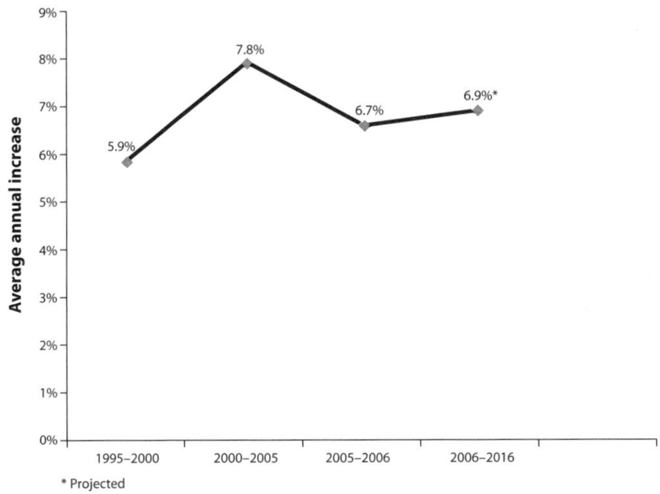

Figure 14.1 Projected Data from *Health, United States*, 2007, p. 378, National Center for Health Statistics; Catlin, A., et al. 2008. National health spending in 2006: A year of change for prescription drugs. Health Affairs 27, no. 1: 14–29; Poisal, J.A., et al. 2007. Health spending projections through 2016: Modest changes obscure Part D's impact. Available at http://content.healthaffairs.org/cgi/content/abstract/hlthaff.26.2.w242 (Accessed August 2008).

20% of the GDP by 2016 (Poisal et al., 2007), up from 16% in 2006. This cost projection coincides with the aging of the baby boomers.

As the U.S. workforce continues to age, employment-based insurance will have a greater number of older adults. A change in the age mix of the workforce is likely to accelerate premium increases (Keenan et al., 2006). Private employers have been gradually shifting costs to the workers, but there is a limit to the extent of cost shifting that workers can endure. Rise in health insurance premiums continues to outpace workers' earnings and inflation in the economy. For example, private insurance premiums increased an average of 6.1% between 2006 and 2007 (Claxton et al., 2007). During this same period, the average weekly earnings of production and nonsupervisory workers on private nonfarm payrolls increased by a mere 3.8%, and the increase in the consumer price index was 3.5% according to data from the Bureau of Labor Statistics. Also, the availability of employer-based health coverage has eroded. Between 2000 and 2007, the percentage of employers that offered health insurance went down from 69% to 60%. Almost all of this decline was in small businesses employing between 3 and 199 workers. Affordability remains the main reason that employers cite for not providing health insurance. Over 70% of the nonoffering firms believe that their employees would rather get an additional $2 per hour in wages as opposed to health insurance (Claxton et al., 2007).

The experience with managed care demonstrates that people are unwilling to accept tight controls from the private sector. To impact unaffordable costs materially, it is necessary to manage utilization, limit reimbursement, and employ some sort of rationing on the supply of health care services. Only the government is in a position to wage war against costs on all three fronts. Fiscally, it is impossible to expand health care and not employ tight mechanisms to control costs. In any event, government intervention will likely become inevitable at some point because government's own expenses for health care will become unsustainable. Unfortunately, a greater degree of competition in health care does not generally address the issue of costs because health care is not governed by free-market principles (see Chapter 1). Politicians, on the other hand, are being fiscally irresponsible when they expand public programs and promise ever-increasing benefits. A recent example is the addition of Part D (prescription drug benefit) to the Medicare program (see Chapter 6). Participants in this program pay premiums that cover only about 25% of the total cost. The bulk of the remaining costs come from taxpayers.

The financing of Medicare is essentially a generation transfer system in which current taxpayers pay for the benefits of current beneficiaries. Any shortfalls in such a financing system must be paid by future generations. According to the 2008 annual report from the trustees of the Medicare and Social Security trust funds, expenditures for Part A benefits have already started to exceed revenues that mainly come from payroll taxes levied on current workers. In other words, Part A is now partially dependent on general tax revenues that were not meant to fund Part A. These deficits are projected to grow, and by 2019, the trust fund reserves will be exhausted (Paulson et al., 2008). Part B and D benefits are paid from a different trust fund which is financed mainly through general taxes. Projected costs over the long term will require increases in enrollee premiums as well as in general tax revenue funding. The entire Medicare program will place an ever-increasing burden on beneficiaries and taxpayers (Paulson et al., 2008).

However, no politician wants to address openly the impending crisis in Medicare, Medicaid, and Social Security—the three major social programs dealing with health and financial well-being in America—and how Americans in the not too distant future will have to face the realities of having to fund these programs by paying more taxes, curtailing benefits, or both. The dilemma is that curtailment of benefits is often not politically feasible. Hence, tax increases will be inevitable. Taxing just the "rich" has never been a solution to such problems wherever in the world it has been tried.

According to a survey of Americans by Blendon et al. (2008) during the presidential primaries in 2007, nearly half of those in support of the Democratic party said there was so much wrong with the health care system that it needed to be completely rebuilt. About two thirds of them said that they wanted to see their presidential candidates propose "a major effort to provide health insurance for all or nearly all of the uninsured," even if it "would involve a substantial increase in spending" (quotes by authors). Most Republican voters, on the other hand, preferred a more limited, less costly expansion. Most Democrats said that government should have primary responsibility for making sure that Americans have health care, whereas the majority of Republicans said that health care coverage should be an individual responsibility. This difference was not driven by the distribution of the uninsured between the two parties' supporters.

As the 2008 presidential race was heating up, once again there was some degree of obsession with the expansion of health insurance on the part of both candidates. Senator Obama made public his stand on health care by stating this (Obama, 2007):

> We now face an opportunity and an obligation to turn the page on the failed politics of yesterday's health care debates . . . My plan begins by covering every American. If you already have health insurance, the only thing that will change for you under this plan is the amount of money you will spend on premiums. That will be less. If you are one of the 45 million Americans who don't have health insurance, you will have it after this plan becomes law.

Obama made a lot of promises and people's expectations have been raised. On the other hand, he carefully avoided giving any indications of how much his plan would cost and how it would be financed except for some vague allusion to his intentions to "tax the rich."

Obama's victory to the presidency will no doubt bring national health insurance to the forefront once again. Control of the House and the Senate in the hands of Obama's party also makes the political environment more favorable to national health insurance than it has been for some time. It is doubtful, however, that President Obama will be able to deliver on his promise to provide health insurance to all Americans. As just pointed out earlier, Americans are deeply divided on the government's role in health care, which makes a major reform in health insurance coverage highly unlikely. The nation is in a recession which can deepen. Economic recovery is not likely to be as fast as many expect. One main reason for this grim outlook is the massive spending of borrowed money that the U.S. government has committed to plow into the financial system in an effort to avert a more severe economic crisis than what has become apparent so far. Tax cuts for 95% of Americans and massive social expansions at the same time that Obama has promised are fiscally impossible dreams. On the other hand, if the current recession deepens and a large number of middle-class Americans become unemployed and lose their employer-sponsored health coverage, Americans could well look to the government for health care. After all, the government has already set the precedence to bail out private institutions. The question would be: why not bail out private individuals as well?

What we are likely to see, however, is some incremental reforms such as expansion of the State Children's Health Insurance Program (SCHIP) to cover adults in low-income families that have children. SCHIP is due for renewal in 2009. Another possible reform could be packaging taxpayer-financed health insurance with unemployment benefits. In the long run, however, rising costs of health care must be controlled for any future expansions of health services to remain viable. Price control is perhaps the "answer" that politicians would offer. But again, price controls were tried during the 1970s, and they failed to accomplish the objective of reducing costs.

TRENDS IN HEALTH INSURANCE

From Defined-Benefit to Defined-Contribution Plans

Currently, the majority of employers offer what is referred to as a *defined-benefit* plan. One or more health insurance plans are preselected by the employer. In the defined-benefit arrangement, consumers have no financial incentives to be prudent purchasers of health insurance, and patients are almost totally removed from the cost of care. In the future, however, the consumer of health insurance and health care is likely to bear more responsibility. The defined-contribution approach holds this promise. Defined-contribution health insurance products that make use of Internet technologies are receiving growing attention (Christianson et al., 2002).

Under a *defined-contribution* plan, employers commit to a fixed-dollar amount for health benefits. The fixed-dollar amount is paid to the employees, who then pay for the health care plan they select, in contrast to the current practice of committing to a fixed health benefits package with preselected health plans for all employees. Actually, the model for a defined-contribution approach is already being used for retirement benefits. In the 1980s, a shift occurred in retirement benefits when employers began moving away from defined-benefit (or pension) plans toward defined-contribution (or savings) plans (White, 2001). Many employers see adoption of the defined-contribution approach for health care benefits as compatible with the need to give employees a greater role in purchasing health insurance, as well as health care services (Christianson et al., 2002).

Currently, a defined-contribution mind-set appears to be developing, but as of yet, employers are not willing to pull away. If the employer contributions are large enough to purchase at least a basic health insurance plan, this could possibly reduce the number of uninsured. A number of startup companies have already emerged to capture the defined-contribution market if and when it becomes mainstream. Internet-based e-health plans will enable consumers to tailor plans according to individual needs, obtain instant quotes, and make online purchases.

High-Deductible Health Plans

High-deductible health plans (HDHPs) are discussed in Chapter 6. Employers, particularly very large businesses, have gradually started to embrace these plans. These plans can be purchased at a lower cost than regular managed care plans. Both high deductibles and health savings accounts (HSAs) or health reimbursement arrangements (HRAs) that are used in conjunction with high-deductible plans put greater responsibility on the consumer about judicious use of health care services. Expansion of HSAs is the preferred approach of the Republican party to expand health insurance coverage.

Tax Credits

Tax credits can work in conjunction with HDHPs and HSAs. McClellan and Baicker (2002) argued that tax credits for the purchase of health insurance would enable millions of Americans to purchase private health insurance. A variation of this approach is to issue the tax credits in advance in the form of vouchers to enable people, particularly the poor, to purchase insurance. Congress created the Health Coverage Tax Credit (HCTC) by passing the Trade Adjustment Assistance Reform Act of 2002. The law, however, applied only to workers who lost their jobs due to trade and to retirees over the age of 55 who lost their employer coverage. The HCTC makes health coverage more affordable by paying 65% of health insurance premiums for individuals who are eligible for the tax credit.

High-Risk Pools

Tax credits would still leave some people uninsured, particularly those who are considered high risk because of severe illnesses or chronic conditions. High-risk pools target population groups that are unable to purchase health insurance on their own because of poor health. At least 30 states operate high-risk pools that enable hard-to-insure people to purchase subsidized coverage. In almost all cases, premium rates are capped at 125% to 150% of the average market rate. Deductibles are generally $1,000 or less, and an 80:20 co-insurance is common.

OPTIONS FOR COMPREHENSIVE REFORM

The last attempt to bring in national health care was made by President Clinton. Past proposals that can be reconsidered in the future have included a single-payer system, managed competition, and employer-based play-or-pay programs. Employer mandates, used in Hawaii, are a variation of these proposals. Double mandates have recently been adopted in Massachusetts. Assuming that a major reform of the U.S. health care system does occur in the future, the single-payer proposal is the least likely to be adopted.

Single Payer

The *single-payer* approach comes closest to resembling the Canadian system. A single-payer health program would place the responsibility of financing health care with one entity, most likely the federal government. One major advantage of such a system is that all Americans and lawful residents would be entitled to benefits regardless of individual or family income. Private insurance plans and government entitlement programs (Medicaid, Medicare, TRICARE, and the Federal Employee Health Benefits Program) would no longer be necessary under a single-payer system, although the market for some private insurance would remain for those desiring coverage beyond what a basic government plan might offer. Health care providers would be reimbursed on a fee-for-service scale with tight government controls on reimbursement. Hospitals, nursing homes, and other institutional facilities would be given an annual prospective budget to provide all required care. Under such a system, controls are generally extended to ration health care services, particularly the availability and use of costly technology.

Managed Competition

The Health Security Act proposed during the Clinton presidency was largely based on the principles of managed competition. The program would have guaranteed every citizen the right to receive a comprehensive package of health care benefits. Administration of such a program envisioned competition between health insurance purchasing cooperatives and managed care plans. Financing for the proposed program was based on cost sharing between employers (80%) and employees (20%).

Play-or-Pay

Employer-based play-or-pay was introduced as a Senate bill in 1989 to help achieve universal coverage. Under this type of system, employers must provide health insurance for employees (play) or pay into a public health insurance program. If the employer chooses to pay, financing is through a payroll tax paid by the employer and the employee, very similar to the way Social Security and Medicare taxes are currently handled through payroll deductions. Because an employer-based system is already in place, this type of plan would be less disruptive than a single-payer system.

Employer Mandates

Employer mandates require employers to help pay for coverage for their employees. Despite the seeming appeal of an employer mandate, only Hawaii has implemented this type of reform. The ability of states to adopt employer mandates has been thwarted by the federal Employee Retirement Income Security Act (ERISA), which exempts self-insured businesses from state insurance regulations and taxes. Hawaii is the only state that received a Congressional exemption from ERISA for its employer mandate because Hawaii enacted its mandate legislation in 1974, before ERISA itself was enacted. Employer mandates have met with vehement and aggressive opposition from employers, especially small businesses (Andersen et al., 1996).

Double Mandates

Double mandates require an employer mandate, discussed above, and an additional individual mandate that requires everyone to have health insurance or face legal penalties. This is the model adopted by Massachusetts.

Health insurance mandates in Massachusetts require all employers with more than 10 workers to offer at a minimum a Section 125 cafeteria plan. Such a plan enables employees to get tax exemption on the purchase of a health insurance plan. For example, the employer can contribute toward the purchase of health insurance on a defined contribution basis. The employee can then choose from among several different plans available through a state health insurance exchange. Contributions made by employers are not taxable to the employee, and the worker's portion of the expense is tax deductible. If a state resident fails to purchase health insurance, the penalty could be over $900 per year. Massachusetts subsidizes the premium cost for those at or below 300% of the federal poverty level and pays the full premium for those at or below the federal poverty level.

NATIONAL AND GLOBAL CHALLENGES

To restrain the mounting burden of health care spending, wellness and disease prevention will have to be incorporated into the delivery of health care. On the other hand, the demands of chronic care as well as new and resurgent infectious diseases must also be incorporated into medical practice. New health care roles are required to coordinate the needs of people with chronic illnesses. Health care institutions and private practitioners need to coordinate their efforts with public health agencies to identify emergent diseases and contain the spread of infection.

Future of Wellness, Prevention, and Health Promotion

Because of the changing causes of death, disease patterns, and the economic burden of disease, the emphasis of health care in the future will move from acute care to preventive care. Large employers in particular have started to promote employee health. Employers are taking a long-term view and proactively identifying employees and dependents with health risk factors and supporting health promotion strategies to reduce health risks through smoking cessation, weight reduction, and stress management programs (Coile, 2002, p. 14). Hospitals and managed care plans will have to continue to be the leaders in integrating wellness and health promotion into medical care delivery. The shift in focus under managed care from acute services to prevention and wellness will change those who provide care and how care is provided.

Challenges Posed by Chronic Illnesses

During the course of one century, the United States and most other nations have made significant gains in health status and life expectancy, mainly by conquering communicable diseases. However, with a higher life expectancy, such chronic disorders as heart disease and lung cancer have become the major causes of death. Medical science can prolong life, but it has thus far been unable to curb physical deterioration associated with the aging process or reverse the course of cardiovascular, oncotic (cancerous), and degenerative diseases.

Despite a dramatic rise in chronic conditions and ensuing disabilities, the existing health care system focuses primarily on addressing acute illnesses. The health care delivery system of the future will have to be configured to meet the impending challenges posed by chronic diseases. Even though the first wave of baby boomers will not likely need professional long-term care services until 2025, the system must be reformed before that time comes. Long-term care faces some major challenges, according to a report by Miller and Mor (2006). Less than 10% of the elderly have private long-term care insurance. Hence, most middle-class Americans are not prepared to meet long-term care expenses. Medicare and Medicaid pay for roughly 60% of all long-term care costs. As mentioned earlier, these programs will be financially unsustainable without major reforms. Less costly community-based services need to be expanded to minimize institutionalization. Medicaid funding, for example, is heavily tilted toward payment for institutional rather than home-based services. Care coordination through interoperable information technology systems is necessary to track patients' care across hospitals, nursing homes, home health agencies, and physicians' offices.

Some recommendations for making the current system more adaptable to address chronic care include patient education, programs to develop and improve self-coping skills, computerized tracking and reminder systems, and organized approaches to follow-up (Wagner et al., 2001), the goal being to promote healthy aging in communities. Physicians need to adopt disease-specific health maintenance and wellness strategies. At least two major areas need to be addressed to accomplish such goals: (1) Reimbursement systems must change to compensate providers for delivering services that improve the efficacy and efficiency of chronic care. Nonphysician providers such as nurse practitioners and community health nurses can play a vital role in the delivery and coordination of chronic care. (2) Health care professionals, including physicians, need to receive appropriate training in the management and coordination of the special needs of people suffering from chronic illnesses.

Infectious Diseases and Challenges of Globalization

The much-needed shift toward care for chronic disease and disability does not mean that infectious disease prevention and control efforts will be unnecessary in the future. In fact, intensified efforts will be required to combat emergent and resurgent infectious diseases. For instance, the sudden appearance in the early 1980s of a previously unknown disease we now know as AIDS challenged the widely held belief that infectious diseases were under control. Since then, other deadly bacterial infections such as Lyme disease have appeared. Even though some of the newer infections have not created the type of panic that AIDS did, the scientific community is baffled by some ordinary bacterial infections that have turned lethal. Another cause for concern is that certain strains of bacteria have become antibiotic resistant because of the inadvertent overuse of antibiotics, which presents fresh challenges in the fight against infectious diseases, both new and old.

New forms of influenza virus have periodically raised alarms in the United States. Hantavirus, which is believed to have originated in Korea, has caused some lethal infections in the United States. National public health alerts made news headlines in 2002 when encephalitis cases in New York were attributed to the West Nile virus, which then traveled 3,000 miles west to California. In 2003, severe acute respiratory syndrome (SARS), which is highly contagious and is believed to have originated in China, led to travel advisories and other precautions as the virus spread to several countries, including the United States.

These examples demonstrate that infectious diseases and health care must be viewed from a global perspective. The HIV/AIDS epidemic, for instance, has so far made its greatest impact on the African continent. The African epidemic received little attention from the United States until very recently when it was recognized that the epidemic posed increasing risks to U.S. interests because of increasing globalization. Immigration of people from other countries to the United States, international travel to and from the United States, and shipments coming to the United States from other countries have made it increasingly possible for deadly infections to cross international boundaries. HIV/AIDS, hepatitis C, and other infectious diseases, some currently known and some yet unknown, will pose growing threats to U.S. interests, particularly as the AIDS crisis is expected to spread rapidly through India, Russia, China, and Latin America, which comprise almost 40% of the world's population (Gow, 2002).

The global aspect of infectious diseases emphasizes the need to link together the nation's foreign and public health policies. Globalization presents social and economic opportunities from which nations can benefit, but it also holds the potential for global catastrophe. International cooperation, sharing of information, and technical and financial assistance will be necessary to avert any major health mishaps that could affect millions of people worldwide.

BIOTERRORISM AND THE TRANSFORMATION OF PUBLIC HEALTH

Historically, in the United States, the medical establishment relegated public health to a level of unimportance. The dichotomous systems of illness care and public health created two distinct cultures that have often been at odds with one another (Keck & Scutchfield, 1997). However, public health has always been about protecting the population's health. More recently, emphasis on homeland security has lifted public health to a new level of respect and recognition as an instrument to protect the public against new threats to well-being. Actually, the interest in public health in America has been like a seesaw, going up during times of danger to people's health and safety and coming down when no dangers loom. The importance of public health and deficiencies in the existing public health system received national attention during terrorism-related attempts to bring about an anthrax epidemic in October 2001, soon after the terrorist attacks and destruction of the World Trade Center in New York City on September 11, 2001. Since then, a heightened awareness of potential threats posed by chemical and biological weapons and low-grade nuclear materials has prompted public officials nationwide to review and revamp the system. Most experts believe that the threat of terrorism on American soil will remain in the foreseeable future. The nation's central public health agency, the Centers for Disease Control and Prevention (CDC), will continue to play a vital role in recognizing emerging threats and developing measures to contain any unexpected outbreaks. Public health agencies at local, state, and federal levels are already in the process of identifying infrastructure weaknesses and reevaluating plans to protect the American public (Baker & Koplan, 2002). Public health must prepare for threats other than those posed by "imported" infectious diseases (discussed earlier) and the possible use of chemical, biological, and nuclear agents for the purpose of inflicting harm. Safeguarding the nation's food and water supplies is equally important.

A major challenge and responsibility of public health agencies in a radically changing world is to forge partnerships with communities and all levels of government. The future effectiveness of public health will involve cooperation among public health agencies at the federal, state, and local levels; other agencies of the government such as the Department of Justice and the Food and Drug Administration; private and public organizations such as hospitals, clinics, and nursing homes; private practitioners such as physicians and nurses; volunteer agencies such as the American Red Cross; civil defense agencies such as police and fire departments; businesses; and individuals and groups within communities.

FUTURE OF THE HEALTH CARE WORKFORCE

Health care delivery influences and is influenced by the characteristics of the health care workforce. Some of the factors influencing the workforce are a decline in inpatient hospital care, an increasing elderly population, and more women and minorities entering the health care workforce. The future health care workforce will also be affected by individual career choices and enrollments in training programs and immigration of trained foreign workers in areas of high labor demand. Shortage of nurses is one of the dominant issues today. However, there is debate over whether this shortage will continue. Currently, pharmacists, technicians, and rehabilitation therapists are also in short supply (Coile, 2002).

Supply of Physicians and Nurses

Even though the aggregate number of physicians in the United States will continue to increase, two main factors suggest that the demand for physicians is likely to outpace supply (Department of Health and Human Services, 2005): (1) A greater proportion of elderly in the population and (2) the changing age-specific per capita physician utilization rates, with those age 45 and above using more services.

Compared to primary care physicians, the number of specialists has continued to increase. There has been a remarkable drop in the number of medical graduates who pursue residencies in primary care. This will further compound the imbalance that already exists in the numbers of generalists and specialists. Such an imbalance continues to focus on technology-driven acute care and is an impediment to moving health care delivery toward a chronic care model needed to address future health care needs of a growing elderly population. Already, nearly one in five Americans (56 million) is medically disenfranchised, not for a lack of health insurance, but for inadequate or no access to primary care physicians because of a shortage of such physicians (National Association of Community Health Centers/The Robert Graham Center, 2007).

Nursing shortages in the past have been cyclical. Widely publicized labor shortages attract students to nursing schools, and enrollments drop when shortages subside. However, the current nurse shortage can be traced to several years of decline in nursing school enrollments nationwide. Although beginning in 2003, nursing school enrollments began to increase, by most accounts, the current nursing shortage will persist in the future. Experts differ on how severe the shortage is expected to be.

Training in Geriatrics

Based on current trends, a shortage of health care professionals trained in geriatrics is a critical challenge. This problem is compounded by the shortage of faculty in colleges and universities who are trained in geriatrics. The elderly use the majority of home health care services and nursing home care, about half of hospital inpatient days, and approximately a quarter of all ambulatory care visits. The growth of the elderly population will impose increasing challenges on a health care delivery system that has thus far ignored the need for specialized training in geriatrics. Many elderly patients suffer from chronic conditions. Their care is complicated by the presence of comorbidities, the use of multiple prescription drugs, and an increased prevalence of mental conditions and dementia. Evidence shows that care of older adults by health care professionals prepared in geriatrics yields better physical and mental outcomes without increasing costs (Cohen et al., 2002a). Current trends in the education and training of health care professionals show the future demand will far outstrip the supply of physicians, nurses, therapists, social workers, and pharmacists with specialized training in geriatrics.

Workforce Diversity

Women continue to enter the workforce in large numbers, which will likely affect health services delivery. Although further research and time will clarify what impact the feminization of the workforce will have, health services managers should be prepared to improve the work environment to accommodate the needs of female workers. Examples include day care services and flexible work schedules. MCOs are likely to select women for their staff physicians, nurses, social workers, and case managers. Female physicians are often thought to prefer managed care to private practice because MCOs are more likely to provide secure income and regular work hours.

The increase in the proportion of nonwhites, particularly in the most populated cities and states, is another change. Already, the states of California, Texas, New York, New Jersey, and Florida have significant minority populations. It is further estimated that somewhere near the middle of this century, more than half of U.S. citizens will be nonwhite (U.S. Census Bureau, 2001, p. 17). Consequently, the health care workforce in the future will be much more diverse, ethnically and racially. Preparation of a culturally competent health care workforce is a growing challenge. The term *cultural competence* refers to knowledge, skills, attitudes, and behavior required of a practitioner to provide optimal health care services to persons from a wide range of cultural and ethnic backgrounds. Development of cultural competence is necessary because most future health care professionals will be called on to deliver services to many patients with backgrounds far different from their own. To do so effectively, health care providers need to understand how and why different belief systems, cultural biases, ethnic origins, family structures, and many other culture-based factors influence the manner in which people experiencing illness comply with medical advice and respond to treatment. Such variations have implications for outcomes of care (Cohen et al., 2002b).

NEW FRONTIERS IN CLINICAL TECHNOLOGY

Technological progress is behind much of the growth in the health services industry. The Institute for the Future (2000) predicted that eight types of medical technologies would especially affect patient care over the next 10 to 15 years: rational drug design, advances in imaging, minimally invasive surgery, genetic mapping and testing, gene therapy, vaccines, artificial blood, and xenotransplantation.

Rational drug design is a step beyond the painstaking and costly random search for new pharmaceuticals, which is characterized by trial and error. Now scientists can study the structure and composition of a receptor or enzyme and actually design new chemicals or molecular entities that bind to the receptors or enzymes. Rational drug design will shorten the drug discovery process. The chief candidates for this process are drugs to treat neurological and mental disorders and antiviral therapies for HIV/AIDS, encephalitis, measles, and influenza.

Imaging technologies present an enhanced visual display of tissues, organ systems, and their functions. Current research focuses on four areas: (1) finding new energy sources and focusing an energy beam to avoid damage to adjacent tissue and minimize residual damage, (2) using microelectronics in digital detectors and advances in the contrast media for a finer detection of abnormalities, (3) having faster and more accurate analysis of images using three-dimensional technology, and (4) making improvements in display technology to produce higher resolution displays.

The latest advances in *minimally invasive surgery* include image-guided brain surgery, minimal-access cardiac procedures, and the endovascular placement of grafts for abdominal aneurysms. The overall impact of minimally invasive procedures on cost efficiency and the patients' quality of life (from faster recovery) assures the growth of this technology as well as the growth of ambulatory surgicenters.

Genetic mapping has enabled the identification of a wide range of genes that can cause complex diseases such as diabetes, cancer, heart disease, and Huntington's and Alzheimer's diseases. The discovery of genetic susceptibility to certain diseases will improve preventive techniques. The term *genometrics* is used for the association of genes with specific disease traits.

Gene therapy is a therapeutic technique in which a functioning gene is inserted into targeted cells to correct an inborn defect or to provide the cell with a new function. The future challenge in this area is to develop methods that discriminately deliver enough genetic material to the right cells. Cancer treatment is receiving much attention as a prime candidate for gene therapy because current techniques (surgery, radiation, and chemotherapy) are effective in only half the cases.

Vaccines have traditionally been used on a preventive (prophylactic) basis to prevent specific infectious diseases such as diphtheria, smallpox, and whooping cough. However, the therapeutic use of vaccines in the treatment of noninfectious diseases such as cancer has opened new fronts in medicine. At the same time, the development of new vaccines for emerging infectious diseases remains on the research agenda. Making today's vaccines safer for wide-scale preventive use against bioterrorism, in which agents such as smallpox and anthrax may be used, will also be an ongoing challenge.

Research will continue on the development of fluids, including *artificial blood*, which in many instances could be used to substitute for real blood in transfusions, particularly under wartime conditions and during natural disasters when supplies may fall short.

The transplantation of organs has been one of the greatest medical advances of the last century. It treats a life-threatening chronic disease by replacing the diseased organ. However, a critical shortage of transplantable tissues remains a major concern. *Xenotransplantation*, in which animal tissues are used for transplants in humans, is a growing research area. New knowledge and methods in molecular genetics, transplantation biology, and genetic engineering look promising.

EVIDENCE-BASED HEALTH CARE

Practice variations—geographic variations in the practice of medicine without clinical justification—have both quality and cost implications. There is little evidence that high-spending providers deliver better outcomes. The goal of evidence-based medicine (EBM) is to increase the value of medicine. Even though consumers, as well as practitioners, often fear that reducing costs translates into lower quality, this is not necessarily true. Quality of care can be improved while reducing costs—thus increasing the value of medical care—by reducing misuse and overuse (Slawson & Shaughnessy, 2001). The tools for the practice of EBM have been developed for several years, mainly in the form of clinical practice guidelines. Evidence-based practice guidelines are intended to represent "best practices" and "proven therapies."

On the other hand, the use of guidelines is not widespread in the medical community. Even though the research community has known about clinical variations since the 1970s, and evidence has mounted since then, relatively little has been done to translate this research into actual practice. Many physicians think that guidelines and protocols are either too simple or too complicated, promote "cookbook care," lack creditable authors or evidence, are biased, decrease flexibility, reduce autonomy, and are not applicable to the practice population (Oeyen, 2007).

Future strategies are needed to improve guidelines and protocols, and their adherence. At least six recommendations can be made for the future:

1. Practitioners, payers, and policy makers need to become stakeholders.
2. Computer-based models will have to be developed to incorporate EBM into medical decision making. Models that are easily usable and understandable are essential.
3. Robust research designs, using clinical trials where applicable, should be the backbone of EBM.
4. Guidelines and protocols must be revised and kept current to incorporate subsequent scientific evidence.
5. Future practice guidelines must incorporate economic analysis. Mounting health care expenditures will pressure society to make rational choices about when certain types of services become unwarranted because costs begin to exceed the expected benefits from certain treatments.
6. Financial incentives, including provider payments and patient cost sharing, must be restructured. Reimbursement methods should focus on paying for best achievable outcomes and the most effective care over the course of treatment instead of paying for units of service (Gauthier et al., 2006).

In the future, EBM will also transcend what physicians do and will incorporate all caregivers. For example, the practice of nursing, pharmacology, and other disciplines allied with the practice of medicine will be governed by EBM. Eventually, EBM will become the standard that will govern the multidisciplinary process of health care delivery.

CONCLUSION

Social, cultural, technological, and economic changes will determine the future direction of health care. A lack of access for the uninsured and cost inflation will continue to haunt the system. In the short run, there will be greater cost shifting from the employers to the employees. A defined contribution from employers is likely to replace the existing defined-benefit program. To what extent this shift will occur and to what extent employers may actually abdicate their responsibility to be directly involved in purchasing health insurance will depend largely on the state of the economy and labor markets, and on any system-wide reforms, if and when a sweeping change in the health care delivery system is supported by the majority of middle-class Americans.

The vast infrastructure of managed care will not be easily dismantled. Instead, it is more reasonable to assume that in a changing environment managed care itself will have to evolve because employers and public bureaucrats will exert renewed pressure to bring about certain desired changes. Managed care in the future will have to focus on managing the financial risk of an increasing number of people with potentially debilitating chronic illnesses and also the sickest people in society.

Under growing cost pressures, wellness and public health will be more strongly emphasized. Increased challenges will also be posed by a rapidly growing elderly population that requires care for chronic ailments and long-term care. Physicians and other health care professionals will need training in geriatrics to function more effectively in a chronic care environment.

In a changing health care system, a major challenge and prime responsibility of public health agencies is to forge partnerships between communities and all levels of government. Developing needed infrastructures has also become critical because of increased threats of bioterrorism and outbreaks of new infectious diseases.

The composition of the health care workforce will also undergo changes because of the increasing elderly population, and more women and minorities entering the health care workforce. Despite recent efforts to bring about some parity, the problems associated with surplus physicians, an imbalance between the numbers of generalists and specialists, and physician shortages in primary care will continue. As minority populations continue to increase and the workplace becomes increasingly diverse, health care managers face the challenge of preparing a culturally competent health care workforce.

New frontiers will be opened in the application of clinical technologies. Evidence-based medicine will proliferate as clinical practice guidelines become more firmly anchored in research-based evidence and incentives are created for caregivers to use them.

REFERENCES

American Public Health Association. 2004. Universal health coverage a must by 2010, advocates say. *The Nation's Health* 34 (2):1, 18.

Andersen, R., et al. 1996. Introduction and overview. In R. Andersen, et al. (eds.). *Changing the US Health Care System: Key Issues in Health Services, Policy, and Management* (pp. 1–12). San Francisco: Jossey-Bass Publishers.

Baker, E. L., and J. P. Koplan. 2002. Strengthening the nation's public health infrastructure: Historic challenge, unprecedented opportunity. *Health Affairs* 21 (6):15–27.

Blendon, R. J., et al. 2008. Health care in the 2008 presidential primaries. *New England Journal of Medicine* 358 (4):414–422.

Carvin, A. 2000. Mind the gap: The digital divide as the civil rights issue of the new millennium. *Multimedia Schools* 7 (1):56–58.

Christianson, J. B., et al. 2002. Defined-contribution health insurance products: Development and prospects. *Health Affairs* 21 (1):49–64.

Claxton, G., et al. 2007. *The Kaiser Family Foundation and Health Research and Educational Trust Employer Health Benefits 2007 Annual Survey*. Menlo Park, CA: Henry J. Kaiser Family Foundation and Chicago, IL: Health Research and Educational Trust.

Cohen, H. J., et al. 2002a. A controlled trial of inpatient and outpatient geriatric evaluation and management. *New England Journal of Medicine* 346 (12):906–912.

Cohen, J. J., et al. 2002b. The case for diversity in the health care workforce. *Health Affairs* 21 (5):90–102.

Coile, R. C. 2002. *Futurescan 2002: A Forecast of Healthcare Trends*. Chicago: Health Administration Press.

Department of Health and Human Services. 2005. *Physician Workforce Policy Guidelines for the United States, 2000–2020*. Washington, DC: Department of Health and Human Services.

Draper, D.A., et al. 2008. Massachusetts health reform: High costs and expanding expectations may weaken employer support. *Issue Brief No. 124*. Washington, DC: Center for Studying Health System Change.

Gauthier, A., et al. 2006. *Toward a High Performance Health System for the United States*. New York: The Commonwealth Fund.

Gow, J. 2002. The HIV/AIDS epidemic in Africa: Implications for US policy. *Health Affairs* 21 (3):57–69.

Institute for the Future. 2000. *Health and Health Care 2010: The Forecast, the Challenge*. San Francisco: Jossey-Bass Publishers.

Keck, W., and F. D. Scutchfield. 1997. *The Future of Public Health*. Albany, NY: Delmar Publishers.

Keenan, P. S., et al. 2006. The "graying" of group health insurance. *Health Affairs* 25 (6):1497–1506.

McClellan, M., and K. Baicker. 2002. Reducing uninsurance through the nongroup market: Health insurance credits and purchasing groups. *Health Affairs* Web Exclusive (October 23, 2002). Retrieved from http://content.healthaffairs.org/cgi/content/abstract/hlthaff.w2.363v1.

Miller, E. A., and V. Mor. 2006. *Out of the Shadows: Envisioning a Brighter Future for Long-Term Care in America.* Providence, RI: Brown University.

National Association of Community Health Centers/The Robert Graham Center. 2007. *Access Denied: A Look at America's Medically Disenfranchised.* Washington, DC: National Association of Community Health Centers/ The Robert Graham Center.

Obama, B. 2007. Speech in Iowa City, IA, May 29, 2007. Retrieved August 2008 from http://www.barackobama.com/issues/healthcare/.

Oeyen, S. 2007. About protocols and guidelines: It's time to work in harmony! *Critical Care Medicine* 35 (1):292–293.

Paulson, H. M., et al. 2008. *A Summary of the 2008 Annual Reports: Social and Medicare Boards of Trustees.* Retrieved August 2008 from http://www.ssa.gov/OACT/TRSUM/trsummary.html.

Poisal, J. A., at al. 2007, February 21. Health spending projections through 2016: Modest changes obscure Part D's impact. *Health Affairs* Web Exclusive. Retrieved August 2008 from http://content.healthaffairs.org/cgi/content/abstract/hlthaff.26.2.w242.

Slawson, D. C., and A. F. Shaughnessy. 2001. Using "medical poetry" to remove the inequities in health care delivery. *Journal of Family Medicine* 50 (1):51–65.

Sloane, T. 2008. Mass. reform has the blues. *Modern Healthcare* 38 (15):20.

U.S. Census Bureau. 2001. *Statistical Abstract of the United States, 2001.* Washington, DC: U.S. Census Bureau.

Wagner, E. H., et al. 2001. Improving chronic illness care: Translating evidence into action. *Health Affairs* 20 (6):64–78.

White, B. 2001. The future of health care financing. *Family Practice Management* 8 (1):31–36.

Index

t denotes tables
f denotes figures